Monoclonal Antibodies in Drug Development

PROCEEDINGS OF THE FIRST
JOHN JACOB ABEL SYMPOSIUM ON DRUG DEVELOPMENT

Monoclonal Antibodies in Drug Development

Edited by

J. Thomas August

The Johns Hopkins University School of Medicine
Baltimore, Maryland 21205

Session Chairmen

Matthew Scharff, Marshall Nirenberg,
Hilary Koprowski, Henry S. Kaplan,
and Mette Strand

American Society for Pharmacology and Experimental Therapeutics
Bethesda, Maryland 20814

Proceedings of the first John Jacob Abel Symposium
on Drug Development, held June 8-10, 1981, at
The Johns Hopkins University School of Medicine,
Baltimore, Maryland 21205

9650 Rockville Pike
Bethesda, Maryland 20814

Printed in the United States of America

Library of Congress Cataloging in Publication Data

John Jacob Abel Symposium on Drug Development (1st : 1982 : Johns Hopkins University School of Medicine)
Monoclonal antibodies in drug development.

"Held June 8-10, 1981, at the Johns Hopkins University School of Medicine, Baltimore, Maryland "--T.p. verso.
Includes bibliographical references.
1. Antibodies, Monoclonal—Congresses. 2. Pharmaceutical microbiology—Congresses. 3. Abel, John Jacob, 1857-1938. I. August, J. Thomas. II. Title. [DNLM: 1. Antigen-Antibody reactions--Congresses. 2. Antibodies, Monoclonal—Congresses. 3. Pharmacology—Congresses. W3 J012J 1st 1981 / QW 575 J65 1981m]
QR186.7.J63 1982 616.07'93 82-13953
ISBN 0-9609094-0-0

Dedication

John Jacob Abel was appointed in 1893 as the first Chairman of Pharmacology at the newly formed School of Medicine of the Johns Hopkins University. The name of the new department was significant: "Materia medica" previously designated only studies of the clinical efficacy of available drugs. "Pharmacology" encompassed the experimental study of basic biochemical and physiological interactions of cells and organ systems with natural and foreign substances.

The basis of Abel's program throughout was a vigorous effort in fundamental research. "It was experiments of this type--born from the interaction of chemistry, physics, and physiology--that demonstrated . . . and buttressed the view that pharmacology must encompass and exploit basic science . . . ." These efforts led Abel to found the *Journal of Biological Chemistry* in 1905 (with Dr. Christian Herter) and the *Journal of Pharmacology and Experimental Therapeutics* in 1909.

This Symposium is dedicated to the memory of John Jacob Abel.

"Monoclonal Antibodies: The Basis for a New Pharmacology" is the title of one of the manuscripts in this symposium (Haber, p. 22). It remains to be proven that this prediction is correct, but there is no lack of enthusiasm for the concept.

The basis of this enthusiasm, the gift of Köhler and Milstein to biomedical research, is the ability of scientists to control and apply one of nature's biological wonders: the antibody response to foreign molecules. The essence of this procedure is to obtain a clonal population of cells producing a single antibody molecule. Provided that a substance is antigenic, an investigator can now produce an immortal cell that secretes a highly specific and sensitive chemical probe to identify, purify, and characterize the target antigen. This may be accomplished within a few months with virtually any strong antigen. Moreover, because the clonal hybridoma cell line is selected to react with a specific antigen defined by the selection technique employed, such pure antibody probes can be prepared from impure or crude mixtures of antigens. Herein is one of the great advantages of the monoclonal technology: the ability to prepare a specific chemical probe to a defined antigen selected from a complex mixture of antigens, without prior purification or even identification of the antigen. This may apply to individual antigenic sites within a single molecule, such as antigenic epitopes or domains within a protein (Parham, p. 61), or to a specific molecule within a complex structure, such as a differentiation antigen on the cell surface (Hughes and August, p. 49). Many of the initial concerns relating to the function of monoclonal antibodies, possible problems of affinity or specificity, have now been put aside. Provided the appropriate selection procedure is applied in identifying the desired immunoglobulin, molecules of high affinity (10^9 to $10^{10}M^{-1}$) and strict specificity are readily obtained. This biological approach thus rivals, and even exceeds, chemical or physical procedures for the specific detection and quantitative analysis of molecules.

A further advantage of a biological system is the possibility of genetic manipulation. Antibodies can be "tailor-made" by the selection of mutant immunoglobulins for specific functions (Scharff, p. 3). The frequency of spontaneous heavy chain switch or gene modification in hybridomas is on the order of 10^{-5} to 10^{-4}; with mutagenesis, between 0.1% and 1.0% of the hybridomas will contain deletions. Therefore, modified immunoglobulins may readily be obtained. Scharff reminds the reader that some problems persist. One obvious *sine qua non* is that the desired target be antigenic. Antigens in crude mixtures must give rise to a reasonable frequency of responder B cells. The problem is that the yield of variable hybridomas in the usual fusion reaction is about 10^{-5}. Therefore, beginning with 10^8 cells, a cell producing antibodies against a given antigen must comprise at least 0.1% of the splenocyte population, or a large number of fusions may be necessary. If the antigen is relatively pure, there are chemical modifications that can be used to make the most molecules reasonably antigenic.

One major application of monoclonal antibodies is to cancer biology. The search for tumor-specific antigens continues, and a number of new cell suface proteins and glyco-sphingolipids have been described (Koprowski, p. 130; Kennett et al., p. 91; Hakomori et al., p. 177). It has become increasingly clear that even monoclonal antibodies exhibiting a very restricted pattern of binding to tumor cells often react with more than one cell type (Kennett et al., p. 91; Brown et al., p. 120). The biochemical basis for these cross reactivities is unknown. Alternative possibilities that must be examined are that different cell types contain the same molecule, the same antigenic determinant is present in different molecules, or that different antigenic determinants are cross-reactive. Despite this problem, antigens have been identified that are either tumor-specific, tumor-enriched, or tissue-specific. Research is now directed at the therapeutic efficacy of such monoclonal antibodies. A prototype demonstration of monoclonal antibodies recognizing tumor-specific antigens and their application to therapy is the use of anti-idiotype antibodies directed against the hypervariable sequence of immunoglobulins produced by clonal populations of B cell lymphomas (Levy et al., p. 108). Other initial trials of monoclonal antibody therapy are in progress with a number of model and human tumor systems. IgG2a monoclonal antibodies acting with effector cells, probably macrophages, *in vivo*, are cytolytic to the targeted cell (Koprowski, p. 130; Badger and Bernstein, p. 151). There also is widespread effort to enhance cytotoxicity by conjugating the monoclonal antibody to toxic compounds (Scheinberg et al., p. 159; Uhr et al., p. 172; Hakomori et al., p. 177). One new approach, applicable both for targeting and treatment of tumors, is to conjugate the antibody with a radiometal chelate capable of accepting a variety of isotopes (Scheinberg et al., p. 159). Indium-chelate conjugated antibodies were shown to provide high resolution tumor imaging of relatively small tumors. These conjugates may also include metal isotopes releasing alpha particles of high energy, short path lengths, and short half-life. Such a conjugated antibody could selectively kill neighboring cells with high efficiency and thus eliminate modified cells that may escape killing by a drug acting only on the target cell.

Other important applications of monoclonal antibodies are to infectious diseases, bacteria, viruses, and parasites. This research will permit more rapid diagnosis of infectious organisms (Polin and Harris, p. 203) and will lead to the identification and characterization of antigens involved in the host immune response to the organism. Extensive results already have been obtained with the malaria and schistosoma parasites (Rener et al., p. 217; Strand et al., p. 223).

This symposium series has been organized to focus on recent advances in biology and chemistry as they apply to pharmacology, particularly to drug development. The organizers are indebted to representatives of the pharmaceutical and chemical industries for the generous support that makes this series possible.

J. Thomas August

Sponsors

Supported by major funding from:

Becton Dickinson and Company
Central Research Laboratories/3M Center
Dow Chemical U.S.A.
Hoffmann-La Roche, Inc.
Richardson-Merrell, Inc.
Smith Kline and French Laboratories
The Burroughs Wellcome Fund
The Upjohn Company

Additional contributions from:

Abbott Laboratories
A.H. Robins Company
Endo Laboratories (subsidiary of E.I. du Pont de Nemours and Company)
Flow Laboratories, Inc. (subsidiary of Flow General Inc.)
McNeil Pharmaceutical
Merck Sharp and Dohme Research Laboratories
Ortho Pharmaceutical Corporation
Pfizer Central Research
Stuart Pharmaceuticals (Division of ICI Americas, Inc.)
Syntex Research (Division of Syntex (U.S.A.) Inc.)

William S. Aronstein	The Johns Hopkins University School of Medicine, Baltimore, Maryland
J. Thomas August	The Johns Hopkins University School of Medicine, Baltimore, Maryland
Irwin Bernstein	University of Washington, Seattle, Washington
Joseph P. Brown	Fred Hutchinson Cancer Research Center, Seattle, Washington
Carlo Croce	The Wistar Institute of Anatomy and Biology, Philadelphia, Pennsylvania
P. Daryenezia	The National Heart, Lung, and Blood Institute, National Institutes of Health, Bethesda, Maryland
Joseph M. Davie	Washington University, St. Louis, Missouri
Otto Gansow	Michigan State University, East Lansing, Michigan
Walter Gerhard	The Wistar Institute of Anatomy and Biology, Philadelphia, Pennsylvania
Edgar Haber	Massachusetts General Hospital, Boston, Massachusetts
Sen-itiroh Hakomori	University of Washington, Seattle, Washington
Edward N. Hughes	The Johns Hopkins University School of Medicine, Baltimore, Maryland
Henry S. Kaplan	Stanford University School of Medicine, Stanford, California
Roger H. Kennett	University of Pennsylvania School of Medicine, Philadelphia, Pennsylvania
Hilary Koprowski	The Wistar Institute of Anatomy and Biology, Philadelphia, Pennsylvania
Ronald Levy	Stanford University Medical Center, Stanford, California
Alban Linnenbach	The Wistar Institute of Anatomy and Biology, Philadelphia, Pennsylvania
Thomas J. McKearn	University of Pennsylvania School of Medicine, Philadelphia, Pennsylvania

J. Moskal	The National Heart, Lung, and Blood Institute, National Institutes of Health, Bethesda, Maryland
Marshall W. Nirenberg	The National Heart, Lung, and Blood Institute, National Institutes of Health, Bethesda, Maryland
Amy P. Norden	The Johns Hopkins University School of Medicine, Baltimore, Maryland
Robert Nowinski	University of Washington, Seattle, Washington
Peter Parham	Stanford University School of Medicine, Stanford, California
Richard Polin	University of Pennsylvania School of Medicine and Children's Hospital of Philadelphia, Philadelphia, Pennsylvania
Joan Rener	Laboratory of Parasitic Diseases, National Institutes of Health, Bethesda, Maryland
Matthew Scharff	Albert Einstein College of Medicine, Bronx, New York
David A. Scheinberg	The Johns Hopkins University School of Medicine, Baltimore, Maryland
Stuart Schlossman	Sidney Farber Cancer Institute, Boston, Massachusetts
M. Schneider	The National Heart, Lung, and Blood Institute, National Institutes of Health, Bethesda, Maryland
Mette Strand	The Johns Hopkins University School of Medicine, Baltimore, Maryland
D. Trisler	The National Heart, Lung, and Blood Institute, National Institutes of Health, Bethesda, Maryland
Jonathan W. Uhr	University of Texas Southwestern Medical School, Dallas, Texas

CONTENTS

IV
Applications to Drug Delivery Systems

V
Applications to Bacteria, Viruses, and Parasites

I
The State of the Art

MONOCLONAL ANTIBODIES: THE PRODUCTION OF TAILOR-MADE SEROLOGICAL REAGENTS

D.E. Yelton, P. Thammana, C. Desaymard, and M.D. Scharff

Department of Cell Biology
Albert Einstein College of Medicine
1300 Morris Park Avenue
Bronx, New York 10461

Immunological assays have been used for years to detect, quantify, and localize small amounts of antigen in complex biological mixtures. The various uses of antibodies in the research laboratory are too numerous to categorize but range from detecting mutant enzymes in bacteria to analyzing the causes of malignancies in man. In the diagnostic laboratory immunologic assays are used routinely to determine levels of hormones, enzymes, plasma proteins, and drugs in the blood; to identify and classify microorganisms in body fluids and tissue samples; and for many other diagnostic tasks. In addition, antibodies have been used therapeutically in man to immunize passively against infectious agents, as antidotes to toxins, and to prevent the rejection of transplanted tissue.

Antibodies are so useful because special structural characteristics allow them to bind tightly and specifically to one of many possible antigens and simultaneously to carry out a few effector functions. The amino-terminal or variable part of each antibody contains sequences, called hypervariable regions, that fold to generate a unique antigen binding site (Fig. 1). Current estimates suggest that an individual can make between a million and a billion different antibody molecules, each with different variable-region sequences, and that the genetic mechanisms required to generate this diversity are unique to the immunoglobulin genes. On the other hand, antibodies must carry out only a few effector functions such as complement fixation and binding to macrophages. These functions are mediated by the carboxy-terminal or constant part of the molecule (Fig. 1), which is much more highly conserved than the amino-terminal part of the molecule. In fact, antibodies have only eight possible constant regions, each of which represents an immunoglobulin class or subclass that can carry a subset of effector functions. Whether antibodies are used as scientific probes, diagnostic reagents, or therapeutic tools, both antigen binding and biological function are important, and both determine the usefulness of the antibody as a reagent.

All of the uses of antibodies in biology and medicine have been complicated by the difficulty of generating large amounts of specific

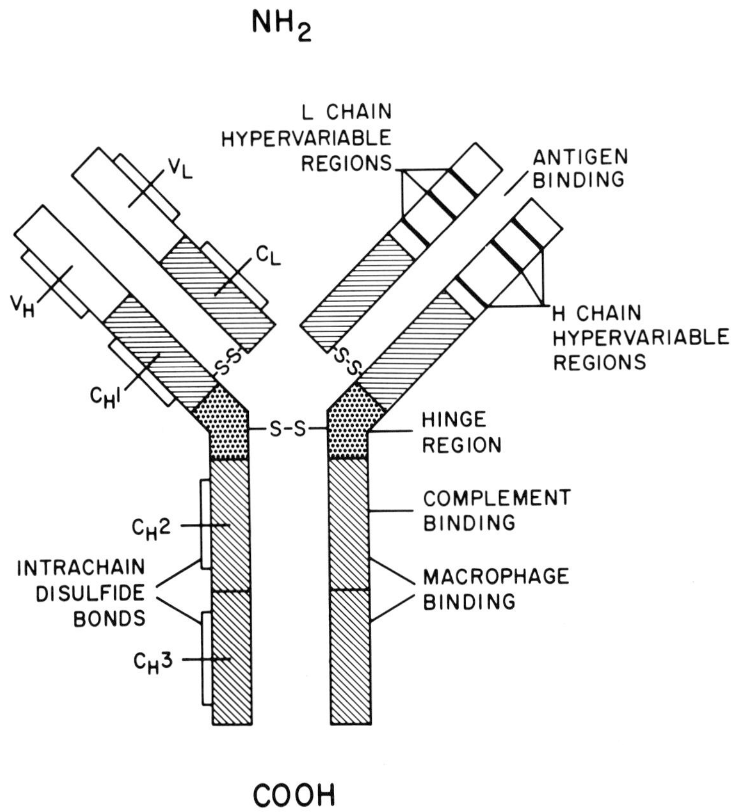

Fig. 1. The structure of immunoglobulin molecules.

antisera by conventional immunization (Table 1). Upon immunization, most individuals or animals respond with the production of different antibodies containing many different variable regions, each covalently linked to some or all of the constant regions. Because of each individual's unique history of past exposure to environmental antigens and because of the complexity of the cellular events and interactions that make up the normal immune response, the production of specific serological reagents is extremely unpredictable. Most antigen preparations are impure, and immunization results in varying amounts of antibody directed against contaminating substances. Even if a purified antigen is readily available, animals or humans immunized with it will generate a very heterogeneous array of antibodies that differ in affinity, cross reactivity with structurally related antigens, and effector functions. Such unpredictability and heterogeneity are obvious when one compares the antisera obtained from different animals or individuals and even when one compares different bleedings of the same animal.

These unavoidable differences in antisera have made it difficult to standardize immunoassays and to accumulate large amounts of antisera that can be used as reference reagents. This is especially true if the antigen is a weak immunogen and does not induce production of large amounts of antibody in recipients or if the antigen is impure or poorly characterized. Tumor antigens provide an example of these problems (1). The biology of malignancy has led investigators to believe that there are chemical differences in the surface components of malignant and normal cells. To confirm this and to obtain a simple way of identifying malignant cells, such cells have been injected into heterologous hosts such as rabbits. The rabbit produces antibodies against the many surface and intracellular components foreign to it. The resulting antiserum is then absorbed extensively with normal cells, preferably with those having the same genetic constitution as the malignant cells. Any residual (unabsorbed) antibody is assumed to be tumor-specific, an assumption that can be confirmed by examining the antibody's reactivity with other malignant and normal cells. Because of the many antigens present and their relatively poor immunogenicity, the amount of residual tumor-specific antibody is small and, after it is used in the experiments required to confirm its specificity, there is usually not enough antibody left to share with other investigators or to use in clinical trials. While some of these problems have been overcome by immunizing large animals and pooling sera, in the end there is never enough antibody, and this has discouraged many investigators from pursuing the problem.

While the heterogeneity and unpredictability of the immune response result from its inherent complexity, the problem can be thought of as arising from the polyclonality of the normal antibody response. Each antibody-forming cell and its progeny make antibodies with identical variable regions, and many different clones of cells respond to a given antigen, resulting in many different antibodies. One potential solution to the heterogeneity of the immune response was to reproducibly stimulate only one of the many clones that could produce antibody reactive with a given antigen. An animal

Table 1. Problems with conventional immunization

1. Unpredictability of the immune response
2. Immunogenicity of minor contaminants
3. Heterogeneity of even highly specific antibodies
    a. Affinity
    b. Cross reactivity
    c. Effector functions
4. Supply often limited

does this when it develops multiple myeloma, a malignancy in which a single antibody-forming cell undergoes malignant transformation, proliferates in an uncontrolled fashion, and produces very large amounts of a single antibody molecule. Many investigators attempted to induce production of such monoclonal antibodies by manipulating conventional immunization or by exploiting the myeloma model (2), but until recently these attempts were not successful enough to be applied to the routine production of antisera. However, as a result of some seemingly unrelated studies on the somatic cell genetics of immunoglobulin production, a technique is now available for making monoclonal antibodies.

In 1975, Köhler and Milstein (3) fused cultured mouse myeloma cells to spleen cells from a mouse immunized with sheep red blood cells and showed that some of the resulting hybrids made homogeneous antibodies that reacted with immunizing antigen. This technology was quickly and successfully applied to many other antigens (2). Since each hybrid or "hybridoma," as it has come to be called, is the clonal progeny of the fusion of the genetic material from a single myeloma and a single antibody-forming cell, it synthesizes structurally identical antibody molecules. Furthermore, the hybridoma retains the properties of the malignant myeloma parent in that it grows continuously in culture, can be frozen and recovered as a viable antibody-producing cell, and can be injected into recipient animals where it produces a tumor. Such tumor-bearing animals accumulate large amounts of the antibody in their blood and ascites fluid. Thus, a hybridoma is the source of homogeneous antibody molecules that are available in very large amounts and for an apparently unlimited period of time, with the result that it is now possible to generate large amounts of a well-defined and chemically homogeneous serological reagent and to replenish the supply of the identical reagent whenever it is needed.

The basic methodology for obtaining hybridomas is illustrated in Fig. 2 (4). The technological details have been published by many laboratories (5-7). Mice or rats are immunized according to many different schemes, none of which is so obviously superior that it has replaced the others. With good immunogens, most investigators have not found it necessary to use extensive hyper-immunization. Many workers believe that the animals with the highest levels of antibody are likely to provide the most antibody-forming hybrids. We believe that it is useful to allow the serum level of antibody to fall off to very low levels before the final injection of antigen which precedes the fusion. Most workers agree that the final injection of antigen should be in saline and is best given intravenously, although if this is not possible, intraperitoneal injections seem to work almost as well. We usually boost a few animals, bleed them 48 h after administering the antigen, and 24 h later remove the spleens from the one or two animals with the best antibody response. A single suspension of nucleated spleen cells is mixed with cultured mouse myeloma cells in the presence of polyethylene glycol (8), an agent that promotes the fusion of cell membranes. As a result of random fusion of myeloma and spleen cells, hybrids are formed between myeloma cells, spleen cells, and myeloma and spleen cells (Fig. 2). This mixture of cells is

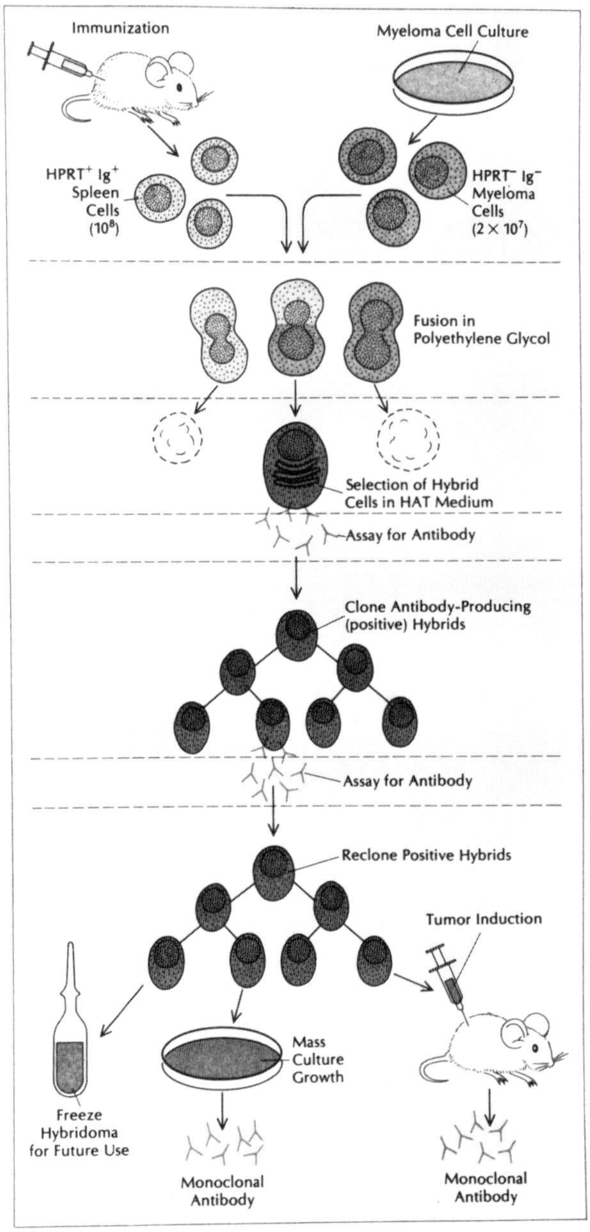

Fig. 2. The production of monoclonal antibodies. (Reprinted with permission from Ref. 4).

plated out in a selective medium containing hypoxanthine, aminopterin, and thymidine (HAT) (9). The myeloma cells used for fusion contain an enzyme defect ($HPRT^-$) that prevents their growth in the presence of aminopterin. The normal spleen cells do not grow in culture but do contain normal enzyme so that hybrids between spleen and myeloma cells survive and grow. A number of methods have been described for carrying out the fusion and propagating the surviving hybrids (5-7). When well-immunized animals and optimum conditions are used, on the average about 500 hybrids are obtained from each mouse spleen. At least in our experience, none of the many variations in the procedure seems to significantly and routinely increase the yield of hybrids. We prefer to plate out the mixture of fused and unfused cells immediately in HAT medium in 96-well microtiter plates at concentrations (5×10^4 cells in 0.1 ml) that will give us one hybrid in every two to three wells. Others clone directly into agar (10) or distribute in larger wells (3). Within two to four weeks, hybrid clones become grossly visible. At this time the clones must be screened for antibody (Fig. 2). Since it is impractical to propagate all of the hybridomas, it is absolutely essential that a rapid and reliable screening assay be perfected before a fusion is carried out.

A convenient radioimmunoassay for antigens that can be absorbed to polyvinyl microtiter dishes is illustrated in Fig. 3. This assay is identical to the one originally developed by Norman Klinman and his colleagues (11) except that it uses an endogenously labelled rat monoclonal antibody specific for mouse kappa chains as a developing reagent (12). The antigen is absorbed to the wells of the polyvinyl plate, medium from the hybridoma is added to the well, and unbound antibody is removed by washing. The ^{14}C- or ^{35}S-labelled monoclonal anti-mouse kappa chain is then added to the well, and after appropriate washing, the wells are cut out and counted in a scintillation counter. Because almost all mouse antibodies contain kappa chains, this monoclonal provides an almost universal screening reagent. The benefit of using endogenously labelled antibody is that it can be generated by incubating the hybridoma cells with ^{14}C amino acids or ^{35}S-methionine. The medium containing the antibody is dialyzed to free it of unincorporated radioactivity and is then used without purification. The nonspecific background is 50-200 cpm, and antibody-producing hybridomas result in the binding of 20-100 times more radioactivity than the background (12). We use this same assay to titer the sera of immunized animals. The rat monoclonal can be purified and iodinated or enzyme-linked if one wishes to use an ^{125}I or Elisa assay.

The one additional technological advance that has gained general acceptance is the use of non-immunoglobulin-producing myeloma cells (13,14) as the malignant parent in the fusion. If a myeloma producing either heavy and light chains or only light chains is used, the antibodies produced will contain mixtures of myeloma and antibody polypeptide chains that may have specificity or affinity different from that of the spleen cell antibody. If chromosome segregation results in the loss of the spleen cell heavy or light chain, the hybridoma will continue to produce antibody that differs from the predominant antibody produced by the original clone (15). This change may go unrecognized. If, on the other hand, a non-producing myeloma is used, loss of a single chain will result in the loss of antibody production; this will be easily recognized, and fresh cells can be recovered from the freezer.

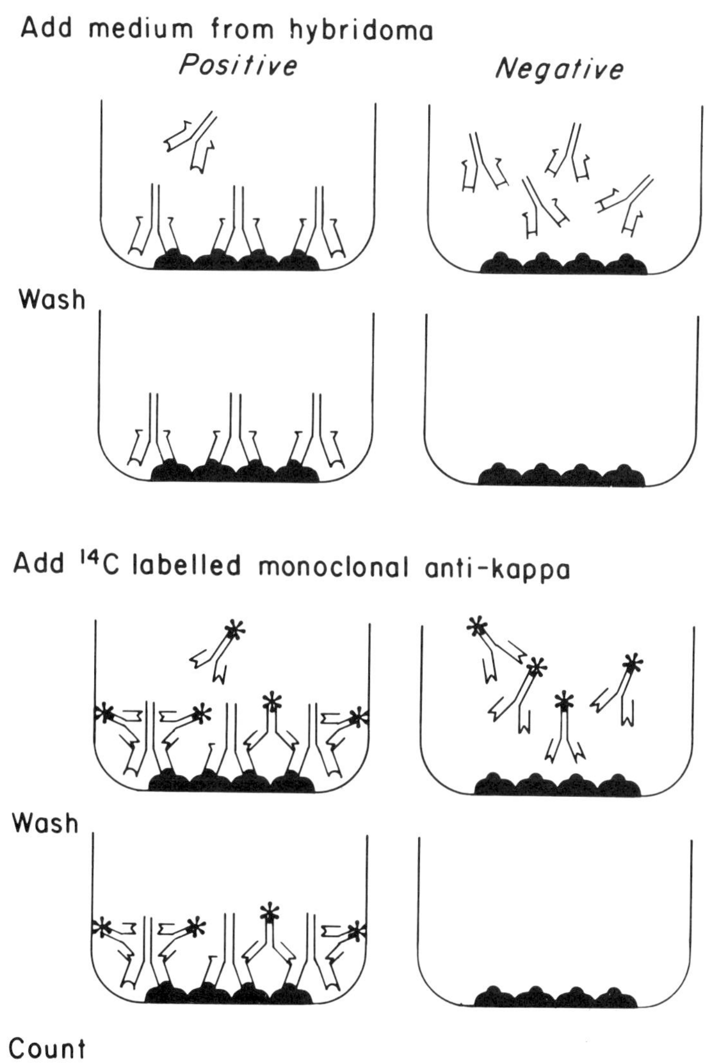

Fig. 3. A radioimmunoassay for detecting mouse monoclonal antibodies using endogenously labelled monoclonal rat anti-mouse kappa chain antibodies.

Once the antibody-producing hybridomas have been identified, they are cloned to ensure that they are really monoclonal and to eliminate any non-producing variants that may have arisen from early chromosome segregation (Fig. 2). If only a few antibody-forming hybrids are obtained, cloning, screening the subclones for antibody, and freezing them away are easily done. However, if many fusions are carried out or if one or a few fusions are very successful, the processing of the positive hybridomas is very time consuming. Most investigators have learned to be very selective about the hybridomas that they keep. Hybrids with low antibody titers are unstable, are low producers, or produce very low-affinity antibody and should be discarded unless these properties are desired. If particular specificities, cross reactivities, or effector functions are required, these should be screened for early, and only those hybridomas with the desired properties should be retained. If care is taken not to keep too many hybridomas, the whole process from immunization to freezing should take three to four months.

As hybridoma technology has been applied to many antigens, its obvious benefits have been realized (Table 2). Very large amounts of monoclonal antibodies can be obtained. The tissue culture fluid from a high-producing monoclonal can contain as much as 100 μg of antibody/ml, and ascites fluid provides concentrations as high as 10 mg/ml. Stable hybridomas continue to produce the same antibody for months or even years in culture and can be recovered from the freezer years after they have been frozen away. Once a hybridoma has been generated and its antibody fully characterized, it is relatively inexpensive to generate additional antibody whenever it is needed. The monoclonal antibodies are homogeneous and predictable, although, as will be discussed below, variants do arise so that it is important to periodically check the specificity of the antibody.

It is important to remember that monoclonal antibodies are not necessarily monospecific. They may be highly restricted in their

Table 2. Benefits of monoclonal antibodies

1. Very large amounts can be generated
2. Available when needed; available indefinitely
3. Homogeneous and predictable
   - Not necessarily monospecific
     1) may be more restricted
     2) may reveal new cross reactivities
        - cannot be absorbed away
        - cross reactivities reliable
4. Pure antibodies from impure antigens, or even from unknown antigens

specificity or they may cross react extensively. In fact, cross-reacting monoclonals may be very useful because they reveal truly shared antigenic determinants. Some of the cross reactions revealed by monoclonal antibodies were not previously seen with conventional antisera, because such antisera had to be absorbed to be usable or because the cross reactivities were attributed to contaminating antigens. One of the most important benefits of the hybridoma technology is that pure antibodies can be obtained from impure or even unknown antigens; excellent examples are described in this monograph, especially in the chapters dealing with differentiation and tumor antigens.

A final and unique benefit of monoclonal antibodies is that they can be tailor-made for each individual use. If many hybridomas are available that react with a particular antigen, individual monoclonals with particularly desirable properties can be selected (Table 3). For example, if one is dealing with a surface antigen and wants a

Table 3. Methods for tailor-making monoclonal antibodies

1. Selecting for various
   a. Specificities
   b. Affinities
   c. Biological activities
      Subclass-restricted
2. Inducing mutations to change effector function
   a. Precipitation or aggregation
   b. Complement fixation
   c. Binding to Fc receptors
   d. Placental transfer
   e. Half-life in the serum

cytotoxic antibody, then a high affinity monoclonal of the IgM class will be most useful and can be screened for and preserved. If one wishes to use a fluorescence-activated cell sorter to purify and passively transfer cells bearing the antigen, it will be desirable to have a non-cytotoxic antibody such as an IgG_1 antibody. If the goal is to purify the surface antigen by affinity chromatography and recover it in its native form, a low affinity monoclonal might be selected so that the antigen can be eluted from the column under mild conditions. If the goal is to do phylogenetic studies or to identify all of the viruses in a particular group, then monoclonals with considerable cross reactivity rather than highly specific monoclonals might be chosen.

For therapeutic or diagnostic purposes, it may not be sufficient to select from among an existing battery of monoclonal antibodies. For example, attaching a cytotoxic or radioactive agent to a monoclonal in order to kill or identify tumor cells may be difficult to achieve, because antibody may associate through its constant region with complement or Fc receptors on phagocytic cells. The usual solution is to digest the antibody with papain to produce Fab fragments. However, an alternative is to induce a mutation in the hybridoma cell that will result in the deletion of the carboxy-terminal region of the monoclonal antibody. One relatively simple technology for identifying such mutations in myelomas and hybridomas has been described (16), and we and others have shown that such mutations may occur as frequently in hybridomas as they do in myelomas (17-19). With mutagenesis, between 0.1 and 1.0% of the hybridomas will contain such deletions (18). We have isolated such mutant monoclonal antibodies and have shown that they no longer fix complement or bind to Fc receptors (17,18). Some mutant monoclonal antibodies that assemble only into HL molecules contain a single antigen-binding site and will not form aggregates with circulating antigen (18). These may be useful in preventing immune-complex disease, which is sometimes associated with passive immunization. It is also possible to change serum half-life and the ability to pass through the placenta by inducing such mutations. We and others have been able to isolate monoclonals that have changed the class or subclass they are expressing while retaining the same variable regions and specificity (20,21). Thus it seems possible that the genetic manipulation of monoclonal antibodies may allow us to develop even more effective diagnostic and therapeutic tools.

While hybridoma technology is clearly successful and has already led to important, useful observations, a few technical problems persist (Table 4). Obtaining monoclonal antibodies against weak immunogens continues to be difficult. Investigators do sometimes try

Table 4. Persisting technical problems with the hybridoma technology

1. Difficulty in obtaining monoclonals against weak immunogens
2. Problems inherent in homogeneity
   a. Limited biological function
   b. Sensitivity to inactivation
3. Species limitation
4. Labor-intensive

to obtain monoclonals despite low antibody titers in the immunized animals and are occasionally successful either by chance or because they are willing to screen a very large number of hybrids. Nevertheless, we have not seen any reports of techniques that allow routine enrichment ten-fold or more for antibody-forming cells prior to cell fusion.

A second problem that results directly from the benefits of the technology is that some monoclonal antibodies are inactivated by small changes in pH or show changes in their affinity and specificity with changes in their environment (22). Another effect of the homogeneity of monoclonal antibodies is that any given monoclonal has a limited range of biological activities because it contains only one constant region.

A final, persisting problem is that it is still not possible to generate monoclonal antibodies from all species. This species-restriction depends to some degree on the availability of malignant cell lines that allow the continued expression of immunoglobulin and do not cause the segregation of the spleen cell chromosomes. For example, mouse myeloma cells can be fused to rat spleen cells (and vice versa) because there is no selective loss of rat chromosomes in such a fusion. However, when mouse myeloma cells are fused to rabbit spleen cells, the rabbit chromosomes are lost so quickly that it is very difficult to isolate hybrids that are still producing rabbit antibodies (23). Human hybrids can be generated because there are human myelomas that serve as the malignant parent in the fusion.

Hybridoma technology has revolutionized the use of antibodies and immunological assays in biology and medicine. It is now possible to obtain very large amounts of homogeneous antibody and to replenish the supply of useful monoclonal antibodies indefinitely. Furthermore, rare antibodies that were previously available only in small amounts can now be reproduced and used widely. By careful selection or by the induction of mutations, monoclonal antibodies can be tailor-made for specific diagnostic or therapeutic tasks. These benefits have resulted in the application of immunology to new basic and clinical problems, many of which will be described in the following chapters of this monograph.

Acknowledgments

Aspects of this work were supported by grants from the National Institutes of Health (AI 10702 and AI5231), National Science Foundation (PCM77-25635), and American Chemical Society (NP-317). D.E. Yelton is a Medical Scientist Trainee supported by Grant 5T 32GM 7288 from the National Institute of General Medical Sciences. C. Desaymard is a Chargee de Recherche Inserm on leave and supported in part by a Fogarty International Fellowship.

References

1. Greaves, MF, G Brown, NT Rampson and T Lister (1975). Antisera to acute lymphoblastic leukemia cells. Clin Immunol and Immunopathol **4**, 67-84.
2. Yelton, DE, and MD Scharff (1981). Monoclonal antibodies: A powerful new tool in biology and medicine. Annu Rev Biochem **50**, 657-680.
3. Köhler, G, and C Milstein (1975). Continuous cultures of fused cells secreting antibody of predefined specificity. Nature (Lond) **256**, 495-497.
4. Yelton, DE, S Roberts and P Thammana (1981). Hybridomas as a source of antibodies. Hosp Pract **16**, 61-66.
5. Kwan, S-P, DE Yelton and MD Scharff (1980). Production of monoclonal antibodies. **In** Genetic Engineering, pp 31-46. JK Setlow and A Hollander, eds. Plenum Press, New York.
6. Herzenberg, LA, and C Milstein (1978). Cell hybrids with antibody forming cells and T-lymphomas with T cells. **In** Handbook of Experimental Immunology, Vol 2, pp 25.1-25.13. M Weir, ed. Blackwell Scientific Publications, Oxford.
7. Kennett, RH, TJ McKearn and KB Bechtol, eds (1980). Monoclonal Antibodies: Hybridomas: A new dimension in biological analyses. Plenum Press, New York.
8. Gefter, ML, DH Margulies and MD Scharff (1977). A simple method for polyethylene glycol-promoted hybridization of mouse myeloma cells. Somatic Cell Genet **3**, 231-236.
9. Littlefield, JW (1976). Selection of hybrids from mixtures of fibroblasts *in vitro* and their presumed recombinants. Science **145**, 709-710.
10. Sharon, J, SL Morrison and EA Kabat (1979). Detection of specific hybridoma clones by replica immunoadsorption of their secreted antibodies. Proc Natl Acad Sci USA **76**, 1420-1424.
11. Pierce, SK, and NR Klinman (1976). Allogeneic carrier-specific enhancement of hapten specific secondary B cell responses. J Exp Med **144**, 1254-1262.
12. Yelton, DE, C Desaymard and MD Scharff (1981). The use of monoclonal anti-mouse immunoglobulin to detect mouse antibodies. Hybridoma **1**, 5-11.
13. Schulman, M, CD Wilde and G Köhler (1978). A better cell line for making hybridomas secreting specific antibodies. Nature (Lond) **276**, 269-270.
14. Kearney, JF, A Radbruch, B Liesegang and K Rajewsky (1979). A new mouse myeloma cell line that has lost immunoglobulin expression but permits the construction of antibody secreting hybrid cell lines. J Immunol **123**, 1548-1550.
15. Milstein, C, K Adetugbo, NJ Cowan, G Köhler, DS Secher and CD Wilde (1977). Somatic cell genetics of antibody-secreting cells: studies of clonal diversification and analysis of cell fusion. Cold Spring Harbor Symp Quant Biol **41**, 793-803.
16. Coffino, PR, R Baumal, R Laskov and MD Scharff (1972). Cloning of mouse myeloma cells and detection of rare variants. J Cell Physiol **79**, 429-440.
17. Yelton, DE, WD Cook and MD Scharff (1980). Somatic variants in mouse myeloma and hybridoma cell lines. Transplant Proc **12**, 439-442.
18. Yelton, DE, P Thammana, C Desaymard, S Roberts, S-P Kwan, A Giusti, DJ Zack, RA Pollock and MD Scharff (1982). Monoclonal antibodies: the production of tailor made reagents. **In** From Gene to Protein: Translation into Biotechnology. WJ Whelan and J Schultz, eds. Academic Press, New York, in press.
19. Köhler, G, and M Schulman (1980). Immunoglobulin M mutants. Eur J Immunol **10**, 467-476.
20. Thammana, P, and MD Scharff. In preparation.
21. Neuberger, MS, and K Rajewsky (1981). Switch from hapten-specific immunoglobulin M to immunoglobulin D secretion in a hybrid mouse cell line. Proc Natl Acad Sci USA **78**, 1138-1142.
22. Mosmann, TR, M Gallatin and J Longnecker (1980). Alteration of apparent specificity of monoclonal (hybridoma) antibodies recognizing polymorphic histocompatability and blood group determinants. J Immunol **125**, 1152-1156.
23. Yarmush, ML, FT Gates, DR Weisfugel and TJ Kindt (1980). Identification and characterization of rabbit-mouse hybridomas secreting rabbit immunoglobulin chains. Proc Natl Acad Sci USA **77**, 2899-2903.

A HUMAN MYELOMA MUTANT PERMITTING THE ISOLATION OF HUMAN MONOCLONAL ANTIBODIES

Alban Linnenbach, Hilary Koprowski, Zenon Steplewski
and Carlo M. Croce
The Wistar Institute of Anatomy and Biology
Philadelphia, Pennsylvania 19104

George Eisenbarth and Richard Jackson
Duke University
Durham, North Carolina 27705

William Hall
Rockefeller University
New York, New York 10021

Monoclonal antibodies of rodent origin can be produced by obtaining hybrids between cells of mouse myeloma lines and B cells derived from animals immunized with a given antigen (1,2). The production of B cell hybrids that secrete human monoclonal antibodies has not been practical, because human chromosomes segregate in mouse x human hybridomas (3,4), and it is unlikely that these hybrids retain both of the human chromosomes carrying the active genes for immunoglobulin heavy and light chains (3,4). The karyotype of human x human hybrids is more stable (5). To obtain human B cell hybrids that secrete human antibodies for long periods of time, we isolated a mutant of the human GM1500 B cell line derived from a patient with multiple myeloma. GM1500 cells (10^7) were selected for hypoxanthine phosphoribosyltransferase (HPRT) deficiency. Two mutant colonies were obtained. One such mutant, GM1500 6TG-A1-2, is resistant to 15 μg/ml of 2-amino-6-mercaptopurine (6-thioguanine) and does not revert to the $HPRT^+$ phenotype, continues to secrete γ and κ chains (Fig. 1, lane 1), and can be grown as ascites in nude mice. Upon fusion with lymphocytes from human donors and subsequent selection in HAT medium (6), permanent, stable hybridomas can be obtained that secrete large amounts of human monoclonal antibody for a considerable period of time. We have succeeded in producing human x human hybridomas secreting: 1) anti-measles virus antibodies (7) and 2) anti-pancreatic islet-cell antibodies (8).

Anti-measles virus antibodies. Human monoclonal antibodies to measles virus were derived from a 19-year-old female suffering from subacute sclerosing panencephalitis (SSPE), a disease caused by a measles virus infection of the brain. Measles virus was recovered from a brain fragment obtained from the patient. Serum from the patient had extremely high titers of anti-measles virus antibodies (7). Ficoll-purified lymphocytes from 10 ml of peripheral blood were fused with the human myeloma mutant in the presence of polyethylene glycol 1000 and distributed into 24 wells of a Linbro FB-16-24 TC plate. Growth of hybrids in 20 wells was apparent after two to three weeks. Cloned hybrids were screened for the expression of human immunoglobulin chains and for the ability to immunoprecipitate measles virus proteins (9).

As shown in Fig. 1, six hybrid clones, including the two that reacted with measles virus (see Fig. 2), expressed the human μ chains, as determined by immunoprecipitation of the immunoglobulins secreted by the hybrids with rabbit anti-μ antiserum (3,4). Some hybridomas also expressed a light chain (L) that migrated differently from the light chain expressed by the GM1500 lines. The clone of the hybridoma illustrated in lane 6 (Fig. 1) lost the ability to produce the light chain expressed by GM1500 cells. The hybridomas' culture fluid in lane 7 was immunoprecipitated with both anti-human μ- and anti-human γ-chain antisera. The hybrid expressed two heavy chains: the γ chain of the GM1500 parent and the μ chain of the human SSPE B-cell parent.

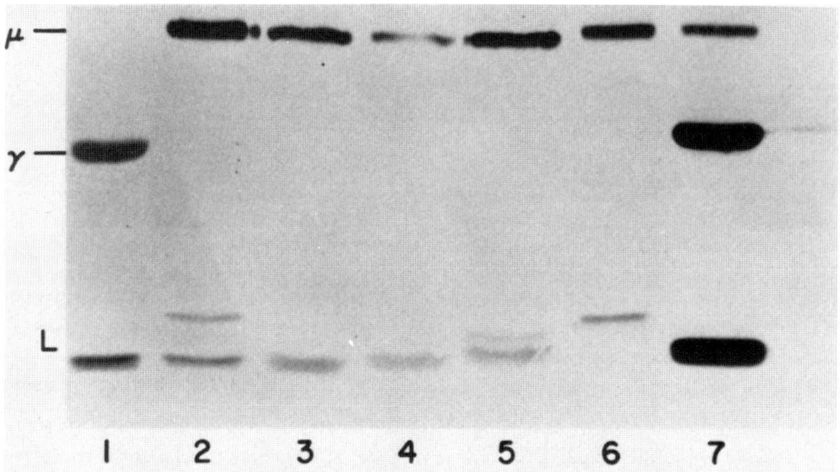

Fig. 1. Immunoprecipitation and 10% SDS-polyacrylamide gel electrophoresis of secreted human immunoglobulin chains produced by hybridomas derived from an SSPE patient. Hybridoma cultures were labeled with 100 μCi ^{3}H-leucine (70 Ci/mmol) ml^{-1} for 12 h. The human immunoglobulin chains were immunoprecipitated with rabbit anti-human heavy chain antigen using established procedures, then separated by 10% SDS-polyacrylamide gel electrophoresis. Lane 1, immunoprecipitates of the immunoglobulin produced by GM1500 6TG-A1-2 cells after reaction with an anti-human γ antiserum; lanes 2-6, immunoprecipitates of immunoglobulin chains secreted by human x human hybridomas after reaction with anti-human μ antiserum; lane 7, immunoprecipitate of immunoglobulin chains secreted by hybridoma D3 after reaction with anti-human μ and γ antiserum.

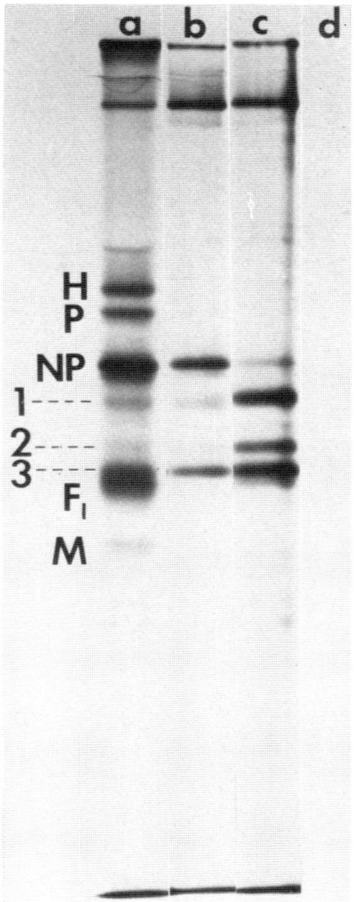

Fig. 2. Polyacrylamide gel electrophoretic analysis of the measles virus polypeptides precipitated by the various monoclonal antibodies. (a) Virus polypeptides precipitated by convalescent serum of a patient with atypical measles were used as markers. The polypeptides are as follows: H, the virus hemagglutin; P, a polypeptide associated with the internal nucleocapsid structure; NP, the major structural polypeptide of the nucleocapsid; F, the polypeptide responsible for cell fusion and hemolytic activities; M, the non-glycosylated membrane polypeptide. Bands, 1, 2, and 3 are not unique virus polypeptides but represent proteolytic cleavage fragments of the NP polypeptide. (b) Virus polypeptides precipitated by antibody D3. (c) Polypeptides precipitated by antibody C5. (d) Culture fluid from the human GM15006TG-A1-2 cell line. Culture fluids of b, c, and d were concentrated 20-fold by freeze-drying before use. The procedures used in immunoprecipitation, similar to those described elsewhere, were as follows: Lysates of virus-infected CV-1 cells labeled with ^{35}S-methionine were used as antigen. Aliquots (25 µl) were mixed with 100 µl concentrated culture fluid and incubated at 37°C for 90 min, then at 4°C for 4 h. Rabbit total anti-human antibody (25 µl) was then added and the incubation period repeated. Precipitated polypeptides were collected by centrifugation in an Eppendorf centrifuge for 20 min at 10,000 rpm. The visible pellet was resuspended and washed three times. After the final washing, the pellet was suspended in lysis buffer, boiled for 3 min, and electrophoresed on a 10% SDS-polyacrylamide gel. After fluorography, the dried gel was exposed to Cronex X-ray film.

The specificity of the antibodies for measles virus was determined by immunoprecipitation using methods similar to those described elsewhere (9). Culture fluids from hybrids D3 and C5 precipitated only the virus nucleocapsid polypeptide (NP) and varying amounts of its cleavage fragments (Fig. 2). The antibodies in the culture fluids seemed to be specific for this one polypeptide, NP, which is the major polypeptide of the virus nucleocapsid (9). NP is extremely sensitive to proteolytic cleavage (9). Thus the long incubation periods used in the immunoprecipitation procedure could be partly responsible for the high level of cleavage of the polypeptide. The level of cleavage is particularly evident in Fig. 2c. The specificity of the antibodies for NP was confirmed by the demonstration that subclones of hybrid clone D3 could also precipitate this polypeptide (Fig. 3b).

Anti-pancreatic islet-cell antibodies. Type 1 insulin-dependent diabetes mellitus (IDDM) is characterized by the destruction of pancreatic beta cells and the presence of anti-islet antibodies early

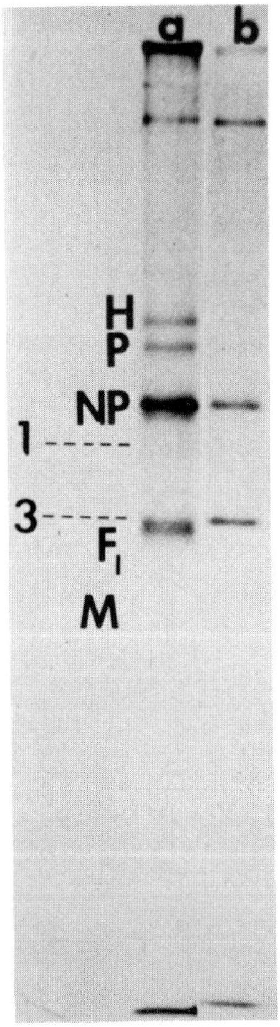

Fig. 3. Lane a represents the virus polypeptides precipitated by the same atypical measles serum as in Fig. 2a. (b) Polyacrylamide gel electrophoretic analysis of the measles virus polypeptides precipitated by culture fluid from subclone D3M2. The conditions of the experiments were as described in the legend to Fig. 2, except that culture fluid was unconcentrated.

in the course of the disease (10). We obtained 10 ml of blood from an 8-year-old female who had had IDDM for 11 months. The lymphocytes were purified and fused with GM1500 6TG-A1-2. After two to three weeks, hybrids were observed in 22 out of 24 seeded wells. One of the culture supernatants, B6, contained antibody that bound selectively to the cytoplasm of islet cells as opposed to acinar cells on Bouin's fixed human pancreatic sections (Fig. 4). Culture fluids from the myeloma cell line did not give immunofluorescence (not shown). This antibody, as well as naturally occurring anti-islet

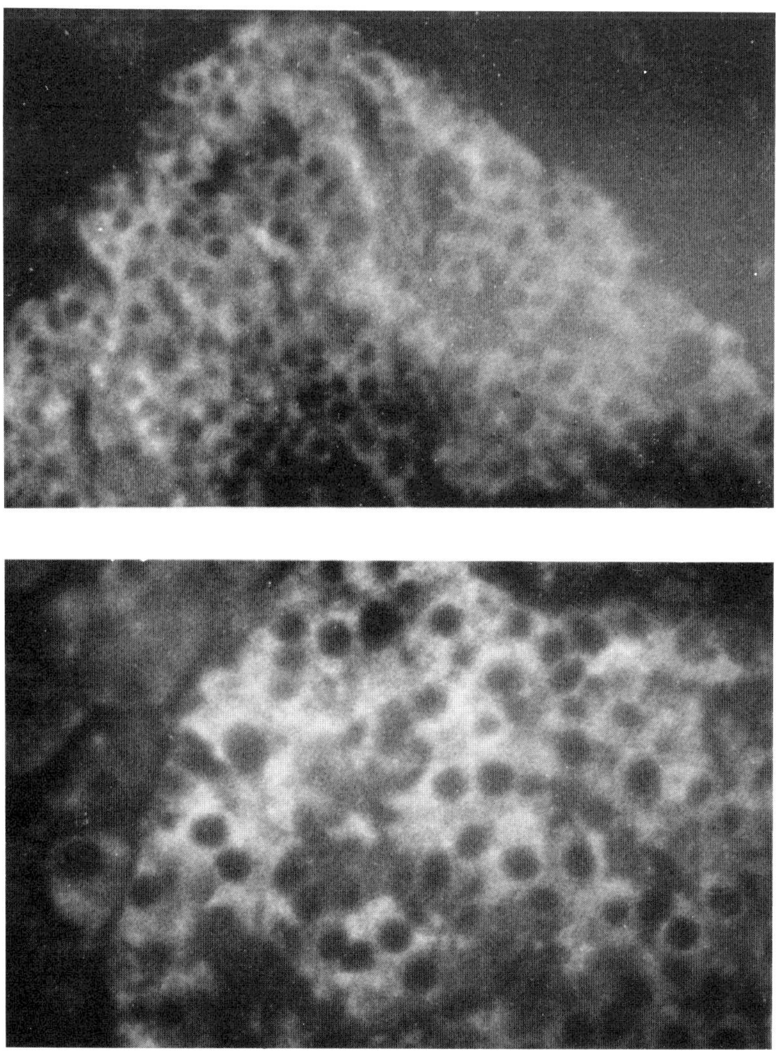

Fig. 4. Indirect immunofluorescence illustrating the binding of antibody B6 to Bouin's sectioned human pancreas. The top panel is magnification at 250X, the bottom panel at 400X.

antibodies, binds not only to insulin-containing cells but also to glucagon- and somatoslatin-containing cells. Clones from the culture have been stably producing IgM antibodies for more than a year as determined by immunoprecipitation and SDS-polyacrylamide gel electrophoresis (Fig. 5, lanes 3-6). The availability of milligram quantities of monoclonal antibody B6, purified from culture supernatant using affinity chromatography, will permit us to investigate the nature of the antigen as well as the role of the auto-antibody in the development of diabetes.

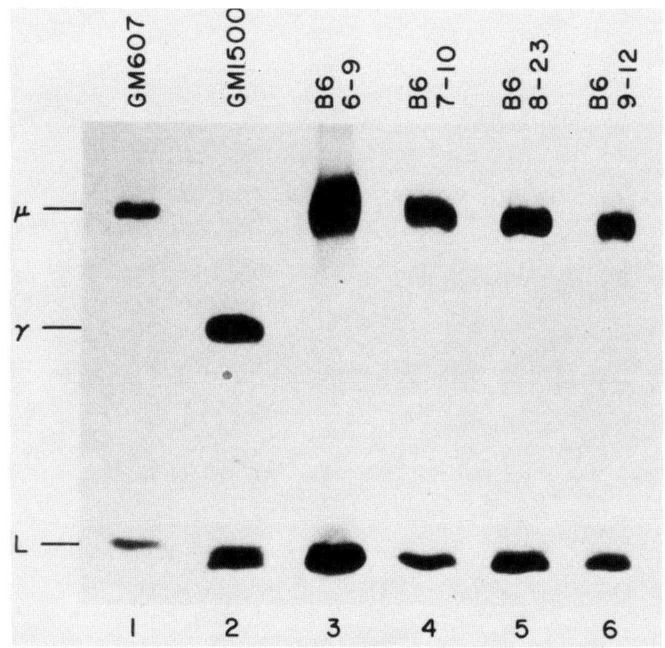

Fig. 5. Immunoprecipitation and polyacrylamide gel analysis of human immunoglobulin chains secreted by hybridomas derived from an IDDM patient. GM607 is an IgM-producing human myeloma cell line.

Thus far, the isolation of the human myeloma mutant cell line GM1500 6TG-A1-2 has made possible the *in vitro* reconstruction of a patient's antibody response to a pathogenic virus and of a patient's auto-antibody response in an auto-immune disease. Yet another possibility could be the cloning of patients' anti-tumor antibodies. The ability to produce human monoclonal antibodies is an important step towards the application of hybridoma technology to human immunotherapy. One possible application could be the use of anti-auto-antibodies in the treatment of auto-immune diseases.

References

1. Köhler, G, and C Milstein (1975). Continuous cultures of fused cells secreting antibody of predefined specificity. Nature (Lond) **256**, 495-497.
2. Koprowski, H, W Gerhard and CM Croce (1977). Production of antibodies against influenza virus by somatic cell hybrids between mouse myeloma and primed spleen cells. Proc Natl Acad Sci USA **74**, 2985-2988.
3. Croce, CM, M Shander, J Martinis, L Cicurel, GG D'Ancona, TW Dolby and H Koprowski (1979). Chromosomal location of the genes for human immunoglobulin heavy chains. Proc Natl Acad Sci USA **76**, 3416-3419.
4. Croce, CM, M Shander, J Martinis, L Cicurel, GG D'Ancona and H Koprowski (1980). Preferential retention of human chromosome 14 in mouse x human B cell hybrids. Eur J Immunol **10**, 486-488.
5. Croce, CM, and H Koprowski (1974). Postitive control of transformed phenotypes in hybrids between SV40-transformed and normal human cells. Science **184**, 1288-1289.
6. Littlefield, JW (1964). Selection of hybrids from matings of fibroblasts *in vitro* and their presumed recombinants. Science **145**, 709-710.
7. Croce, CM, A Linnenbach, W Hall, Z Steplewski and H Koprowski (1980). Production of human hybridomas secreting antibodies to measles virus. Nature (Lond) **288**, 488-489.
8. Eisenbarth, GS, A Linnenbach, R Jackson and CM Croce (1981). Antibody B6: A human monoclonal anti-islet antibody. Clin Res **29**, No 2, 404A.
9. Hall, W, RA Lamb and PW Choppin (1979). Measles and subacute sclerosing panencephalitis virus proteins: Lack of antibodies to the M protein in patients with subacute sclerosing panencephalitis. Proc Natl Acad Sci USA **76**, 2047-2051.
10. Lendrum, R, G Walker and DR Gamble (1975). Islet-cell antibodies in juvenile diabetes mellitis of recent onset. Lancet **1**, 880-883.

MONOCLONAL ANTIBODIES: THE BASIS FOR A NEW PHARMACOLOGY

Edgar Haber, M.D.

Cardiac Unit and Department of Medicine
Massachusetts General Hospital
Boston, Massachusetts 02114

The exponential acceleration of our understanding of immunology emphasizes an opportunity of which we have long been aware but which we have been unable to exploit fully. The products of the immune system, of which humoral antibodies are the most accessible, provide an incredible diversity of highly selective recognition sites. The number of molecules that can be differentiated by antibodies exceeds by many orders of magnitude the recognition potential of all the drugs with which the medicinal chemist has been able to provide us. Until the last five years, however, the inherent heterogeneity and lack of reproducibility of antibodies has restricted their application beyond the field of immunoassay. Even here, attempts at commercial distribution of reagents have resembled a cottage industry, for when a particular antiserum from an optimal donor was exhausted, the test had to be revised and restandardized. The advent of monoclonal antibodies produced by somatic-cell fusion has already vastly extended the application of the products of the immune system, but I believe that we are only seeing the beginning of a new pharmacology based on the remarkable properties of the antibody combining site.

In the following sections I shall examine the enhanced role of monoclonal antibodies in immunoassay, their application in the reversal of drug intoxication, their potential as imaging agents *in vivo*, and their value as probes of physiologic receptors.

Monoclonal Antibodies to Drugs: A Selective Approach to Immunoassay

The conventional approach to the production of an antibody suitable for immunoassay of drug concentration begins with immunization of an animal with a drug-protein conjugate, followed by testing of the antisera with respect to affinity and specificity at various times after immunization. Each antiserum (whether obtained from the same animal at different times after immunization or from different animals) has a unique spectrum of affinities and specificities for the mixture of antibodies that it contains. Some specificities, however, tend to be dominant, and it is often very difficult to find antibodies that effect a desired resolution, such as between a drug and its metabolite or among closely related compounds. For example, even after many years of effort, a method has not been found that reliably produces antibodies that differentiate between the octapeptide, angiotensin II, and its heptapeptide metabolite (1,2) although antibodies that differentiate between this hormone and its decapeptide precursor, angiotensin I, are readily produced in most immunizations. Thus, in addition to the problem that most antisera present as mixtures of antibodies rather than as single reagents, the problem of preference in the production of certain sets of antibodies (immunodominance) often defeats the investigator. The incredible power of selection possible with monoclonal antibodies should allow one to overcome these difficulties. An example of this remarkable selectivity is seen in a set of monoclonal antibodies specific for the drug digoxin.

Digoxin, one of a large group of cardiac glycosides, is the drug most frequently prescribed for patients with congestive heart failure. Cardiac glycosides are composed of a steroid, or agylcone portion, and from one to four sugar molecules (Fig. 1). The pharmacological activity resides in the aglycone portion of the molecule, and the sugar residues modify water solubility and potency.

Digoxin is an uncharged, chemically well-defined hapten, sufficient in size to occupy most of the antibody combining site. For this reason, cardiac glycosides which include 64 structurally related analogs (3,4) are suitable for a detailed study of antibody specificity. The rigid four-ring structure common among all cardiac glycosides and other steroids does not allow for major conformational changes as functional groups are substituted at various positions on the steroid backbone. Through an analysis of antibody affinity for related glycosides, the detailed specificity of antibodies can be defined readily. Certain heterogeneous antibodies raised to digoxin have been shown to be very selective in that they discriminate between digoxin and digitoxin, which differ from each other by the presence or absence of a single hydroxyl group at position 12 on the steroid backbone (Fig. 1) (5). This specificity is very commonly found, however (Table 1, sheep antidigoxin sera), to the exclusion of others that might be of value or interest in studying cardiac glycosides and their metabolites. Thus we sought to examine a repertoire of monoclonal anti-digoxin antibodies (6,7).

Three high-affinity monoclonal antibodies specific for digoxin have been produced successfully by somatic-cell fusion. Each antibody has been analyzed for its affinity and fine specificity for digoxin and related cardiac glycosides. Two of the antibodies, Dig 26-10 (subclass IgG_{2a}) and Dig 35-20 (subclass IgG_1), have a high affinity (10^9 M^{-1}) for digoxin, while the third, Dig 25-54 (subclass IgG_1), has an affinity that is an order of magnitude lower (10^8 M^{-1}) (Table 1). As demonstrated in Table 2, both Dig 26-10 and Dig 35-20 are as capable of quantitating digoxin in human sera as the sheep anti-

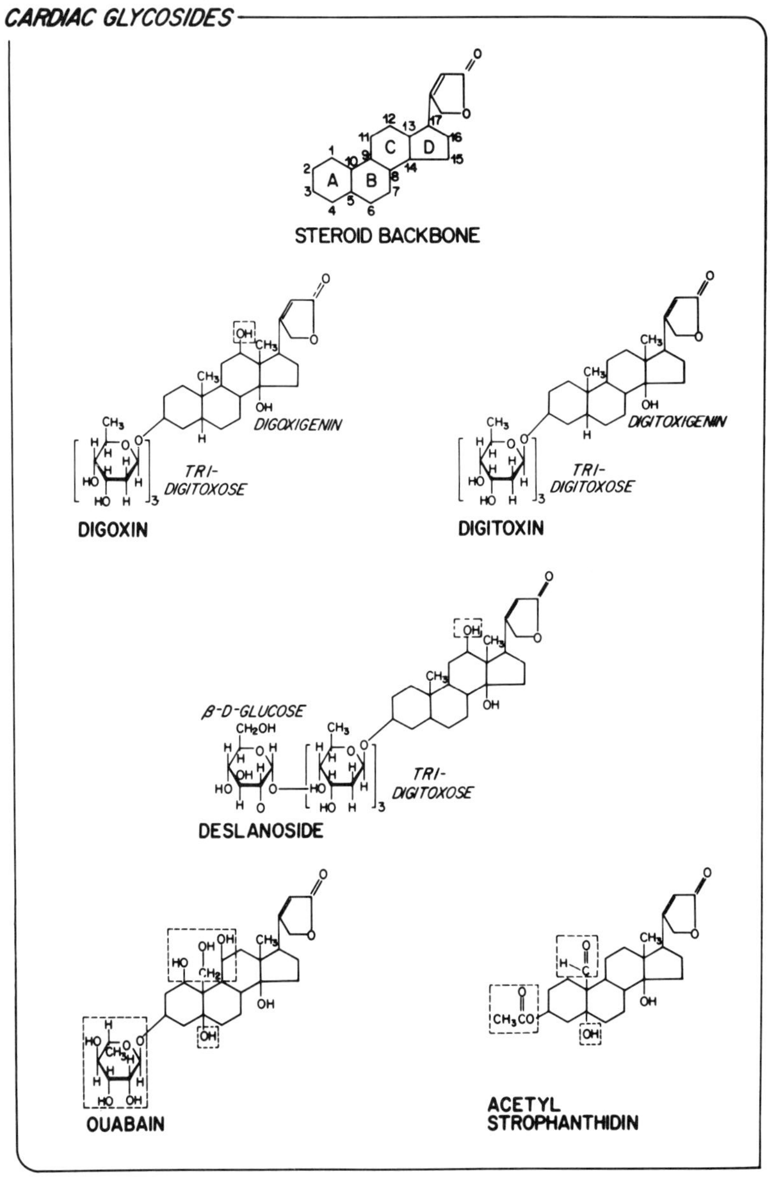

Fig. 1. Structures of digoxin and related cardiac glycosides.

digoxin antisera raised in this laboratory and commercially produced heterogeneous anti-digoxin antibodies (Corning, New York). High-affinity monoclonal antibodies, which can be obtained in essentially unlimited supply, are particularly attractive as standard reagents in clinical assays for digoxin.

Each of these three antibodies demonstrates a unique specificity pattern (Table 3). Based on the results from inhibition of related cardiac glycosides, the following general conclusions can be stated. None of the monoclonal anti-digoxin antibodies is specific for the digitoxose moiety because all of the hybridoma antibodies are reactive towards digoxin and digitoxigenin. Unlike the sheep antisera, all three monoclonal antibodies are equally reactive to digoxin and to digitoxin; hence, none is specific for the hydroxyl at position C12 of the steroid ring (Fig. 1). Since the unsaturated lactone ring structure is common to all the cardiac glycosides tested, differences in specificity cannot be attributed to this part of the molecule. Where there are major differences in the functional groups substituted on rings A and B of the steroid structure (Fig. 1), major differences in relative affinities for the cardiac glycosides occur. For example, the molecular structures of rings A and B of ouabain and acetyl strophanthidin differ significantly from those of digoxin, digitoxin, and deslanoside (compare respective structures of Fig. 1 with each other and with Table 3). Thus, the differences in relative affinities parallel these structural changes (i.e., all three antibodies are less reactive toward ouabain than they are to digoxin, digitoxin, or deslanoside).

Table 1. Hybridoma affinity constants for digoxin

Hybridoma clone	H-chain isotope	Affinity constant $K_0(M^{-1})^a$ — Culture media	Affinity constant $K_0(M^{-1})^a$ — Antibody purified from ascites
25-10	γ_{2a}	8.5×10^9	4.7×10^9
	Fab		1.2×10^9
25-54	γ_1	2.6×10^8	5.2×10^8
35-20	γ_1	1.9×10^9	1.3×10^9
Sheep anti-digoxin sera			1.2×10^{10}

[a]Affinity constants (K_0) were determined in an RIA that utilizes (^{3}H)digoxin and dextran-coated charcoal to adsorb free digoxin (Smith, TW, 1972. J Clin Invest **51**, 1583). Data were plotted according to a modified Sips equation (Nisonoff, A, and D Pressman, 1958. J Immunol **80**, 417). Correlation coefficients varied from r = 0.989 to 0.999. (By permission of Academic Press, Inc., modified from: Haber, E, in press. Monoclonal antibodies to drugs: new diagnostic and therapeutic tools. In Monoclonal Antibodies in Clinical Medicine. AJ McMichael, ed.)

In addition to being examined with respect to these general trends, each hybridoma antibody may be further analyzed individually with regard to its specific recognition of antigenic determinants. Dig 25-54, for example, has a lower affinity for digitoxigenin because it requires 54 times as much digitoxigenin as digoxin to achieve 50% inhibition (Table 3). This reduced affinity for digitoxigenin implies that the digitoxose sugar moiety plays a role in binding to the Dig 25-54 combining site. Dig 25-54 also bound ouabain and acetyl strophanthidin with affinities reduced by at least two orders of magnitude

Table 2. Monoclonal antibodies tested in a clinical assay for digoxin[a]

RIA used:	^{125}I-RIA kit[b]	(^{3}H)Digoxin-RIA[c]		
Antidigoxin Ab:	Supplied by Corning	Sheep antisera	Dig 26-10	Dig 35-20
Digoxin/ml sera:	ng/ml	ng/ml	ng/ml	ng/ml
Patient Number				
4601	2.6	2.8	2.6	ND[d]
4605	0.9	1.2	0.8	ND
4615	0.4	0.8	0.8	ND
4617	0.8	1.0	0.7	ND
5875	1.3	1.4	1.6	ND
5876	1.3	1.1	1.2	ND
5884	1.2	1.6	1.6	ND
9708	4.4	4.8	5.4	6.0
9717	2.5	2.3	2.1	1.9
9761	2.0	1.5	ND	1.6

[a]Monoclonal antibodies Dig 26-10 and Dig 35-20 were compared to the sheep anti-digoxin sera and to anti-digoxin antibody provided in a commercially available kit for their ability to quantitate digoxin in patients' sera.

[b]The commercially available ^{125}I-RIA kit for digoxin was obtained from Corning (New York).

[c]This (^{3}H)digoxin RIA is the clinical dextran-coated charcoal RIA described in section 1.

[d]ND, not done.

(By permission of Academic Press, Inc., modified from: Haber, E, in press. Monoclonal antibodies to drugs: new diagnostic and therapeutic tools. In Monoclonal Antibodies in Clinical Medicine. AJ McMichael, ed.)

(Table 3). Both ouabain and acetyl strophanthidin are characterized by extensive substitutions on the A and B rings of the steroid portion of the digoxin molecule (positions 1, 5, 10 and 11 and 5 and 10, respectively) not found on digoxin or digitoxin (Fig. 1) that would be likely to cause steric hindrance to an antibody combining site ordinarily fitting the A and B rings of digoxin.

The specificity of monoclonal antibody Dig 35-20 is similar to that of Dig 25-54 because substitutions in rings A and B similarly cause the molecule to bind less tightly to the antibody (Table 3). However, since there is essentially no difference in the relative affinity of Dig 35-20 for digoxin and digitoxigenin, the digitoxose sugar groups have no role in binding to this antibody in contrast to Dig 25-54 (see above).

Dig 26-10, as Dig 35-20, apparently does not distinguish between glycosides with or without digitoxose since no significant difference in binding to digoxin and digitoxigenin was observed (Table 3). The specificity of Dig 26-10, as that of Dig 35-20 and Dig 25-54, probably resides in rings A and B, but unlike the other two monoclonal antibodies, Dig 26-10 does not discriminate between digoxin and acetyl strophanthidin; yet ouabain is not well bound. The essential difference between ouabain and acetyl strophanthidin, with respect to the steroid nucleus, is the presence of hydroxyl groups at positions 1 and 11 on the A and C rings, respectively. The hydroxyl at 1 has an α orientation, that at 2, a β orientation. This brings these two structures quite close together in three-dimensional space and allows one to visualize steric hindrance to the antibody combining site of 26-10 if it were to bind to the upper part of rings A and B, yet miss position 12 (since it does not differentiate between digoxin and digitoxin), as well as not including the lower part of the A and B rings that contain the substitutions that differentiate digoxin from acetyl strophanthidin.

In many years of study of conventionally obtained digoxin-specific antisera, the kind of molecular discrimination provided by these monoclonal antibodies has not previously been observed. Such antibodies provide powerful tools for the study of the fine structure of organic molecules. Because of their desirable high affinity, they also offer the possibility of producing a world standard reagent for immunoassay.

The Sandwich Immunoassay Utilizing Two Monoclonal Antibodies

At times, even careful and extensive screening of antibody-producing clones does not provide the requisite specificity. An example will be given in which two monoclonal antibodies were needed to effect the requisite resolution in an immunoassay (8,9).

Monoclonal antibodies recognize a single antigenic determinant,

Table 3. Specificity of hybridoma antibodies for various cardiac glycosides relative to digoxin[a]

Hybridoma clone or antisera	Cardiac glycoside inhibitors					
	Digoxin	Digitoxin	Digitoxigenin	Deslanoside	Acetylstrophanthidin	Ouabain
Dig 25-54	1.0	1.8	54.0	4.3	>100	>100
Dig 35-20	1.0	4.6	2.7	3.7	110	333
Dig 26-10	1.0	1.3	3.7	2.6	1.50	66
Sheep anti-dig serum	1.0	152.0	860.0	ND[b]	ND	>10^5

[a]Inhibition of binding to (^{3}H)digoxin by a series of cardiac glycosides was determined for each hybridoma antibody and for a standard sheep anti-digoxin serum. The assay system used was the dextran-coated charcoal RIA (Smith, TW, 1972. J Clin Invest **51**, 1583). The values reported here are amounts of inhibitor required to give 50% inhibition relative to the amount of cold digoxin that gave 50% inhibition.

[b]ND, not done.

(By permission of Academic Press, Inc., modified from: Haber, E, in press. Monoclonal antibodies to drugs: new diagnostic and therapeutic tools. **In** Monoclonal Antibodies in Clinical Medicine. AJ McMichael, ed.)

which should allow for enhanced specificity of recognition, and thus should allow selection of an antibody specific for the epitope that defines the difference between two very similar molecules. Yet it appears that cross reactivity is often seen. With monoclonal antibodies this is probably a manifestation of the sharing of parts of an epitope by two antigens. A method that entails the combination of two antibodies that recognize different epitopes on the same molecule should enhance specificity markedly. The differentiation between cardiac- and skeletal-muscle myosin appears to offer a good test case. The molecules are different structurally, yet elicited antibodies (mixtures), and most monoclonal antibodies we have tested, exhibit varying degrees of cross reactivity. When an assay is constructed so that two different monoclonal antibodies must bind to the same antigen, the resultant cross reactivity observed corresponds, as might be expected from theoretical considerations, to approximately the product of the two fractional cross reactivities.

Cardiac myosin light chains are structurally (10,11) and immunologically (12,13) different from skeletal- and smooth-muscle myosin light chains and thus may provide a unique cardiac-specific antigen. Unfortunately, there is sufficient immunologic similarity between myosin light chains from various tissues such that antibodies that uniquely recognize one and not the others have not been obtained (12,13). The sera of 25 rabbits immunized with human cardiac-myosin light chains were examined by us at varying times after immunization. Cross reactivity between cardiac- and skeletal-muscle light chains varied between 10 and 100%. An antiserum could not be found that would provide the specificity requisite for use in clinical assay. A solution to this problem uses monoclonal antibodies that recognize two different epitopes on the same antigen and thus markedly enhances the resolution possible in immunoassay. Examples of the varieties of antigenic specificities found are depicted in Fig. 2. Antibody 3C7 typifies the most common type. There is complete identity of reactivity between cardiac- and skeletal-myosin light chains, indicating recognition of common antigenic determinants. Antibody 2B2 is representative of a less frequent type. These monoclonal antibodies demonstrate a partial cross reactivity between skeletal- and smooth-muscle light chains. Perhaps only a part of a common antigenic determinant is recognized. The least common monoclonal response is typified by 1E6. This antibody shows no evidence of cross reactivity between skeletal- and smooth-muscle light chains and thus recognizes the unique determinants of the cardiac light chain, providing the basis for the development of an entirely specific immunoassay for cardiac cell damage.

Three monoclonal antibodies that exhibited varying degrees of cross reactivity between cardiac- and skeletal-muscle light chains were selected for study. When immobilized on Sepharose, each bound ^{125}I-cardiac myosin light chains effectively, allowing ready determination of cross reactivity with skeletal-muscle light chains utilizing a solid-phase competitive radioimmunoassay. Increasing concentration of either unlabeled cardiac or skeletal light chains resulted in decreased binding of ^{125}I cardiac light chains (Table 4, top). Antibody 1C5 proved to be fully cross reactive, 4F10 17.5% cross reactive, and 2B9 25% cross reactive. The antibodies appear to possess varying affinities for myosin light chains, with the most cross-reactive antibody, 1C5, providing the greatest sensitivity in measurement.

Table 4 (bottom) demonstrates the enhanced specificity inherent in an assay where two antigenic determinants (epitopes) are independently measured. One monoclonal antibody is immobilized by covalent linkage of Sepharose. When exposed to an antigen mixture, only those molecules recognized by that antibody will adhere. A second antibody, labeled with ^{125}I, is then added. It will bind only to those antibody molecules that are both immobilized and possess the epitope for which it is specific. Thus immobilized radioactivity represents the recognition of two different epitopes on the antigen molecule. It

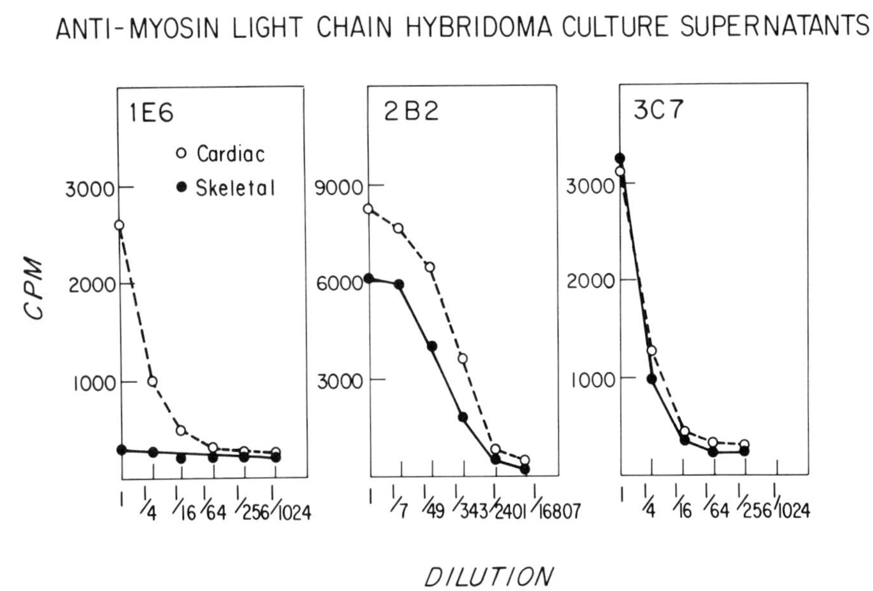

Fig. 2. Binding of hybridoma antibodies to cardiac- or skeletal-muscle light chains immobilized on plastic microtiter plates. Dilution of the cell-culture supernatant is plotted against counts/min of ^{125}I-labeled goat-(anti-mouse) Fab antibody bound to the plate that recognizes the myosin light chain-specific antibody. (By permission of Raven Press from: Haber et al., 1981. Resolving antigenic sites and purifying proteins with monoclonal antibodies. **In** Monoclonal Antibodies in Endocrine Research. RE Fellows and G Eisenbarth, eds.)

can be seen from Table 4 that when a fully cross reactive antibody (1C5) is combined with a partially cross reactive antibody (2B9 or 4F10), there is no change in cross reactivity measured in the combined sandwich assay. However, the combination of two partially cross reactive antibodies results in a significantly lower cross reactivity. Seemingly the resultant cross reactivities in the sandwich assay approximate the product of the individual cross reactivities of the component antibodies.

This form of dual recognition requires that epitopes not be overlapping and that they be sufficiently distant from one another to prevent steric hindrance between two antibodies. A logical consequence of the last argument is that the use of the same antibody, both immobilized to Sepharose and labeled, should result in no apparent binding of the label. This is demonstrated in Fig. 3. When antibody 2B9 is both immobilized on the support and labeled, no radioactivity remains on the solid support after washing.

Table 4.

Competitive assay utilizing labeled antigen

Antibody	Measured fractional cross reactivity
1C5	1.00
4F10	0.17
2B9	0.25

Bi-determinant assay utilizing labeled second antibody

Antibodies	Calculated cross reactivity	Measured cross reactivity
1C5 and 2B9	0.17	0.17
1C5 and 4F10	0.25	0.25
2B9 and 4F10	0.037	0.043

(By permission of Academic Press, Inc. from: Haber, E, in press. Monoclonal antibodies to drugs: new diagnostic and therapeutic tools. **In** Monoclonal Antibodies in Clinical Medicine. AJ McMichael, ed.)

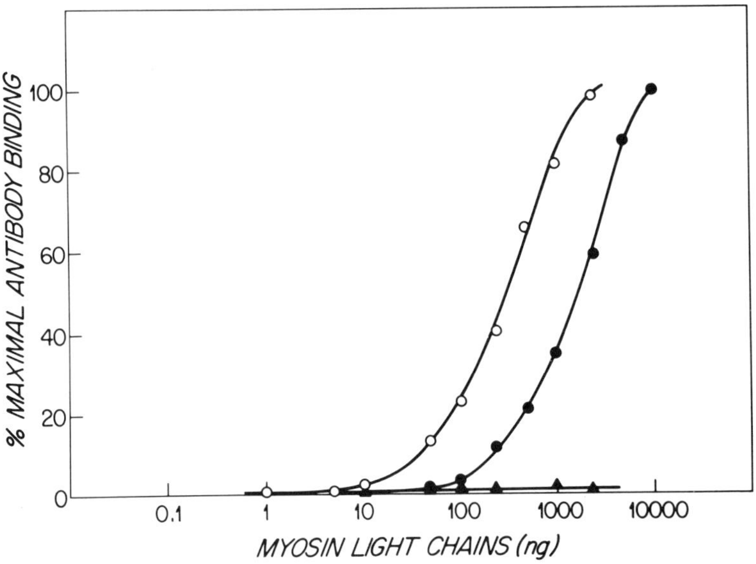

Fig. 3. Binding of ^{125}I-labeled second antibody to antigen that had first been bound to Sepharose-immobilized antibody. Percent maximal labeled antibody binding in antigen excess is plotted against the amount of cardiac- or skeletal-muscle light chain added. Skeletal-muscle light chains (●), cardiac-muscle light chains (O) measured with antibody 2B9 immobilized on Sepharose and antibody 1C5 labeled. Cardiac-muscle light chains (▲) measured with antibody 2B9 immobilized on Sepharose and antibody 2B9 labeled. (By permission of Pergamon Press from: Katus et al., in press. Increased specificity in human cardiac myosin radioimmunoassay utilizing two monoclonal antibodies in a double sandwich assay. Molec Immunol.)

Reversal of Drug Intoxication With Antibodies

The digitalis glycosides are of great value in the treatment of congestive heart failure and consequently are frequently used in clinical medicine. Unfortunately, they are characterized by a very close toxic-therapeutic ratio. Digitalis intoxication is one of the most frequent adverse drug reactions reported. There is no specific antidote, and the cardiac arrhythmias that are a feature of digitalis intoxication are not uncommonly fatal.

We reasoned that if an antibody specific to the digitalis glycosides had a higher affinity for the drug than for the physiologic receptor, it should be possible to transfer the ligand from the receptor to the antibody simply by mass action. For optimal effectiveness diffusion distances should be minimal, and the antibody should be in high concentration in the extracellular fluid in proximity to the receptor.

It would also be desirable to remove the antibody-drug complex rapidly from the body. If a conventional antibody preparation is utilized, all of these goals may not be achieved optimally.

Intact antibody has a number of troublesome properties when used as a drug. When the source is a heterologous species, it is an immunogen: after the first use, an immune response develops that may result in anaphylaxis, serum sickness, or at best accelerated elimination. Antibody is only eliminated by metabolism, with the half-life for endogenous immunoglobulins measured in days or weeks, depending on the species and the immunoglobulin isotype. If immune complexes form, elimination is more rapid by the reticuloendothelial system. The presence of immune complexes may adversely affect renal function, and the activation of the complement system may likewise be undesirable. The immunoglobulin molecules that bind two moles of antigen per mole may be cleaved into smaller fragments by the enzyme papain (14). The resultant Fab bind one mole of antigen each, whereas the Fc contains the complement binding site. Fab has a number of desirable properties when compared with the intact molecule, IgG: equilibrium distribution in extracellular fluid is achieved more rapidly, the volume of distribution is greater, and the fragment is eliminated with a far shorter half-life (15). In addition, when injected intravenously, Fab is less immunogenic than IgG (15). The immune complexes that may be formed are smaller than those that cause nephrotoxicity (comprising a single antigen molecule with several Fab attached), and complement cannot be fixed because the relevant binding sites on the Fc have been lost.

Digoxin-specific antibody was purified from sheep antiserum utilizing immobilized ouabain. Fab was then isolated after papain cleavage (16). After demonstration of safety and effectiveness in animal studies, clinical investigations were initiated. At the time of this writing, 17 patients with life-threatening digitalis intoxication have been studied. The patients ranged in age from infants to septuagenarians, and in each case a dramatic reversal of the signs and symptoms of intoxication occurred (17-19).

The recently reported history of a patient is typical of the group (18). The individual was a 34-year-old woman who took 20 mg of digitoxin, a massive overdose, with suicidal intent. On admission to the hospital she appeared to be well except for nausea, but she soon lapsed into a series of life-threatening arrhythmias that included multiple episodes of ventricular fibrillation (treated with countershock), as well as asystole (treated with ventricular pacing). At the time the antibody Fab became available to the physicians treating her, she was in shock and was aneuric, and she exhibited dilated pupils. The patient's serum potassium was elevated, a grave prognostic sign in digitalis intoxication (20). Within an hour after the intravenous administration of antibody Fab, her atrioventricular conduction had returned, and she was soon in normal sinus rhythm. No further dysrhythmias occurred. The patient was discharged from the hospital without sequellae several days later. Figure 4 demonstrates the initial marked increase of serum digitoxin concentration in this patient as tissue-bound drug equilibrated with the antibody (antibody-bound drug is pharmacologically inactive), followed by rapid clearance of both drug and Fab. It should be noted that the half-life of digitoxin in man is normally 3.5 days, with hepatic metabolism of the drug being the major source of removal. It is apparent that excretion has been markedly accelerated by the antibody Fab, the half-life seemingly being reduced to about 12 h. Figure 5 shows that both antibody and Fab appear in the urine largely within the first day after Fab administration.

The digitalis glycosides in most common use are digoxin and digitoxin. They differ very little from one another in their chemical structure, yet most antibodies differentiate between them with differences in affinity of 50- to 100-fold as indicated in the first section above, and in Table 3 (21). It would be desirable to use an antibody that bound both digoxin and digitoxin with equal affinity.

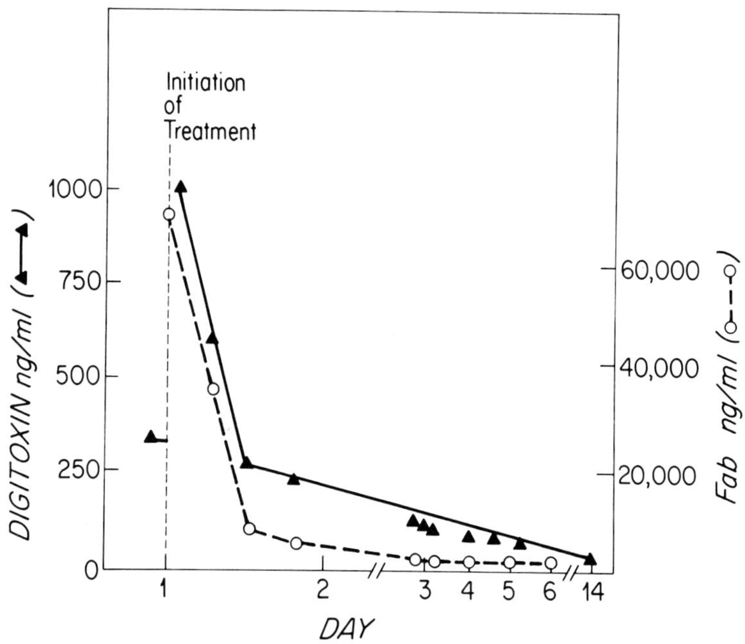

Fig. 4. Blood levels of digitoxin and Fab after intravenous administration of antibody Fab to a 34-year-old woman suffering a series of life-threatening arrhythmias as a result of a massive overdose (20 mg) of digitoxin. Within an hour of intravenous administration of antibody Fab, atrioventricular conduction had returned. (By permission of Academic Press, Inc., from: Haber, E, in press. The antibody combining site: A basis for a new pharmacology. **In** Contributions of Chemical Biology to the Biomedical Sciences. A Dean, AN Schechter and RF Goldberger, eds.)

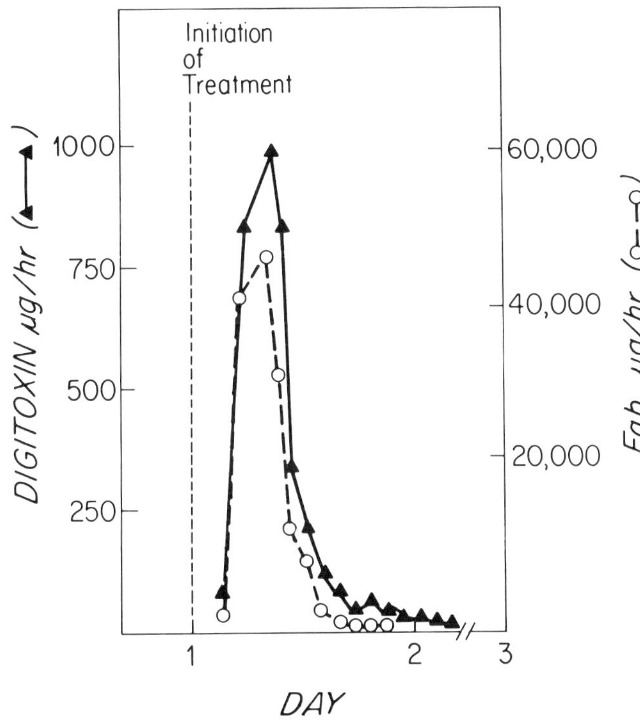

Fig. 5. Urinary excretion rates of digitoxin and Fab following intravenous administration of antibody Fab to a 34-year-old woman suffering from digitalis intoxication (20 mg). (By permission of Academic Press, Inc., from: Haber, E, in press. The antibody combining site: A basis for a new pharmacology. **In** Contributions of Chemical Biology to the Biomedical Sciences. A Dean, AN Schechter and RF Goldberger, eds.)

The monoclonal antibody 26-10 (described above) had an affinity of 5×10^9 for digoxin and a nearly equal affinity for digitoxin (Table 3) (6). Since a monoclonal antibody is a homogeneous protein that recognizes only a single aspect of an antigen molecule, it appears that the hydroxyl group is not a part of the antigenic recognition site of this molecule. This antibody, which can be produced in quantities essentially without limit, has been shown to reverse digoxin intoxication in experimental animals.

It should be apparent that this approach could be applied to many other drugs or toxins. Of particular interest is accelerating the excretion of a substance that is normally metabolized slowly. Fab is capable of altering the route of disposal from hepatic metabolism to renal excretion (22).

Antibodies as Imaging Agents

The hallmark of cell death is loss of membrane integrity: when there is no longer a physical separation between inside and outside, the cell ceases to exist. This principle is commonly employed in clinical practice in diagnosing tissue infarction. Intracellular enzymes or other proteins (see the second section above) are lost to extracellular fluid, and their increased concentration in the blood may be used as a measure of tissue necrosis. An alternative approach is the inward diffusion of a marker that is normally excluded from cells. We have selected myocardial infarction as a model and radioactively labeled myosin-specific antibody as a marker.

Myosin is the principal protein of the cardiac cell. The covalent structure of the entire molecule, as of the light chains (see second section above), is unique to the heart (23), allowing the development of antibodies that differentiate between cardiac and either skeletal- or smooth-muscle myosins. In the intact organism, cardiac myosin is protected from extracellular fluid by the cell's plasma membrane. When cell death occurs and the membrane breaks down, myosin is exposed to extracellular fluid. It is then available to react with labeled antibodies or antibody fragments.

A visual demonstration of this phenomenon is seen in Fig. 6. The figure shows a scanning electron micrograph of part of a neonatal mouse cardiac myocyte that had been rendered ischemic by prolonged exposure to nitrogen and had then been incubated with 1-μ diameter, polystyrene spheres covalently bound to myosin-specific antibody. Myofibrils are seen protruding from a hole in the cell membrane. Antibody-coated microspheres clearly bind to the myofibrils. Not only is myosin very insoluble in physiological fluids so that membrane breakdown does not result in antigen loss, but it also persists for considerable periods after ischemic necrosis (24). This should allow identification of infarcted myocardium for days to, perhaps, several weeks after the initial event.

In our initial exploration of this concept, we used a canine myocardial infarction model (25). The left anterior descending coronary artery was ligated, and four h later ^{125}I-labeled, myosin-specific antibody or antibody fragments were injected intravenously. At varying times subsequent to the injections, animals were killed, the hearts perfused with triphenyltetrazolium chloride, and the myocardium examined (26). Figure 7 (left) shows a section of a heart treated in this way. The light area represents a largely subendocardial infarction. The central panel of the figure is a tracing of the slice superimposed on an autoradiograph. The exposed area corresponds to the infarct as revealed by the triphenyltetrazolium stain. The right panel shows specific radioactivity in the area of the infarct relative to myocardium on the posterior wall. It is apparent that the major concentration of radioactivity is in the subendocardial region, with lesser concentration in the subepicardial region that had been

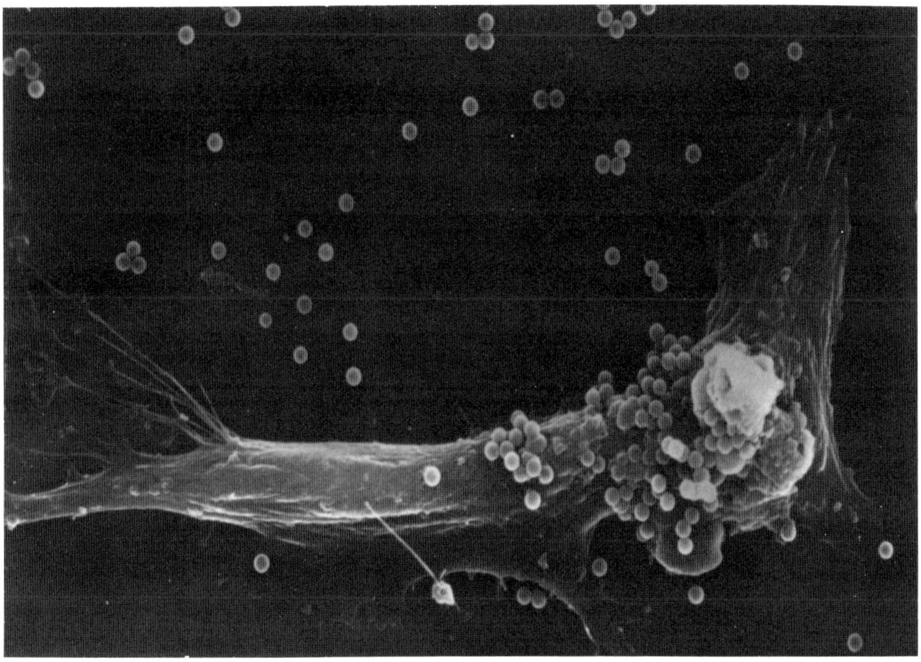

Fig. 6. Scanning electron micrograph of an ischemic neonatal mouse myocyte (magnification 2400x). The spheres adherent to the cell are covalently bonded to myosin-specific antibody. Non-ischemic cells do not bind significant numbers of spheres. (By permission of the British Medical Association from: Haber, E, in press. Immunological probes in cardiovascular disease. Brit Heart J.)

subjected only to spotty necrosis as indicated in the triphenyltetrazolium stain.

Microautoradiographs showed that individual necrotic myocytes could be identified and differentiated from adjacent viable cells (27). To demonstrate that antibody concentration was specific and not simply the result of passive diffusion of a macromolecule into infarcted cells, specific antibody labeled with ^{131}I and nonimmune globulin labeled with ^{125}I were injected simultaneously into the coronary arteries (26). At the center of the infarct, the antibody concentrated 34-fold in relation to normal myocardium, while the nonimmune globulin was only 7-fold in excess. In normal tissue, as expected, concentrations were equal. When compared to a marker of relative flow--the distribution of radioactive microspheres that had been injected into the left atrium--it was clear that the concentration of labeled antibody was inversely related to relative blood flow

(25,26). There seems to be sufficient collateral circulation in this ischemic model to provide for delivery of antibody, even to the regions of minimal blood flow. It would be very desirable to apply this method to the detection, localization, and quantification of myocardial infarcts in the living subject.

Optimal imaging with a gamma or positron camera requires the labeling of antibodies with radionuclides of appropriate half-life and affinity. We have accomplished this by covalently linking diethylene triamine pentaacetic acid (DTPA) to antibody or antibody fragment and then binding cationic radionuclides by chelation (28). Successful images have been obtained using the following radionuclides linked to antibody: ^{111}In-DTPA-Ab Fab (28), ^{68}Ga-DTPA Fab (29), and ^{99m}Tc-DTPA-Ab Fab (28). An example of a positron image of an anterior infarct in a living dog using ^{68}Ga-labeled antibody is shown in Fig. 8 (left). The positron imaging technique allows for tomographic reconstruction, and thus, the heart is visible on cross section in the ^{13}N-ammonia image in the center panel of Fig. 8. (Ammonium ion is a potassium analog and concentrates in normal tissue.) On the left side of this image there is clearly less density, reflecting the region of infarction. Superimposition of the ^{13}N and the ^{68}Ga images (right panel) showed that the antibody was concentrated directly in the area of diminished ammonium ion uptake. The potential for applying this method to the evaluation of myocardial infarcts in a clinical setting seems very great indeed because it provides for a method of great specificity and resolution.

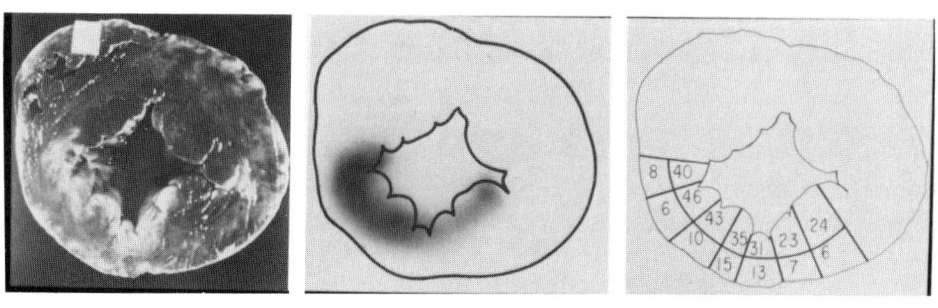

Fig. 7. Histochemically delineated myocardial infarction in a ventricular slide (left panel) seen as white or lighter-colored regions, and normal myocardium seen as darker regions. The corresponding macroautoradiograph is shown in the center with the outline of the ventricular slide. The right panel shows relative antibody uptake in the indicated areas. Ratios of antibody uptake were determined as specific radioactivity in relation to normal posterior ventricular myocardium. (By permission of the American Heart Association, Inc., from: Haber, E, and BA Khaw, 1979. Antibodies as imaging agents. Proc N Engl Cardiovasc Soc, Vol. II, 31-38.)

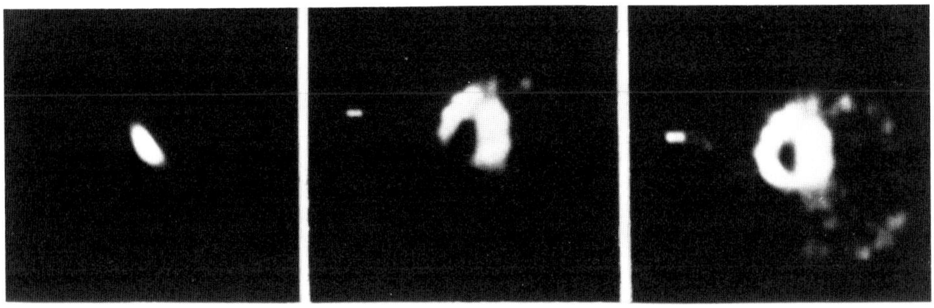

Fig. 8. ^{68}Ga and $^{13}NH_4^+$ were obtained sequentially utilizing a positron camera; 5 mCi of $^{13}NH_4^+$ was administered intravenously to a dog that had a prior four-hour occlusion of the distal segment of the left anterior descending artery and was imaged (center); 30 min later 1 mCi of ^{68}Ga was injected into the same artery and imaged (left panel). The right panel is a composite of both images. (By permission of the American Heart Association, Inc., from: Haber, E, and BA Khaw, 1979. Antibodies as imaging agents. Proc N Engl Cardiovasc Soc, Vol. II, 31-38.)

Antibodies to Drugs as Receptor Probes

The hormone receptors of the cell's plasma-cell membrane are present in a very small number of copies (10,000 to 50,000 per cell), which makes their isolation exceedingly difficult. Antibodies to partially purified receptor preparations have been elicited (30), but their utility is limited because these preparations of necessity contain antibodies to other membrane constituents. The ligands for these receptors, however, are usually readily available in quantity. Agonistic substances are often either peptides of modest size or organic compounds, both readily synthesized. For some receptors, a variety of antagonists has been created in the organic chemist's laboratory. Could an antibody for the receptor be obtained by utilizing the ligand (agonist or antagonist) as a template?

The vast diversity of antibody combining sites provides the potential for creating a complementary fit to a molecule of almost any shape. If a figurative plaster mold could be cast upon the surface of the ligand that bound to the receptor, then a second mold made from the first one should have a perfect fit to the receptor. The well-known immunologic principle of raising antibodies specific for another antibody's combining site (anti-idiotypic antibodies) may be utilized as the vehicle for molding the desired shape. The first antibody must bind the ligand generally in the same way as the receptor does, and thus the same atoms of the ligand may be utilized in the interatomic interactions with antibody as with the receptor. There are two ways of achieving this short of depending on serendipity. When conventional immunization is employed, many antibodies to the immunogen are formed, each binding to it in a somewhat different manner. The antibodies of this polyclonal response may be fractionated by the use of ligands of different structure. By virtue of being receptor ligands, they are all capable of binding to the receptor and must have some common structures, but if appropriately selected, structures irrelevant to binding are not shared. Those components of the polyclonal antibody mixture that bind to all possible ligands must be most similar to the receptor. The most practical way of achieving fractionation with polyclonal antibodies is through the use of sequential affinity chromatography. However, when monoclonal antibody techniques are employed, it is simply necessary to use selection techniques that will identify those antibodies that have the property of binding to all possible ligands. This general approach has now been applied to the insulin receptor (31).

A wide variety of structurally different β-antagonists is available; all, however, share a common structure, a propanolamine side chain (Fig. 9). Rabbits were immunized with an alprenolol-protein conjugate (32). The resulting antiserum was passed over an acebutolol-affinity column and the fall-through volume discarded. Elution of the affinity column was carried out with l-propranolol and the eluant antibody characterized after the l-propranolol had been removed by dialysis. Figure 10 demonstrates the specificity profile of this antibody fraction. Several β-adrenergic antagonists as well as agonists are bound with considerable affinity, in some cases similar to that of the receptor. This fraction also resolved l and d stereoisomers of isoproterenol (not shown). Thus the antibody fraction could be considered as a qualitative, but not a strictly precise, quantitative model for the β-adrenergic receptor.

Antibodies specific for the combining sites of the first antibody set were then raised by immunization of allotypically matched rabbits (33). The immunogen was identical to the immunoglobulins of the recipient animals except for the variable region of the molecule. Because of tolerance to self-determinants, the immunized animals made antibodies only to unique structures on the immunogen (anti-idiotypes). Table 5 shows the inhibition of binding of a labeled β-adrenergic antagonist, (^3H)alprenolol, to several kinds of binding sites by the anti-idiotypic antibody. Binding of the ligand, alprenolol, to the idiotype (the first generation antibody that had been raised in response to alprenolol) is largely inhibited by anti-idiotype (second generation antibody). Of greater interest is the inhibition of the specific binding of alprenolol to a plasma-membrane preparation of several different organs in two different animal species. Scatchard analysis shows the binding of the anti-idiotype to be competitive with

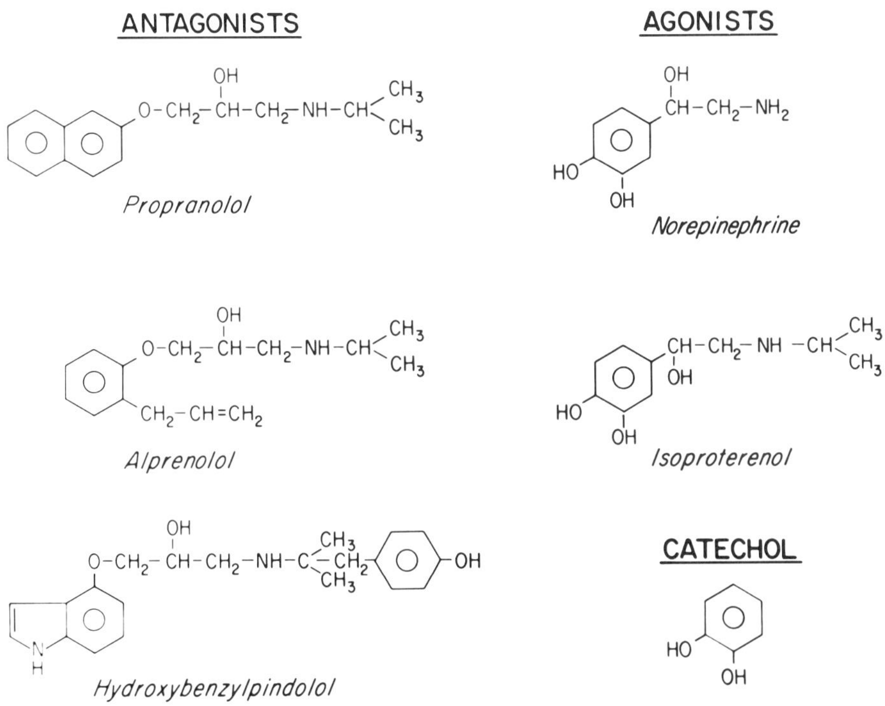

Fig. 9. Structures of β-antagonists and agonists. Note the common propanolamine side chain. Catechol, which is neither agonist nor antagonist, does not possess this structure. (By permission of Academic Press, Inc., from: Haber, E, in press. The antibody combining site: a basis for a new pharmacology. **In** Contributions of Chemical Biology to the Biomedical Sciences. A Dean, AN Schechter and RF Goldberger, eds.)

β-adrenergic antagonists. The anti-idiotype also appears to be an inhibitor of adenylate cyclase activation by β-adrenergic agonists. Increasing concentrations of isoproterenol progressively inhibit adenylate cyclase production in turkey erythrocyte membranes at an isoproterenol concentration of 5×10^{-7} M. At a higher concentration of isoproterenol (10^{-4}M), less inhibition is observed, suggesting a competitive nature for this interaction as well. Thus the anti-idiotype behaves as a true β-adrenergic antagonist, competing with both agonists and antagonists for the receptor site. The obvious potential uses of such receptor-specific antibodies include the recognition of structural differences among subsets of β-adrenergic receptors (34), a more rigorous examination of their respective physiologic roles utilizing reagents of greater resolution, and the isolation of receptors with antibody affinity chromatography.

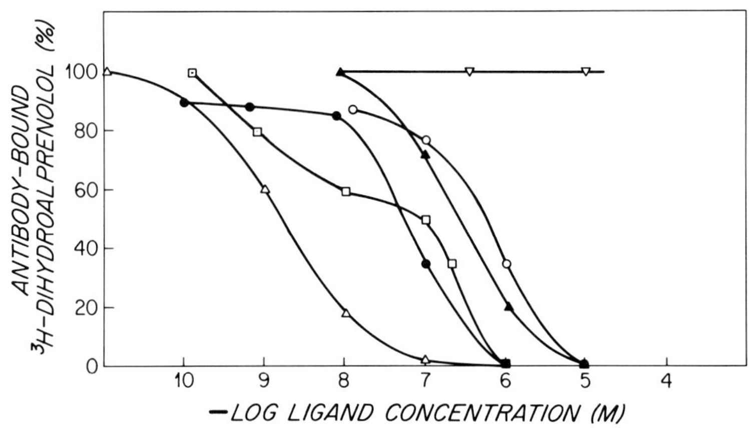

Fig. 10. Competitive inhibition of (-)(^{3}H)dihydroalprenolol binding to unfractionated anti-alprenolol antiserum. Rabbit immune serum (100 μl) was diluted 1:10 in buffer and incubated for 1 h at 25° C with (-)(^{3}H)dihydroalprenolol and increasing concentrations of (±)-propranolol (Δ), (±)-alprenolol (□), (±)-hydroxybenzylpindolol (●), (±)-norepinephrine (O), (±)-isoproterenol (▲), or catechol (∇). Each determination was performed in triplicate and corrected for the nonspecific (-)(^{3}H)dihydroalprenolol binding to rabbit preimmune serum. The results are expressed as a percentage of the total antibody-binding capacity for the tritiated antigen. (By permission of the American Heart Association, Inc., from: Rockson et al., 1980. Anti-alprenolol antibodies in the rabbit: a new probe for the study of β-adrenergic receptor interaction. Circ Res **46**, 808-813.)

Table 5. Inhibition of (^{3}H)alprenolol binding to antibodies and receptors by anti-idiotypic antibody[a]

	Maximal binding with preimmune	In presence of anti-idiotype	Inhibition
	dpm	dpm	%
Original idiotype (alprenolol)	10853 ± 250	488 ± 250	96
Turkey erythrocyte	19643 ± 540	6195 ± 525	68
Canine lung	6385 ± 283	4315 ± 190	34

[a]Specific binding at 4-6 nM (^{3}H)alprenolol.

(By permission of Williams and Wilkins Co., Baltimore, from: Haber, E, in press. Antibodies *in vivo*. Proceedings of the PMA Workshop on Immunological Aspects of Toxicology, 1981.)

Antibodies as Drugs

The development of a new drug is often the result of empiricism, serendipity, or the deliberate modification of an existing natural product. These products of the organic chemist's laboratory are usually characterized by a lack of specificity with a consequent abundance of adverse reactions. If antibodies were the basis of identification of a specific locus of action, one could choose among some 10^{11} different combining sites and thus markedly increase the potential for reacting only with the desired site. Specificity would be enhanced and side reactions diminished. The considerably larger size of the antibody combining site in comparison with conventional drugs allows for the establishment of a larger number of interatomic interactions and thus for both greater affinity and specificity. While some of the advantages of antibodies are obvious, the disadvantages, discussed in part in previous sections, must also be considered. When binding to a specific site is all that is desired, the activation of the biological effects that are an intrinsic part of an immune reaction is undesirable. The smaller Fab that was discussed above as a possible solution to some of these problems still carries with it an entire domain (one half of its mass) that is of no relevance to antigen binding. Fab from a heterologous species, while of diminished immunogenicity, is likely to cause hypersensitivity when used on a long-term basis.

The solutions to these problems are almost at hand. A much smaller fragment of antibody has been produced that retains all the binding energy and specificity of the intact molecule. Fv comprises a single domain and has a molecular size of 25,000 daltons (35). While the pharmacokinetics of Fv have not as yet been examined, I anticipate that this fragment will be very rapidly cleared and distributed. The advent of the hybridoma method will make possible not only the selection and large-scale production of antibodies of uniform properties, but also the reduction or elimination of the potential problem of hypersensitivity since it will be possible, as indicated above, to produce human antibodies. Will the formation of anti-idiotypic antibodies defeat the long-term utility of antibody therapy? I believe that the well-recognized difficulty in raising anti-idiotypes, even when the effort is undertaken with deliberation, indicates that this problem will rarely manifest itself. The next decade will surely see a new pharmacology based on the antibody combining site.

References

1. Oparil, S, GW Tregear and E Haber (1972). Role of the C-terminal sequence of angiotensin I on immunologic reactivity and on conversion to angiotensin II in vivo and in vitro. In Protein and Polypeptide Hormones, pp 262-266. Proceedings

of the 2nd International Symposium, Liege, Belgium. M Margolies and FC Greenwood, eds.

2. Oparil, S, and E Haber (1974). The renin-angiotensin system. New Engl J Med **291**, 389-401, 446-457.
3. Fieser, LF, and M Fieser (1959). Steroids, pp 727-809. Reinhold Publishing Corp, New York.
4. Fullerton, DS, K Yoshioka, DC Rohrer, AHL From and K Ahmed (1979). Digitalis genin activity: side group carbonyl oxygen is a major determinant. Science **205**, 917-919.
5. Smith, TW, VP Butler, Jr and E Haber (1969). Determination of therapeutic and toxic serum digoxin concentration by radioimmunoassay. New Engl J Med **281**, 1212-1216.
6. Margolies, MN, M Mudgett-Hunter, J Novotny and E Haber (1981). Monoclonal antibodies to the cardiac glycoside digoxin. **In** Monoclonal Antibodies and T Cell Hybridomas. G Hammerling, U Hammerling and JF Kearney, eds. Elsevier/North-Holland, New York.
7. Mudgett-Hunter, M, MN Margolies, EM Rosen and E Haber (1980). Hybridoma antibodies to the cardiac glycoside digoxin. (Abstract). Fed Proc **39**, 928.
8. Hurrell, JGR, HA Katus, BA Khaw, E Haber and VR Zurawski (1981). Monoclonal antibodies directed against human myoglobin: characterization and application in a bideterminant radioimmunoassay. J Immunol Methods **45**(3), 249-254.
9. Katus, HA, JG Hurrell, GR Matsueda, P Ehrlich, VR Zurawski, Jr, BA Khaw and E Haber (in press). Increased specificity in human cardiac myosin radioimmunoassay utilizing two monoclonal antibodies in a double sandwich assay. Molec Immunol.
10. Leger, JJ, and M Elzinga (1977). Studies on cardiac myosin light chains: comparison of the sequences of cardiac and skeletal myosin LC-2. Biochem Biophys Res Commun **74**, 1390-1396.
11. Weeds, AG, and B Pope (1971). Chemical studies on light chains from cardiac and skeletal muscle myosin. Nature (Lond) **234**, 85-88.
12. Khaw, BA, HK Gold, JT Fallon and E Haber (1978). Detection of serum cardiac myosin light chains in acute experimental myocardial infarction: radioimmunoassay of cardiac myosin light chains. Circulation **58**, 1130-1136.
13. Trahern, CA, JB Gere, G Krauth II and DA Bigham (1978). Clinical assessment of serum myosin light chains in the diagnosis of acute myocardial infarction. Am J Cardiol **41**, 641-646.
14. Porter, RR (1950). The hydrolysis of rabbit γ-globulin and antibodies with crystalline papain. Biochem J **73**, 119-126.
15. Smith, TW, BL Lloyd, N Spicer and E Haber (1979). Immunogenicity and kinetics of distribution and elimination of sheep digoxin-specific IgG and Fab fragments in the rabbit and baboon. Clin Exp Immunol **36**, 384-396.
16. Curd, J, TW Smith, J-C Jaton and E Haber (1971). The isolation of digoxin specific antibody and its use in reversing the effects of digoxin. Proc Natl Acad Sci USA **68**, 2401-2406.
17. Smith, TW, E Haber, L Yeatman and VP Butler, Jr (1976). Reversal of advanced digoxin intoxication with Fab fragments of digoxin-specific antibodies. New Engl J Med **294**, 797-800.
18. Aeberhard, P, VP Butler, TW Smith, E Haber, D Tse Eng, J Brau, A Chalom, B Glatt, JF Thebaut, B Delangenhagen and B Morin (1980). Le traitement d'une intoxication digitalique massive (20 mg de digitoxine) par les anticorps antidigoxine fractionnes (Fab). Arch Mal Coeur **73**, 1471-1478.
19. Hess, T, P Stucki, J Barandun, G Scholtysik and W Riesen (1979). Treatment of a case of lanatoside C intoxication with digoxin-C specific $F(ab')_2$ antibody fragments. Am Heart J **98**, 767-771.
20. Bismuth, C, M Gaultier, F Conso and ML Efthymiou (1973). Hyperkalemia in acute digitalis poisoning: prognostic significance and therapeutic implications. Clin Toxicol **6**, 153-162.
21. Smith, TW, VP Butler, Jr and E Haber (1970). Characterization of antibodies of high affinity and specificity for the digitalis glycoside digoxin. Biochemistry **9**,

331-337.

22. Ochs, HR, and TW Smith (1977). Reversal of advanced digitoxin toxicity and modification of pharmacokinetics by specific anti-bodies and Fab fragments. J Clin Invest **60**, 1303-1313.
23. Katz, AM (1970). Contractile proteins of the heart. Physiol Rev **50**, 63-158.
24. Fetisova, TV, and IP Zabolotnyuk (1965). Changes in heart muscle and liver proteins in experimental myocardial infarction. Fed Proc **24**, T960-962.
25. Khaw, BA, GA Beller, E Haber and TW Smith (1976). Localization of cardiac myosin-specific antibody in experimental myocardial infarction. J Clin Invest **58**, 439-446.
26. Khaw, BA, HK Gold, RC Leinbach, JT Fallon, W Strauss, GM Pohost and E Haber (1978). Early imaging of experimental myocardial infarction by intracoronary administration of ^{131}I-labeled anticardiac myosin $(Fab')_2$ fragments. Circulation **58**, 1137-1142.
27. Khaw, BA, JT Fallon, GA Beller and E Haber (1979). Specificity of localization of myosin-specific antibody fragments in experimental myocardial infarction: Histologic, histochemical, autoradiographic and scintigraphic studies. Circulation **60**, 1527-1531.
28. Khaw, BA, JT Fallon, HW Strauss and E Haber (1980). Myocardial infarct imaging of antibodies to canine cardiac myosin with Indium-111-diethylene triamine pentaacetic acid. Science **209**, 295-297.
29. Khaw, BA, JT Fallon, W Strauss, HK Gold, HA Katus, B Essington and E Haber (1979). Indium-111 diethylenetriamine pentaacetic acid-antimyosin Fab fragments localization and imaging in experimental myocardial infarction. J Nucl Med **20**, 605.
30. Wrenn, S, and E Haber (1979). An antibody specific for the propranolol binding site of cardiac muscle. J Biol Chem **254**, 6577-6582.
31. Kahn, CR (1976). Membrane receptors for hormones and neurotransmitters. J Cell Biol **70**, 261-286.
32. Rockson, S, C Homcy and E Haber (1980). Anti-alprenolol antibodies in the rabbit: a new probe for the study of β-adrenergic receptor interaction. Circ Res **46**, 808-813.
33. Homcy, CJ, SG Rockson and E Haber (in press). An anti-idiotypic antibody which recognizes the β-adrenergic receptor. J Clin Invest.
34. Burges, RA, and KJ Blackburn (1972). Adenyl cyclase and the differentiation of beta-adrenoreceptors. Nature New Biol **235**, 249-250.
35. Hochman, J, D Inbar and D Givol (1976). An active antibody fragment (Fv) composed of the variable portions of heavy and light chains. Biochemistry **12**, 1130-1135.

II
Identification of Cell Proteins

PURIFICATION OF A MAJOR CELL SURFACE DIFFERENTIATION ANTIGEN OF MOUSE MACROPHAGES AND OTHER MESENCHYMAL CELLS BY MONOCLONAL ANTIBODY AFFINITY CHROMATOGRAPHY

Edward N. Hughes and J. Thomas August

Department of Pharmacology and Experimental Therapeutics
The Johns Hopkins University School of Medicine
Baltimore, Maryland 21205

Macrophages have been assigned a diversity of immune response functions mediated by the cell surface, including phagocytosis, antigen processing-presentation, and the secretion of biologically active molecules (for reviews, see Refs. 1-3). One approach to investigating these cell functions is to identify, characterize, and purify proteins expressed differentially on the macrophage plasma membrane. The development of the Köhler and Milstein technique for monoclonal antibody production to individual antigens of complex biological mixtures has facilitated such analyses (4).

A number of mouse macrophage-associated differentiation antigens have been identified by use of monoclonal antibodies. The immunoglobulin Fc receptor, a glycoprotein of 47,000 to 70,000 daltons, was found on macrophages and β lymphocytes and has been purified by monoclonal antibody affinity chromatography (5,6). Mac-1 antigen, composed of polypeptides of 190,000 *M*r and 105,000 *M*r, was found on all phagocytes (7). Mac-2, a polypeptide of 32,000 *M*r, and Mac-3, of 110,000 *M*r, marked the mononuclear cell lineage of mouse macrophage differentiation (8,9). The leucocyte common or T200 antigen, glycoproteins ranging from 150,000 *M*r to 200,000 *M*r, was also present on macrophages, in addition to being broadly distributed over all leucocytes (10,11). We recently described a collection of monoclonal antibodies that identify three additional mouse cell surface glycoproteins as macrophage differentiation antigens (12). These glycoproteins, of 150,000 *M*r, 130,000 *M*r, and 92,000 *M*r, appeared to differ from any of the other previously described macrophage proteins. A novel feature in the identification of these glycoproteins was that the monoclonal antibodies were derived from rats immunized with plasma membranes of NIH/3T3 cells, a contact inhibited cell line established from NIH Swiss mouse embryos. Thus, the macrophage cell surface glycoproteins binding these antibodies shared, in every case, an antigenic determinant present on the 3T3 cell surface glycoprotein.

One of these newly identified glycoprotein antigens, a molecule of about 92,000 daltons in leucocytes and 80,000 daltons in NIH/3T3 cells, is noteworthy in several respects (13-15). 1) It is a differentiation antigen of mesenchymal cells, including macrophages, monocytes, granulocytes, fibroblasts, and myoblasts, and it is reduced or absent in other lymphoid and nonlymphoid cells. 2) It is a major plasma membrane component, with about 10^6 antibody binding sites per cell, and is distinguished as the predominant iodinated cell surface polypeptide of 3T3 cells and macrophages[1] (14). 3) The molecule on the cell surface was remarkably sensitive to proteolytic cleavage, and treatment of intact cells yielded a water soluble, antigenically active fragment of about 65,000 daltons.[2] 4) It was genetically polymorphic, with the antigenic determinant present on cells of A/J, AKR/J, C3H/HeJ, C57BL/6J, C58/J, NZB, RF/J, SJL/J, SWR/J, and 129/J inbred mice, but absent on cells of BALB/cJ, DBA/1J, DBA/2J, and CBA/J mice (14,15). 5) A single co-dominant gene controlling antigen expression was located on chromosome 2, closely associated with a gene complex encoding the transplantation antigen H-3, the differentiation alloantigen Ly-4, the immune response function Ir-2, and the structural gene for β_2 microglobulin (15). 6) It was uniformly distributed throughout the cell surface, except for the coated pits (16).

Further structural and biological characterization of this molecule will be greatly augmented by the availability of purified glycoprotein. For this purpose we have used the specific monoclonal antibody to purify the glycoprotein by immunoaffinity chromatography. The procedure was simple, rapid, and yielded large amounts of the pure glycoprotein. The molecule was purified about 1700-fold and comprised 0.06% of the total soluble cell protein.

Experimental Procedures

The derivation and characterization of the AMF-15 rat monoclonal antibody has been described (12). The antibody was of the IgG_{2a} subclass and was composed only of rat heavy and light chains. The source of the monoclonal antibody was ascites fluids from athymic BALB/c nu/nu mice (Life Sciences) (17). Immunoglobulins were purified from pooled ascitic fluids by precipitation with solid ammonium sulfate (final concentration 45%) and by chromatography with DEAE-cellulose (Whatman DE-23) (18). Affinity-purified goat IgG anti-rat IgG has been described (12).

NZB ME (clone 35) (19) cells (obtained from the Division of Cancer Cause and Prevention, National Cancer Institute) were grown in 850 cm^2 roller bottles in Eagle's minimal essential medium

[1]Hughes, EN, A Colombatti, and JT August, unpublished observations.

[2]*ibid.*

containing 10% (v/v) fetal calf serum. The NZB ME cell pellets were stored at -70°C for four months without loss of antigenic activity.

The immunological reagents and the conditions for the solid phase radioimmunoassay of the antigen have been described (12).

Sodium dodecyl sulfate/polyacrylamide gel electrophoresis was performed by the method of Baum, Horwitz, and Maizel (20). The reagents for gel electrophoresis were obtained from Bio-Rad Laboratories.

The sources of the other reagents were as follows: cyanogen bromide and 2,6,10,14-tetramethylpentadecane (Aldrich); 1-0-n-Octyl-β-D-glucopyranoside (Boehringer Mannheim); phenylmethylsulfonyl fluoride and Triton X-100 (Calbiochem); Sepharose CL-4B (Pharmacia); guanidine-hydrochloride, sodium deoxycholate, tris-hydroxymethyl-aminoethane, and urea ultrapure grade (Schwarz/-Mann).

Results

Subcellular fractionation studies indicated that the polymorphic glycoprotein bound by the AMF-15 monoclonal antibody was localized primarily on the cell surface (data not shown). Conditions for solubilizing the glycoprotein were studied using different detergents or chaotropic reagents. A plasma membrane fraction, prepared by homogenization and differential centrifugation (21), was treated with the different reagents, and particulate and soluble fractions were separated by centrifugation at 100,000 x *g* for 60 min. Both the supernatant and pellet fractions were analyzed for antigen activity using a solid-phase antibody binding assay (Table 1). Freezing and thawing in a low ionic strength buffer containing a metal chelating agent or treatment with a number of chaotropic reagents at high concentration failed to extract the antigen. These reagents included guanidine hydrochloride, potassium thiocyanate, sodium perchlorate, and urea. The antigen was partially solubilized by treatment with 1.0 M KI. The optimum solubilization was obtained with detergents. More than 50% of antigen activity was released into the high speed supernatant by Triton X-100. Other detergents, including Nonidet P-40, octylglucoside, or sodium deoxycholate, also solubilized antigen activity in a concentration-dependent manner (data not shown). For large scale purification, the cells were treated with a high pH, high ionic strength buffer solution containing Triton X-100 (lysis buffer), as previously described (22).

In a typical purification procedure, 15 ml of packed NZB ME cells were homogenized in a loose-fitting Dounce pestle with 60 ml of cell lysis buffer (5 mM Tris-HCl, pH 9.2, 400 mM KCl, 1 mM EDTA, 1% (w/v) Triton X-100, and 1 mM phenylmethylsulfonyl fluoride). The volume of cell lysis buffer was then adjusted to yield an approximately 2:1 ratio of nonionic detergent to protein (185 ml) (23).

Table 1. Solubilization of antigenic activity

NZB ME cells, described in "Experimental Procedures," were scraped into Dulbecco's modified Eagle medium, collected by centrifugation, and washed three times with Dulbecco's phosphate buffered saline. Aliquots of the packed cells were frozen at -20°C. An aliquot of the frozen cells (12.75 gm wet weight) was thawed at 37°C in 25 ml of 50 mM Tris, pH 8.0, and 1 mM phenylmethylsulfonyl fluoride, and the cells were disrupted at 2°C in a Polytron PY355T for 3 min at a setting of 3. The suspension was then diluted with 40 ml of 50 mM Tris-HCl, pH 8.0, and centrifuged at 600 x *g* for 10 min. The pellet was discarded, and the supernatant was centrifuged at 10,000 x *g* for 30 min. This pellet was suspended in 40 ml of 50 mM Tris-HCl, pH 8.0, and disrupted by homogenizing (Polytron), as described above. The suspension was centrifuged at 10,000 x *g* for 30 min. The supernatant was retained and centrifuged at 100,000 x *g* for 60 min. The high speed pellet was suspended in 50 mM Tris, pH 8.0, and divided into aliquots of 2.0 ml containing 3 mg of protein and each of the different reagents, as listed below. One of the aliquots was three times frozen in solid CO_2/methanol and thawed at 37°C as indicated; the others were incubated for 10 min at room temperature. Each of the treated aliquots was then centrifuged at 100,000 x *g* for 60 min. The pellets, suspended in 400 µl of Dulbecco's phosphate buffered saline, and the supernatants were both dialyzed against 2000 ml Dulbecco's phosphate buffered saline at 4°C. The dialyzed fractions were diluted 10-fold in Dulbecco's phosphate buffered saline, and 20 µl of each fraction was adsorbed to microtiter wells for measurement of antigenic activity by the solid phase radioimmunoassay, as described under "Experimental Procedures." An excess, 50 µl, of AMF-15 hybridoma culture supernatant, and 50 µl of a ^{125}I-labeled goat anti-rat IgG antibody solution (0.25 µg/ml; 44 µCi/µg), were added to each well.

Agent	Antigen	
	Pellet	Supernatant
	cpm ^{125}I-anti-rat Ig antibody bound	
Untreated	13,679	632
5 mM EDTA; freezing-thawing	11,448	103
1.0% (w/v) Triton X-100	3,494	9,607
1.0 M KI	9,519	8,498
0.5 M guanidine-hydrochloride	12,524	1,208
1.0 M KSCN	8,465	941
0.5 M $NaClO_4$	13,520	731
1.0 M Urea	12,097	659

The cell suspension was three times frozen in solid CO_2/methanol and thawed at 37°C, and then centrifuged in the Sorvall SS-34 rotor at 5000 rpm (3000 x *g*) for 5 min at 4°C. The supernatant was collected, dialyzed for 15 h against 4000 ml of column buffer containing 50 mM Tris-HCl, pH 7.6, and 0.2 Triton X-100, with three changes of dialysate, and clarified by centrifugation in the Sorvall T-865 rotor at 37,000 rpm (100,000 x *g*) for 1 h at 4°C. Approximately 85% of the antigenic activity and 75% of total cell protein were solubilized by this procedure (data not shown). This step was designed to extract the antigen in high yield, not to achieve purification. The 100,000 x *g* supernatant was then applied to a column containing nonderivatized Sepharose CL-4B (5 ml packed bed volume/100 ml of supernatant) in order to adsorb aggregated and nonspecifically adherent materials.

A monoclonal antibody affinity column was prepared with AMF-15 coupled to Sepharose CL-4B; all procedures were carried out at 0° to 4°C. Purified AMF-15 antibody in 500 mM NaCl and 200 mM sodium citrate buffer, pH 6.5, was coupled to cyanogen bromide-activated Sepharose CL-4B (200 mg of cyanogen bromide/ml of packed beads) at a ratio of 3 mg protein/ml of packed beads (24). Briefly, 10 ml of Sepharose CL-4B (Pharmacia) was washed with 20 ml of distilled water on a sintered-glass filter. The washed Sepharose CL-4B beads were mixed with 10 ml of distilled water and 20 ml of 2 M sodium carbonate. The suspension was vigorously stirred, and activation was initiated by the addition of 2 g of cyanogen bromide (Aldrich, Milwaukee, Wis.) dissolved in 2 ml of HPLC grade acetonitrile (Fisher, Pittsburgh, Pa.). After 3 min the activated Sepharose CL-4B beads were washed on a sintered-glass filter with 1) 100 ml of 100 mM sodium carbonate-bicarbonate buffer, pH 9.5, 2) 100 ml of distilled water, and 3) 100 ml of 200 mM sodium citrate buffer, pH 6.5. The contact time for each buffer solution was 5 min. The activated Sepharose CL-4B cake was suspended in 6 ml of a solution containing 30 mg of rat monoclonal antibody, 500 mM NaCl, and 200 mM sodium citrate buffer, pH 6.5. The coupling reaction proceeded for 18 h at 4°C in a round-bottom flask with continuous slow stirring. The monoclonal antibody-Sepharose CL-4B beads were then washed with 30 ml of 20 mM sodium citrate buffer, pH 6.5, suspended in 10 ml of 1 M 2-aminoethanol, pH 9.0, and incubated for 4 h at 4°C with slow stirring. After blocking of excess active groups, the monoclonal antibody-Sepharose CL-4B beads were washed on a sintered-glass filter with 50 ml of a solution containing 500 mM NaCl, 100 mM Tris-maleate buffer, pH 6.0, followed by 50 ml of a solution containing 500 mM NaCl, 100 mM Tris-HCl buffer, pH 9.2. The monoclonal antibody-Sepharose CL-4B beads were washed alternately with the low and high pH buffer solutions three more times, and were stored in a buffer solution containing 10 mM sodium azide, 20 mM Tris-HCl, pH 7.6, at 4°C. Determination of the protein concentration of the filtrates indicated that 96% of the antibody preparation was coupled.

A 1.5 cm x 7.5 cm column, containing 15 mg of monoclonal antibody AMF-15 coupled to Sepharose CL-4B, was pre-eluted with 30 ml of a buffer solution containing 100 mM diethylamine, pH 11.5, 30 ml of a buffer solution containing 1 M Tris-HCl, pH 7.6, and 30 ml of column buffer. Approximately 725 mg protein in 200 ml of a 100,000 x *g* NZB cell extract supernatant was applied to the column at a rate of 0.25 ml/min. Most of the protein in the extract passed through the column (Fig. 1). The column was then washed with 50 ml of the column buffer, followed by 50 ml of a borate-salt buffer, pH 8.5 (1 M NaCl, 100 mM boric acid, 25 mM sodium borate, 0.2% (w/v) Triton X-100), to remove proteins adsorbed nonspecifically (25). None of the antigenic activity was eluted by this wash buffer. The column was then eluted at a rate of 0.5 ml/min with 40 ml of a buffer solution containing 100 mM diethylamine and 0.2% (w/v) Triton X-100, pH 11.5. Fractions of 2 ml were collected in tubes containing 0.5 ml of a neutralizing buffer (2 M Tris-HCl, pH 7.6). The antigen

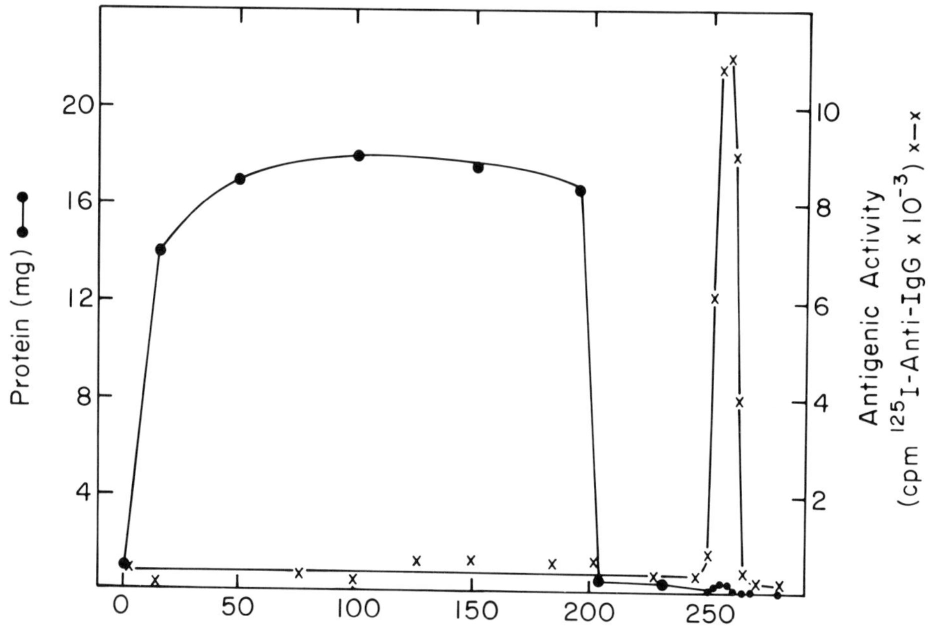

Fig. 1. Monoclonal antibody affinity chromatography of a major cell surface glycoprotein. Approximately 196 ml of the 100,000 x *g* supernatant of a detergent extract of NZB ME cells was applied to the AMF-15 monoclonal antibody-Sepharose CL-4B column. The antibody column was washed and eluted as described in the text. Protein was measured by a modification of the Lowry procedure (26), antigenic activity by the solid phase radioimmunoassay as described under "Experimental Procedures."

eluted as a single, sharp peak of activity together with a small protein peak. Virtually all of the antigen applied to the column was recovered. The active fractions were pooled and concentrated at 4°C to a volume of 1.5 ml by use of a negative pressure dialysis-concentrating apparatus (Micro-Pro Di Con; Bio-Molecular Dynamics, Beaverton, Oreg.). The vacuum dialysis buffer (2000 ml) contained 20 mM sodium phosphate, 100 mM NaCl, and 0.2% (w/v) Triton X-100, pH 8.0.

The concentrated antibody affinity fraction was further purified by molecular sieve chromatography in a 1.6 cm x 87 cm column (200 ml) of Sephacryl S300 Superfine (Pharmacia); the column was eluted with the dialysis buffer, as above. The antigenic activity was recovered as a single symmetrical peak (data not shown), and the fractions containing the antigen were pooled and concentrated as above.

The purity of the glycoprotein was determined by sodium dodecyl sulfate/polyacrylamide gel electrophoresis followed by staining for protein with Coomassie Brilliant Blue R-250 (Fig. 2). A single band of about 80,000 apparent molecular weight was present as the major species in the eluates of both the antibody affinity and S300 columns. The purified glycoprotein represented a very small fraction of the total soluble cell proteins and was not detected among the other polypeptides of similar molecular weight in the crude extract. The diffuse pattern of the glycoprotein may be attributed to heterogeneity in glycosylation and the amount of purified protein, 16 μg, applied to the gel. Analysis of the individual fractions from the Sephacryl S300 column showed that this glycoprotein co-purified with the antigenic activity (data not shown). An immunologically unreactive polypeptide of 38,000 daltons present in the affinity column eluate was removed by Sephacryl S300 chromatography.

A summary of the procedure is shown in Table 2. The quantity of glycoprotein in the crude extract and antibody affinity fractions was measured by radioimmune assay, standardized with the pure glycoprotein. There was no detectable loss of antigenic activity. The concentration of the glycoprotein in crude extracts, as calculated from these data, was 0.06%, with an overall purification of about 1700-fold.

Discussion

The monoclonal antibody affinity chromatography procedure described here provided a rapid and simple means for the preparative purification of a major plasma membrane glycoprotein which is a polymorphic differentiation antigen of mouse macrophages and other phagocytic cells. The procedure also has been applied with equal success to a number of mouse cell surface glycoproteins recognized

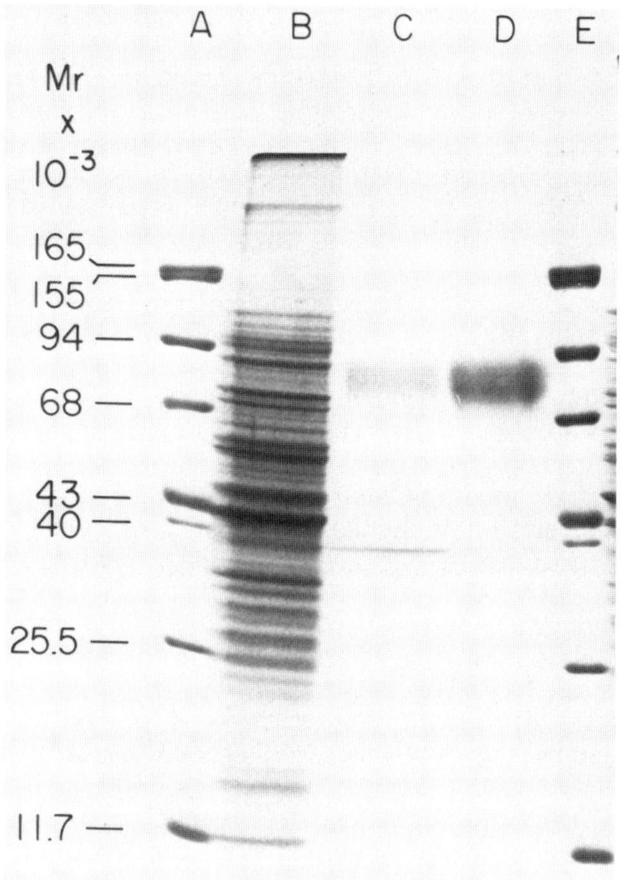

Fig. 2. Electrophoretic analysis of the purified polymorphic glycoprotein. The polymorphic glycoprotein antigen was purified by monoclonal antibody affinity and molecular sieve chromatography in the presence of Triton X-100, as described in the text. The samples were analyzed by electrophoresis in a linear 5% to 20% polyacrylamide gel gradient in the presence of 0.1% sodium dodecyl sulfate (20). The gel was stained with Coomassie Brilliant Blue R-250. B, 125 μg of NZB ME crude extract; C, 15.6 μg of antibody column eluate; D, 16 μg of Sephacryl S300 eluate; A and E, standard proteins: *Escherichia coli* RNA polymerase β', β subunits (*M*r = 165,000, 155,000); phosphorylase a (*M*r = 94,000) bovine serum; albumin (*M*r = 68,000); ovalbumin (*M*r = 43,000); *Escherichia coli* RNA polymerase α-subunit (*M*r = 40,000); chymotrypsinogen (*M*r = 25,500); and cytochrome c (*M*r = 11,700).

Table 2. Purification of an 80,000-dalton differentiation antigen of mouse mesenchymal cells

Purification Fraction	Volume	Total protein[a]	Antigen Protein[b]	Antigen Fraction of total	Antigen Yield
	ml	mg	mg	%	%
Crude extract	196	725	0.4	0.06	--
Antibody affinity	1.4	0.8	0.4	50	95+
Sephacryl S-300	1.5	0.4	0.4	(100)	95+

[a]Protein was measured by a modification of the Lowry procedure (31).

[b]Antigen protein was measured by the solid phase radioimmunoassay as described under "Experimental Procedures," standardized with the pure protein.

specifically by other monoclonal antibodies. We have used the same experimental protocol and the same cell extract to purify five different plasma membrane glycoproteins. In several cases, complete purifications were achieved with a single affinity column step. Moreover, the affinity columns were used several times without detectable loss of antigen binding capacity. A similar procedure has been employed for the purification of rodent and human lymphocyte glycoproteins expressed on the plasma membrane (10,27-30).

A major advantage of using monoclonal antibody affinity chromatography as an early step in the purification of plasma membrane glycoproteins was the bypassing of more traditional procedures of ion-exchange and molecular sieve chromatography. The charge and size heterogeneity of the glycoproteins restricted the efficacy of such methods. The need for the continued presence of detergents to maintain glycoproteins in a soluble form also appeared to handicap the application of conventional procedures. Another advantage of the affinity column was the ease of application to large scale purification. The effective capacity of the AMF-15 monoclonal antibody affinity column was remarkably high, and chromatography of even larger quantities of cell extract resulted in a correspondingly greater amount of purified glycoprotein. In other studies, approximately 2 mg of the purified 80,000-dalton glycoprotein was obtained by passing 3 g of crude extract through the same AMF-15 antibody column. All of the antigenic activity of the extract was recovered in the purified fraction, indicating that the functional capacity of the antibody column had not been exceeded. As the column contained about 15 mg of monoclonal antibody, this amount of antigen approached the maximal capacity. Such high capacity may not be attainable uniformly with all monoclonal antibodies, however, as the capacity of the column can be expected to differ depending upon the affinity of the antibody and the effect of antibody coupling. The reported antigen-binding capacities of other monoclonal antibody affinity columns appeared to differ widely (10,27,28).

The purified glycoprotein was a single component of about 80,000 daltons that was greater than 95% pure by sodium dodecyl sulfate/polyacrylamide gel electrophoresis. The glycoprotein co-purified with the antigenic activity and was quantitatively immunoprecipitated by the antibody; it thus constituted the structure carrying the antigenic determinant recognized by the monoclonal antibody. The preferential solubilization of the antigen by use of detergent was consistent with the characterization of the glycoprotein as an integral membrane component.

The preparative purification of the polymorphic glycoprotein from mouse embryo 3T3 cells showed that this molecule was a major cell surface component. The concentration of the glycoprotein was 0.06% of the total soluble proteins in the cell, or greater if there was less than 100% yield on the purification procedure. From these data it can be calculated that there were at least 2×10^6 molecules of the glycoprotein/3T3 cell. This value is in agreement with the number of antibody molecules bound/3T3 cell in saturation binding studies (13). Because plasma membrane proteins as a group comprise less than a few percent of total cell protein (31), it may be presumed that the glycoprotein accounted for a substantial fraction of plasma membrane protein.

With its high concentration and restricted tissue expression, the polymorphic glycoprotein can be expected to make an important contribution to the molecular architecture and function of the phagocyte cell surface. The purification and characterization of the polymorphic glycoprotein is an important step in elucidating its cell surface organization and its role in the biology of phagocytic cells.

Acknowledgments

We thank Dr. Mette Strand for the critical reading of this manuscript and Dr. J. Lemp (Electro-Nucleonics, Bethesda, Md.) for providing the NZB ME cells. We wish to acknowledge Mr. James Freedy and Mrs. Debra Gilbert for their assistance in these experiments and Ms. Lydia Cumor for the preparation of the manuscript.

This research was supported by National Institutes of Health grant R01 CA19471. E.N. Hughes is a postdoctoral fellow supported by Public Health Service Grant CA-09243, awarded by the National Cancer Institute, Department of Health and Human Services.

References

1. Unanue, ER (1976). Secretory function of mononuclear phagocytes. Am J Pathol **83**, 395-417.
2. Silverstein, SC, RM Steinman and ZA Cohn (1977). Endocytosis. Annu Rev Biochem **46**, 669-722.
3. Zuckerman, SH, and SD Douglas (1979). Dynamics of the macrophage plasma membrane. Annu Rev Microbiol **33**, 267-307.
4. Köhler, G, and C Milstein (1976). Derivation of specific antibody producing tissue culture and tumor lines by cell fusion. Eur J Immunol **6**, 511-519.
5. Unkeless, JC (1979). Characterization of a monoclonal antibody directed against mouse macrophage and lymphocyte Fc receptors. J Exp Med **150**, 580-596.
6. Mellman, IS, and JC Unkeless (1980). Purification of a functional mouse Fc receptor through the use of a monoclonal antibody. J Exp Med **152**, 1048-1069.
7. Springer, T, G Galfre, DS Secher and C Milstein (1979). Mac-1: a macrophage differentiation antigen identified by monoclonal antibody. Eur J Immunol **9**, 301-306.
8. Springer, T (1980). Cell-surface differentiation in the mouse. Characterization of "jumping" and "lineage" antigens using xenogeneic rat monoclonal antibodies. **In** Monoclonal Antibodies, pp 185-217. R. Kennett, T McKearn and K Bechtol, eds. Plenum Press, New York.
9. Springer, T (1981). Monoclonal antibody analysis of complex biological systems. Combination of cell hybridization and immunoadsorbents in a novel cascade procedure and its application to the macrophage cell surface. J Biol Chem **256**, 3833-3839.
10. Sunderland, CA, WR McMaster and AF Williams (1979). Purification with monoclonal antibody of a predominant leukocyte-common antigen and glycoprotein from rat thymocytes. Eur J Immunol **9**, 155-159.
11. Trowbridge, IS (1978). Interspecies spleen-myeloma hybrid producing monoclonal antibodies against mouse lymphocyte surface glycoprotein, T200. J Exp Med **148**, 313-323.
12. Hughes, EN, and JT August (1981). Characterization of plasma membrane proteins identified by monoclonal antibodies. J Biol Chem **256**, 664-671.
13. Hughes, EN, G Mengod and JT August (1981). Murine cell surface glycoproteins: characterization of a major component of 80,000 daltons as a polymorphic differentiation antigen of mesenchymal cells. J Biol Chem **256**, 7023-7027.
14. Mengod, G, EN Hughes and JT August (1981). Murine cell surface glycoproteins: immunochemical analysis of a major differentiation alloantigen of phagocytic cells. Arch Biochem Biophys **209**, 718-722.
15. Colombatti, A, EN Hughes, BA Taylor and JT August (1982). Linkage analysis of the gene for the major trypsin-sensitive membrane glycoprotein of mouse macrophages and granulocytes. Proc Natl Acad Sci USA, in press.
16. Bretscher, MS, JN Thomson and BMF Pearse (1980). Coated pits act as molecular filters. Proc Natl Acad Sci USA **77**, 4156-4159.
17. Potter, M (1972). Immunoglobulin-producing tumors and myeloma proteins of mice. Physiol Rev **52**, 631-719.
18. Medgyesi, GA, G Fust, J Gergely and H Bazin (1978). Classes and subclasses of rat immunoglobulins: interaction with the complement system and with staphylococcal protein A. Immunochem **15**, 125-129.
19. Levy, JA, P Kazan, O Varnier and H Kleiman (1975). Murine xenotropic type C viruses. I. Distribution and further characterization of the virus in NZB mice. J Virol **16**, 844-853.

20. Baum, SG, MS Horwitz and JV Maizel (1972). Studies of the mechanism of enhancement of human adenovirus infection in monkey cells. J Virol **10**, 211-219.
21. Cuatrecasas, P (1972). Affinity chromatography and purification of the insulin receptor of liver cell membranes. Proc Natl Acad Sci USA **69**, 1277-1281.
22. Strand, M, and JT August (1977). Polypeptides of cells transformed by RNA or DNA tumor viruses. Proc Natl Acad Sci USA **74**, 2729-2733.
23. Helenius, A, and K Simons (1975). Solubilization of membranes by detergents. Biochim Biophys Acta **415**, 29-79.
24. March, SC, I Parikh and P Cuatrecasas (1974). A simplified method for cyanogen bromide activation of agarose for affinity chromatography. Anal Biochem **60**, 149-152.
25. Smith, JA, JGR Hurrell and SJ Leach (1978). Elimination of nonspecific adsorption of serum proteins by Sepharose-bound antigens. Anal Biochem **87**, 299-305.
26. Chandrarajan, J, and L Klein (1975). Lowry assay of dilute protein solutions containing high concentrations of Triton X-100. Annal Biochem **69**, 632-636.
27. McMaster, WR, and AF Williams (1979). Monoclonal antibodies to Ia antigens from rat thymus: cross reactions with mouse and human and use in purification of rat Ia glycoproteins. Immunol Rev **47**, 117-137.
28. Parham, P (1979). Purification of immunologically active HLA-A and -B antigens by a series of monoclonal antibody columns. J Biol Chem **254**, 8709-8712.
29. Herrmann, SH, and MF Mescher (1979). Purification of the H-2K^k molecule of the murine major histocompatibility complex. J Biol Chem **254**, 8713-8716.
30. Brown, WRA, AN Barclay, CH Sunderland and AF Williams (1981). Identification of a glycoprotein-like molecule at the cell surface of rat thymocytes. Nature (Lond) **289**, 456-460.
31. Lauter, CJ, A Solyom and EG Trams (1972). Comparative studies on enzyme markers of liver plasma membranes. Biochim Biophys Acta **266**, 511-523.

ANALYSIS OF HUMAN HISTOCOMPATIBILITY ANTIGENS WITH MONOCLONAL ANTIBODIES

Peter Parham
Department of Structural Biology
Stanford University School of Medicine
Stanford, California 94305

Antibodies have been used almost exclusively to study and define gene products of the human, major histocompatibility complex or HLA region. Over the last 20 years serological methods for typing individuals for HLA-A,B,C and DR antigens have been developed using alloantisera obtained from multiparous women. The goal has been to find sera that will uniquely identify each of the different allelic products in the population. One approach has involved comparing the reaction patterns of sera on panels of cells and finding clusters of similar sera that are then used to define antigens. As the analysis becomes more sophisticated the reaction patterns of ostensibly similar sera are compared to find differences that allow splitting of the given HLA antigen. The effect of such an analysis is to accentuate the differences among allelic products and to ignore their similarities. The potential benefits of switching from a complex, serologically defined system in which suitable alloantisera were weak, of limited supply, and difficult to find, to a monoclonal antibody-based HLA typing seemed considerable. Several groups began producing monoclonal antibodies against HLA antigens, analyzing their specificity, and comparing them to the established HLA types (1-20). Their results have raised the following issues:

1) A significant proportion of mouse monoclonal antibodies cannot be used in the standard HLA typing assay because they do not fix complement. Should typing methodology be altered to measure a primary effect, e.g., binding, or should the production of only cytotoxic monoclonal antibodies be our goal? Either of these choices will involve significant technological revamping either by the HLA typing laboratories or by those laboratories making monoclonal antibodies.

2) It is not clear that results obtained with mouse monoclonal antibodies can be related to human allotypes defined by human sera. For this reason the utility of mouse monoclonal antibodies in HLA typing has been seriously questioned. Because human monoclonal antibodies cannot yet be produced by a reproducible and reliable technique, this objection cannot be avoided by the obvious sidestep and must be confronted. In possible therapeutic applications the side effects associated with use of xeno-antibodies must also be considered.

3) Monoclonal antibodies have revealed antigenic complexities of

HLA antigens, suggesting that a simple exchange of alloantisera for monoclonal antibodies with identical specificity will not be possible. Redefinition of the whole HLA system in terms of monoclonally-defined antigenic specificities may be the only option if this technology is to be realistically applied.

It is presently unclear whether monoclonal antibodies will be widely used in clinical histocompatibility testing. If they are not, then pharmacological uses of monoclonal antibodies against human histocompatibility antigens will have no future. Anti-HLA reagents will be useful only if it becomes possible to exploit their polymorphism and to encompass a majority of the different antigenic types found in the population. Production and, more importantly, analysis of such reagents require a commitment from the international HLA typing community.

HLA-A,B,C (Class 1) antigens are found on all tissues whereas HLA-DR (Class 2) antigens show a more restricted tissue distribution, being found on B lymphocytes, macrophages, activated T cells, and thymic epithelium. As site-directing agents, anti-HLA-A,B,C will be most useful in transplantation or where reagents specific for fetal or maternal tissue during pregnancy are required. Anti-HLA-DR reagents may be useful in the treatment or diagnosis of tumors that express these antigens. However, the main issue is not how to apply these reagents but whether sufficient numbers of well-characterized reagents will be available for well-planned trial applications. It is apparent that successful application will encourage production and characterization, and that we are facing a classical chicken-and-egg-situation.

Introduction

Archimedes once said, "Give me somewhere to stand, and I will move the earth" (21).

His sense of frustration is shared by those of us using mammalian antibodies to study mammalian gene products. By the very nature of the immune response antibodies can usually be generated only against structural differences between an injected antigen and the antigenic spectrum of the host. All species commonly used to raise antibodies have a major histocompatibility complex (MHC) homologous to the HLA region. By choosing to use antibodies to study HLA antigens, we are confined in our examination to those parts of these molecules that have changed during mammalian evolution. Thus antibodies provide tools for comparative rather than absolute analysis, although in the manner of Archimedes one might claim that given the appropriate species one would be able to study total protein structure at monoclonal antibody resolution.

As stated above, human alloantibodies have usually been used to study and define the structure of HLA gene products. An alloantibody recognizes a piece of molecular structure found on one but not on another subset of allelic proteins. We call these antigenic determinants and believe they are in general three-dimensional configurations that are the direct consequence of differences in primary structure. In studying HLA antigens with monoclonal antibodies we have found many such antigenic determinants, and we are trying to relate the permutation of antigenic determinants that constitute a given allelic product to the chemical structure and amino acid sequence of the proteins. In considering how our results with monoclonal antibodies relate to HLA typing with alloantisera and amino acid sequences, it is sometimes convenient to consider what the total set of antigenic determinants might be irrespective of whether an animal could be found to make such an antibody. These real or imaginary antigenic determinants can be called structural elements or just structures. Thus a given amino acid substitution in an HLA protein will alter some structures of the molecule and not others. All these differences are potentially detectable by an appropriate monoclonal antibody.

Function of Class 1 MHC Antigens (22-25)

Class 1 MHC antigens exhibit an unprecedented level of polymorphism. This property allowed the immunogenetic discovery that the functions of these molecules are to instruct and to effect recognition of foreign antigens by specific receptors on or in certain classes of T cells. Multiple loci code for these antigens so that each individual expresses a small subset of all the gene products found in the population. Biochemical analysis shows that class 1 antigens are rather conserved protein complexes in which polymorphic variation is subservient to a basic molecular architecture (26,27). Functionally this makes sense. Each individual's immune system functions successfully, independent of the magnitude of polymorphism found in the total population. Therefore each different class 1 gene product must be able to perform the basic function of these molecules. In contributing to that basic function, structures conserved among all species are more important than structures conserved within a species, which are more important than those varying within a species. By functional, serological, and chemical criteria there appear to be no locus-distinguishing features, which implies that 1) the loci are functionally equivalent and that 2) multiple gene products within an individual are advantageous. The high degree of polymorphism also suggests that diversity at the population level is an advantage. To rationalize these phenomena one can suppose that the polymorphic differences fine-tune or modulate the basic functional capabilities of class 1 antigens. Then the repertoire of T cell specificities generated in the context of one product will be slightly different from that generated in the context of another. The immunological repertoire will be increased with the number of different class 1 gene products expressed (28).

If one assumes that antigenic threats faced by organisms are diverse, variable, and capable of evolution, then organisms with the largest immunological repertoire are most likely to survive. However, within a single organism, increasing the immunological repertoire beyond a certain point probably requires a deleterious investment of limited resources. Keeping the individual's repertoire a constant size while allowing further diversification may be accomplished by establishing a larger pool of T cell specificities within the population of which each individual has a subset. Thus the HLA types given by individual A, B, and C antigens are markers for the differences in the fine structure of the immune repertoire. The result is that the number and quality of T cell clones responding to any antigen or pathogen will vary with HLA type so that small but significant differences in the probability of surviving a certain disease or antigenic insult will exist among individuals. All individuals will respond to most antigens, but the size and quality of the response will vary. On the average, individuals have antigens to which they respond relatively well and others to which they respond relatively poorly. The advantage is that within the population some individuals respond well to a greater number of antigens, so that if the population is stressed by any given antigen the possibility that some individuals will survive is much greater. A consequence of this scheme is that all HLA types will be associated with greater or poorer responses to different antigens; this may be correlated with susceptibility or resistance to disease. In general these effects will be small, difficult to measure and will often be lost in the noise generated by other factors. However, in certain instances the presence or absence of a single, specific T cell clone or a small number of them may profoundly affect susceptibility to disease. The high correlation of ankylosing spondylitis with B27 may be an example of this (29,30).

We have made a case for class 1 polymorphism being functionally important in causing subtle differences in the education and action of T cells. For enzymes polymorphic differences often cause small differences in kinetic constants, pH, or temperature dependence that do not affect catalytic activity qualitatively (31). However, the quantitative difference in catalytic activity is possibly advantageous under certain conditions. We suggest that polymorphic HLA differences have similar effects on class 1 functions.

Structure of Class 1 MHC Antigens (26,27)

The HLA-A,B,C genes of the human, major histocompatibility complex code for homologous glycoproteins of 43,000 molecular weight that associate with β_2-microglobulin (32,33). This association is required for expression of the HLA-A,B,C gene products in the plasma membrane and produces dramatic changes in their conformation and antigenic properties (34,35). A triplet of loci--H-2D,K, and L homologous to HLA-A,B,C--in mice provides evidence that gene duplication of a single locus predates the divergence of man and mouse (23). Extension of this argument allows the conclusion that individual loci have been evolving independently for a long time. Thus analogy with the various isotypes of immunoglobulin chains or the α β chains of hemoglobin suggests that locus-specific characteristics do exist, i.e., that all gene products of HLA-A share structural features not found in any HLA-B gene products. Experimental results indicate this is not so. Amino acid sequence analysis shows no locus-specific residues (27), a finding confirmed by our serological studies with anti-HLA-A,B,C monoclonal antibodies. Among the 30 different antibodies we have analyzed, none fulfills the requirements of a locus-specific reagent (36). This contrasts sharply with the repetitive occurrence of monoclonal antibodies that react with all HLA-A,B,C products or with groups of allelic products from different loci (19,20).

Two possible explanations for this discordance are that 1) it was wrong to assume that gene duplication occurred prior to man-mouse divergence--instead, HLA-A,B,C and H-2D,K,L may have arisen from separate gene duplications in the two species; 2) selection on the gene products keeps them similar. At first the latter possibility seems unlikely, because it was their high level of polymorphism, presumably reflecting a lack of selection, that drew attention to the class 1 transplantation antigens. However, the complex serological polymorphism is based on a family of molecules that are rather conserved both within and among species. In man, 80-90% of all residues in the HLA-A,B,C heavy chain are conserved among the known sequences. The residues that show variability are scattered throughout the polypeptide chain with some bias in distribution towards the NH_2 terminal 180 residues. As far as we can tell from the limited sequence information, many of the residues that exhibit variability are constrained, because only a few different amino acids are found. The amino acid sequence of β_2-microglobulin appears invariant within the human population, although one example of a polymorphism has been found in mice (37,38). Because association with β_2-microglobulin is crucial to correct cellular placement (39) and by extension to function of HLA-A,B,C antigens, β_2-microglobulin binding probably provides for strong selection against many mutations in the genes for both β_2-m and HLA-A,B,C heavy chains. This will have the effect of maintaining similarity between all the allelic products of the HLA-A,B,C genes, because all must bind β_2-m. The extent of this effect will depend upon how much of the HLA-A,B,C heavy chain is directly or indirectly involved in the association with β_2-m. Our studies suggest that most of the extracellular portion of HLA-A,B,C heavy chain, that part which is released from the cell by papain, is dependent upon β_2-m for its native three-dimensional structure. Therefore it seems possible that a large proportion of the heavy chain polypeptide is involved in the β_2-m interaction and is equivalently constrained in the products of all three loci. Similar arguments may also explain the lack of β_2-m polymorphism.

In conclusion, we suggest that there are strong selective forces against individuals carrying mutations which prevent a strong association between β_2-m and any of the HLA-A,B,C gene products. Because of the central role played by β_2-m in the structure of the complex and the possibility that much of the heavy chain conformation is affected by β_2-m, severe constraints are placed on the patterns of polymorphic variation attainable. The net result is that many positions in the sequence are conserved within all A,B,C gene products. Selection on the different loci is essentially the same, so that positions varying in one locus will also vary in the others; positions that cannot vary in one locus will not vary in the others.

The Nature of Alloantigenic Sites on HLA-A,B,C Antigens

Let us consider the evolution of HLA-A,B,C antigens in a small, imaginary population having no polymorphism. A mutation first occurs at one locus, e.g., the A locus, in one individual and produces a structural difference in the HLA-A β_2-m complex capable of eliciting a specific alloantibody response. This single mutation gives rise to two alternative structures determined by either the original amino acid (a) or the new amino acid (b) at the residue position where the mutation occurred. As this single mutation spreads through the population, fetal-maternal stimulation will result in production of anti-(b) alloantibodies in appropriate pregnancies. However, anti-(a) will not be produced in any mating combination, even for fathers homozygous for (b) at the A locus, because every individual has the (a) structure in the products of the other two loci, HLA-B and -C. Thus that single mutation generates two different structures, only one of which is a true "alloantigen" because of the existence of multiple, co-dominantly-expressed, homologous genes and the immunological nature of their detection. However, one can predict that subsequent mutations in the B and C loci will break the population's tolerance to the (a) structure, and it will be revealed later as an alloantigen. The simplest case would involve the identical mutation (a)→(b) occurring in the B and C loci. Mating would produce individuals containing the (b) amino acid in all A,B,C gene products and capable of making alloantibodies against the (a) structure. In this simple case the (a) and (b) amino acids would give rise to diallelic antigens, one of which would be found on every A,B,C gene product. Initially (b) would be a low-frequency antigen and (a) a high-frequency antigen, a circumstance that could change depending on the selection operating on these antigens. An important property of alloantigens is that, although mutation is required to produce new alloantigenic determinants, the actual structures recognized by the alloantibodies do not have to result from that mutational change. The example described shows how the original (a) structure can eventually become or later be revealed as a polymorphic alloantigenic determinant (40).

Simple amino acid substitutions of the kind described above probably exist within the HLA-A,B,C system. The number of mutations permissable[1] at a position (x) may also be greater than two so that eventually gene products of the A,B,C loci with amino acids (a), (b), (c), (d) will be found. In this case three antigenic structures (b), (c), (d) that are the direct result of recent mutational change correspond to one (a), which is the original or primordial structure.

Monomorphic and Polymorphic Antibodies

Although β_2-m and ≃ 80% of the A,B,C heavy chain are conserved within a species, differences are found among species at about 30% of those residues. Thus if one makes antibodies between species instead of using alloantibodies to analyze these molecules, additional antigenic determinants of two types are detectable. The first type results from differences in positions that are invariant within a species. These determinants, which are found on all gene products of the A,B,C loci, have been called monomorphic (41). The antibodies that define these determinants recognize each gene product with the same affinity. The clearest example is the human β_2-m determinant recognized by mouse monoclonal antibodies BBM.1, PA2.12, BB7.3, and BB7.4 (21,42).

The second type of antigenic determinant includes those primordial structures still present in sufficiently high frequency among the total gene products that most individuals carry at least one A,B,C product with that particular antigenic determinant. In this situation every individual recognizes the determinant as self, although when analyzed at the level of the gene products there can be considerable polymorphism. These have been called broadly polymorphic structures (19).

If one assumes that β_2-m association eliminates locus diversification of the polymorphism of A,B,C, one has in essence a six-ploid rather than a diploid situation for the A,B,C genes. Producing an alloantibody against any polymorphic structure requires individuals who do not have that structure and are carrying alternative structures at all six gene products. Thus if there is a 50% chance of

---

[1]Permissable mutations are those that will survive selection and become part of the balanced polymorphism.

alternate structures at each locus, the frequency of such individuals is $(1/2)^6 = 1/64$, or slightly less than 2%. If the frequency is 1/10, this becomes $(1/10)^6 = 1$ in 10^6. Thus an antigenic determinant could be present in significant numbers of gene products without being detected readily by alloantisera.

These considerations indicate that a large number of polymorphic antigenic determinants probably have not been detectable with alloantisera. The method of selecting alloantisera for typing compounds the number of such undetected determinants. In general sera that show broad reaction patterns have been discarded in favor of those that react with a small frequency of the population and split existing groupings of antigens. Therefore, a number of these detectable, broadly polymorphic antigenic determinants have been ignored. Monoclonal antibodies of this type are produced with considerable frequency and in general outnumber those recognizing more specific determinants, which suggests that such determinants are present in high frequency and attests to the fact that in most allelic products only some small fraction of the total residues which could have undergone polymorphic variation have in fact done so. Alternatively, the number of mutations is high, but the mutational possibilities are so limited that identical residues or structures do keep reappearing.

A question is raised by these observations: By making monoclonal antibodies across species differences do we preferentially make antibodies against the broad or supertypic differences rather than the specific antigenic determinant? My hunch is that in general the monoclonal antibodies reasonably represent the total number of polymorphic antigenic determinants present. The problem is more that traditional HLA typing has selected only certain polymorphic antigenic determinants and that what are called single HLA types in classical serology may in fact be defined by combinations of antibodies.

Mouse Monoclonal Anti-HLA-A,B,C Antibodies: A Synopsis of Our Results

Our analysis of mouse anti-HLA-A,B,C monoclonal antibodies shows that they fall into three discrete groups according to the types of antigenic determinant they recognize.

Monomorphic antibodies (36). Monomorphic antibodies react with all allelic products of the HLA-A,B,C loci with similar affinity. Thus the structure of the antigenic determinant is probably identical for all the gene products and results from residues conserved within species but differing among them. In this work we always immunized mice with HLA, so that the relevant comparisons are between the structures of HLA and H-2. Examination of 11 HLA and 6 H-2 NH_2 terminal sequences shows that within the first 20 residues three positions, 2, 5, and 17, are of this type. The sequence of human β_2-m microglobulin, which appears to be totally conserved among individuals, has 32 out of 100 residues different from those of mouse β_2-m (38). These could all potentially be involved in monomorphic antigenic sites.

Within the group of monomorphic antibodies a minimum of three fundamental, different reactivities can be distinguished by 1) inhibition experiments with free or HLA-associated β_2-microglobulin, 2) binding to mouse-human hybrids expressing either HLA or human β_2-m associated with the appropriate mouse polypeptide, and 3) examination of the patterns of cross reactivity with cells of other species.

a) **Anti-β_2-m monoclonal antibodies** (e.g., BBM.1). Antibodies similar to BBM.1 occur with regularity, and we have characterized six of them. They bind free β_2-m and HLA-associated β_2-m with similar affinity and are thus directed against an antigenic site that is present and equally accessible in both forms of the molecule. This structure can obviously play no direct role in the association of HLA with β_2-m. We have been unable to distinguish among these antibodies and therefore believe they recognize the same antigenic site. This site shows almost no conservation in evolution. Anti-β_2-m antibodies bind only to cells from humans and our nearest relatives, the African apes, chimpanzees, and gorillas. No binding to any other species, including the Asian apes, has been found. Thus this antigenic site is the result of recent evolution and serves to discriminate humans from almost all other species (43).

When monoclonal antibodies BBM.1 and W6/32 with specificity for both subunits of HLA antigens had been made and characterized, we were able to quantitate the relative amounts of β_2-m and HLA on the surface of different types of cells (42). This was of considerable interest as previous reports indicated an excess of β_2-m presumed to be associated with other membrane proteins. Quantitative binding assays showed β_2-m and HLA present in comparable amounts on most cell types. The exceptions were thymocytes and a thymocyte-like cell line, Molt 4, which both expressed significantly more β_2-m than HLA. It seemed likely that the excess β_2-m was associated with a human analogue of the mouse thymus leukemia antigen (TLA), which was known to be β_2-m-associated. Subsequent studies indicate there may be multiple thymus-specific products associated with β_2-m (44,45).

b) **Anti-HLA antibodies** (e.g., W6/32) (35,36,46). Three antibodies, including W6/32, are inhibited by HLA but not by β_2-m. The inferred specificity for the HLA heavy chain was confirmed by the observation that these antibodies bound to man-mouse hybrid cells having human chromosome 6 in the absence of chromosome 15, but not to hybrids having chromosome 15 in the absence of chromosome 6. These antibodies reacted with all apes and old-world monkeys tested but did not react with most other species tested (47). Unexpected reactions with some other species were observed that did not follow any evolutionary trends (43,48). For example, all three antibodies reacted with a single subspecies of new-world monkey, the Bolivian owl monkey, and with cows and buffalo. W6/32, but not PA2.6 or MB40.5, also reacted with ringtailed lemurs. It was striking that these antibodies reacted with single species out of groups of related species, e.g., ringtailed lemurs but not brown or mongoose lemurs, yet also reacted with evolutionarily distant species such as cows.

A particularly interesting example is seen in the reactivity of W6/32 with owl monkeys. This species, which is widely distributed throughout South and Central America, can be divided into nine races or subspecies on the basis of chromosomal differences (49-51). These have been designated karyotypes I through IX. W6/32 antibody binds to cells of K VI and K VIII animals but not to K I-V cells. BB7.7 binds to cells of all the karyotypes. Immune precipitation experiments showed that W6/32 and BB7.7 both precipitated the same set of owl monkey leukocyte antigens (OMLA) from K VI and K VII cells (52). However, for K I-V cells, BB7.7 precipitated cell surface OMLA heavy chain with owl monkey β_2-m whereas W6/32 precipitated cytoplasmic, β_2-m-free OMLA heavy chain (52). Analogous behavior has been observed for HLA, which binds only rabbit anti-H antibodies when not associated with β_2-m and only W6/32 when associated with β_2-m (39). These results and other studies examining the properties of isolated HLA heavy chain indicate that β_2-m profoundly alters the three-dimensional structure of HLA on association whereas the three-dimensional structure of β_2-m is, to a first approximation, not altered. In owl monkeys W6/32 binds to free OMLA heavy chain in some karyotypes and to the β_2-m-associated heavy chain in the others. Moreover the effects appear to apply to all class 1 OMLA products expressed and not to be allele- or locus-specific. The simplest interpretation of these results is that β_2-m is different in the two groups of owl monkeys and that the difference is sufficient to alter the W6/32 binding site of the OMLA heavy chain. Unlike HLA, the free OMLA heavy chain in cells of all karotypes can probably bind to W6/32, but the binding to the cell surface, β_2-m-associated form is controlled by the type of β_2-m. Evidence to support this hypothesis shows that some W6/32-reactive somatic cell hybrids were obtained by fusing lymphocytes from a W6/32-negative owl monkey with mouse cells. In these hybrids we presumed that the owl monkey β_2-m gene had been lost and that OMLA heavy chain combined with mouse β_2-m to give a W6/32 reactive product.

It is interesting that differences in the β_2-m of the various subspecies of owl monkey may be associated with ongoing speciation in these animals (53). The basic biological function of HLA-A,B,C antigens and their homologues involves the recognition of self. The conservation of β_2-m within species indicates its importance for this function. It is obviously advantageous to the formation of new species if the family of molecules that recognize self can be fundamentally altered so as to be functional only within the context of the new self. This is not easily accomplished by mutations in the HLA genes, as multiple gene products are expressed that are, to a first approximation, functionally equivalent. However, a single alteration in β_2-m can affect the structure of all class 1 antigens and lead to significant functional differences that change the MHC restriction patterns. Thus, as discussed by Sanderson (54), the β_2-m part of the two-subunit structure of class 1 antigens may be an important discriminator of species. This property would be a consequence of the association of the products of one gene (β_2-m) with the products of multiple other genes (HLA-A,B,C) and should not be assumed to be a primary function of the molecule. The analogies with the A,B,C chain are of some interest when considered within a species. Perhaps β_2-m ensures diversification of the immunological repertoire among the population of a species. Each individual functions more or less adequately with the six or fewer HLA-A,B,C antigens it expresses. Thus the high polymorphism of class 1 antigens is not of primary importance to the individual but serves to enhance the survival of the population or species as described above.

If relatively minor polymorphic differences in the HLA-A,B,C chain can produce changes in the repertoire of T cell receptors, it seems likely that changes in the functionally more important parts of a molecule, e.g., β_2-m, will produce even greater changes. Therefore, disease susceptibility in closely related species might show interesting differences based on change in their β_2-m. A lead worth following is the observed susceptibility to malaria of owl monkeys of some karotypes (55). One might postulate that diversity of β_2-m among related species enhances their survival.

c) **Antibodies against combinatorial determinants of HLA and β_2-m** (36). The binding of this group of antibodies is strongly inhibited by preparations of the HLA/β_2-m complex and weakly inhibited by free β_2-m. The difference in the molar amounts of material required to achieve the same amount of inhibition is > 1000. This behavior contrasted with that of the BBM.1 group of antibodies and suggested that structures contributed by both subunits were involved in the antigenic determinant(s). When these antibodies were tested against various man-mouse hybrid cells, binding was found only when genes for both HLA and β_2-m were present. Thus both human components were required to produce the correct antigenic determinant, and hybrid molecules containing either mouse β_2-m or H-2 heavy chain were inactive. Analysis of cross reactions in other species showed two distinguishable reactivities. BB7.5 and BB7.9 reacted only with African and Asian apes whereas BB7.7 and BB7.8 reacted with all apes and monkeys and with a single species of prosimian, the slow loris (43). It is not clear if these two pairs of antibodies recognize spatially separate sites or make different antigen-antibody contacts with part of the same structure. Studies of antibody blocking may clarify this point. For the moment we will consider them as two different antigenic sites as suggested by the clear difference in their patterns of cross reactivity.

Specific polymorphic antibodies (1,2,10,16). The antigenic determinants recognized by these antibodies are, we believe, the direct results of recent evolution within the human species. As a consequence they show no cross reactions with cells of other species and react with a limited number of HLA gene products. It is these antigenic determinants that approximate most closely the HLA antigens defined by HLA typing with human alloantisera. That mouse monoclonal antibodies may not recognize the same antigenic determinants as alloantibodies is not an omnipresent problem, from our experience. In contrast the extra evolutionary distance enables identification of all the allodeterminants and more. However, it is also apparent that monoclonal antibodies cannot and probably will not dispel all of the knotty problems of HLA typing. For example, it was relatively straightforward to produce monoclonal antibodies specific for antigens A2 and B7, which can be readily and uniquely defined with highly specific alloantisera. In contrast immunization with those antigens, e.g., A28,B40, for which it is unusual to find monospecific alloantisera has not so far yielded highly specific monoclonal antibodies. What those experiments produced were monoclonal antibodies with cross reactivities similar to those found in the common alloantisera used to operationally define those antigens. Thus we have made antibodies that react with B7 and B40 or A2 and A28.

It appears that the development of monoclonal serology will parallel that of conventional serology. Some gene products will be easy to define serologically and others will not be. From a protein chemical point of view this is perfectly reasonable. Some mutations that define a new gene product will not result in antigenic differences sufficient for the production of an operationally-monospecific antibody. The result is that all antibodies with specificity for this site will show some degree of cross reaction onto the most closely related gene products. Cross reactivity is, we believe, an intrinsic feature of the HLA system that is related to the homology between the different gene products and cannot always be eliminated by use of monoclonal antibodies. The benefits of analysis with monoclonal antibodies are a proper understanding of the basis of each cross reaction and resolution of the traditional dilemma between complex antigen or complex antibody.

HLA-A2: Analysis of an HLA Antigen with Monoclonal Antibodies

HLA-A2 and HLA-A28 are biochemically distinct from other HLA gene products examined. There are ≃ 40 amino acid differences between the primary structures of A2 and B7, whereas the amino acid sequence obtained from pooled specificities excluding A2 and A28 was the same as that of B7 (27,56). This unique structure probably explains why HLA-A2 has very specific antigenic properties and was the first HLA antigen to be described. Other properties that make HLA-A2 a particularly interesting antigen are its high gene frequency in the population and its sole restriction of T cell responses to the H-Y antigen (57).

Monoclonal antibodies with three different, specific, polymorphic activities have resulted from immunization with HLA-A2 and are listed in Table 1. The first group of antibodies reacts with HLA-A2 and with no other gene products, including HLA-A28 (1,2). One exception to date is that some cells from donor IDF type as A28 but do react with these antibodies. The second type of antibody reacts only with A2 and B17 and does not react with any A28 tested, including that expressed by IDF cells (10). The third type of antibody reacts with A2 and A28, including the A28 of IDF cells (19).

Table 1. HLA typing with monoclonal antibodies

		A2	A28	A28*	B17
Type 1	PA2.1	++++[a]	-[b]	++++	-
Type 2	MA2.1	++++	-	-	++++
Type 3	MA28.1	++++	++++	++++	-

[a] ++++, strong reaction.
[b] -, no reaction.

Type 1 antibodies probably recognize the same A2-specific determinant as mono-specific alloantisera do. Type 3 antibodies recognize the well-characterized cross reaction between A2 and A28. Type 2 antibodies define a cross reaction that was unexpected and not well characterized. Subsequent investigation has shown that this type of antibody can be found in alloantisera. The combined use of these monoclonal antibodies enables unique definition of four different HLA gene products--A2, A28, A28*, B17—although no single antibody is specific for a single gene product (Table 1). The A28 of IDF cells is different from the common A28, because it reacts with type 1, and from A2, because it does not react with type 2, and is a new gene product which we call A28*. As shown in Table 1, we define each gene product in terms of combinations of antigenic determinants. Because of the indirect nature of the cytotoxicity assay used for HLA typing, it is possible that some of the HLA antigens have always been unknowingly defined by a combination of two different antibodies, both of which can react with other gene products. This has been the classical explanation for the cytotoxicity negative absorption positive (CYNAP) phenomenon (21,22). It is therefore of interest to examine whether the three types of antibodies are reacting with distinct antigenic determinants on the surface of the HLA-A2 molecule. Preliminary experiments indicate at least two distinct alloantigenic sites on A2, which is in agreement with a more extensive analysis of B40 (16).

One of the most challenging problems associated with these studies is how to analyze the cross reactions. Simple binding assays show that PA2.1 antibody binds to A2 and A28*, or that MA2.1 binds to A2 and B17. But how similar are the antigenic structures identified by the monoclonal antibodies on these pairs of cross-reacting gene products? It is apparent that one must use more quantitative forms of analysis that allow measuring the strength of binding between antigen and antibody. Trucco et al. used equilibrium binding between cells and radioactively-labelled IgG to estimate binding constants for a number of monomorphic antibodies (57). We have begun to apply their methods for analysis of our polymorphic anti-HLA-A2 antibodies. An experiment to compare the binding of ^{125}I-PA2.1 to A2 and A28* indicates that it binds equivalently to both gene products (Fig. 1), suggesting that the antigenic determinant is identical in the two gene products.[2] Experiments of this kind using bivalent IgG suffer from the drawback that it is often unclear whether an avidity or affinity constant is being measured. A cell is in essence a polymeric antigen; at equilibrium a monoclonal IgG may be bound predominantly through one or two combining sites. If the binding is univalent, affinity is measured, whereas if binding is bivalent then avidity is measured (58). This problem becomes even more complex if IgM antibodies are used. For example, in the experiment shown in Fig. 1, PA2.1 might bind monovalently to a high-affinity site on A2 and bivalently to a low-affinity site on A28*, such that the measured binding constants, one for affinity and the other for avidity, are the same. In that case our interpretation that the sites are identical would be hopelessly wrong. This problem can be eliminated by using Fab fragments so that monovalent binding is enforced and affinity is measured. Unfortunately, a significant proportion of the interesting anti-HLA antibodies are of low affinity, and bivalency is essential to detect binding in a conventional assay. In this case we can either try to derive more sensitive assays that minimize dissociation or be content with measuring avidity. Comparison of Fab with IgG or preferably $F(ab')_2$ will usually indicate whether an antibody is binding monovalently or divalently.

---

[2] Ways, J, unpublished observations.

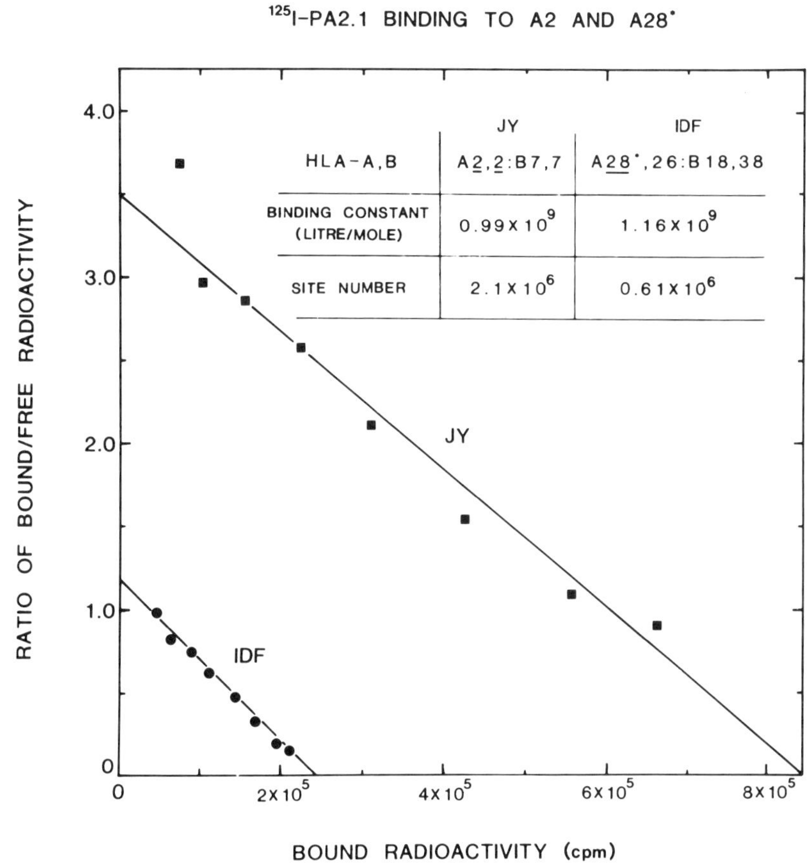

Fig. 1. Measurement of binding constant (avidity) of PA2.1 monoclonal antibody for A2 of JY cells and A28* of IDF cells. Cells (10^6) were incubated with different concentrations of ^{125}I-PA2.1 in a volume of 1 ml at 4°C with constant agitation for 6 h. Free and bound radioactivity were then separated by centrifugation and assayed in a gamma spectrophotometer. The results are plotted as linear transform of the mass action equation for a biomolecular association (J. Ways, unpublished results) (57).

Broadly polymorphic antibodies. These antibodies react with many gene products in the human population and detect polymorphic relationships often not previously characterized using alloantisera. As a group they resemble the public antigens of the mouse H-2 system (23). A particular property unusual in HLA serology is that they often reacted polymorphically with products of different loci (11). It seems likely that many of these antibodies react with evolutionary remnants of class 1 molecules produced as an indirect consequence of mutation. That many of these antibodies cross react extensively and polymorphically with other species supports this hypothesis. It is likely that many of the rat monoclonal antibodies produced by McKearn and co-workers that cross react onto cells of many other species, including humans, are of this type (3,7,13). Characterization of these antibodies can be difficult because the proportion of positive gene products is large, and each cell expresses at least three different class 1 antigens. The frequency of negative cells is often low and can be zero. Thus if a qualitative assay with a relatively small panel of cells is used, many of these broadly polymorphic antibodies will be mistaken as monomorphic. Errors of this type could generate considerable confusion.

Two striking properties of the broadly polymorphic antibodies are the frequency with which they are produced and the diversity of their specificity (19,20). Of 11 antibodies examined, no 2 have identical specificity, whereas in the collection of monomorphic and specific, polymorphic antibodies, repeat specificities are quite common. Often a pair of broadly polymorphic antibodies will appear identical in their reactions on all but one cell tested, but that one difference will be quite clear. Our impression is that these antibodies are sensitive to very subtle changes in the structure of class 1 antigens. It seems possible that most if not all amino acid substitutions will produce detectable differences in the antigenic properties of class 1 antigens. Even simple trace binding assays show that, although this type of antibody binds to many different gene products, it binds with an extensive range of affinities. Thus the antigenic determinant is not identical on all the positively reacting gene products; rather, there is a range of structures, many of which will give detectable binding reactions. The true character of broadly polymorphic antibodies that react with human cells can be discovered by examining the antibodies' reactions with individuals of other species (43).

In general the affinities of anti-HLA-A,B,C antibodies with HLA homologous in other species will be lower than for HLA. Therefore, in species at a greater evolutionary distance from man the number of positive reactions decreases for broadly polymorphic antibodies. Thus an antibody that reacts with 29 out of 30 human cells tested may react with only 15 out of 30 rhesus monkey cells. This is never observed with monomorphic antibodies, which always show similar reactions with all members of a species (43).

It seems probable that Bw4 and Bw6 are antigenic determinants that fall within the group discussed here. These determinants are found on a relatively large number of gene products, and the relevant alloantisera do cross react significantly with other species. In HLA typing, these antibodies have been extraordinarily useful because they often distinguish between highly cross-reactive pairs of alleles. This property, displayed by broad antisera which split many pairs of cross-reactive antigens which are themselves relatively noncross-reactive, was also demonstrated for the monoclonal antibody MB40.1 (11). For Bw4 and Bw6 it is as though an older diallelic polymorphism has been conserved during the evolution of the set of B locus alleles.

Alternatively, this may be the result of convergent evolution caused by the rather limited diversity acceptable at many of the polymorphic positons in the amino acid sequence (11). It is possible that many of the broadly polymorphic antigenic determinants definable by monoclonal antibodies will contribute to HLA serology as Bw4 and Bw6 have done. We reemphasize the probability that monoclonal antibodies reacting with only one gene product will be the exception rather than the rule and that this is a biologic fundamental rather than the product of insufficient work. It is imperative that these antibodies not be ignored despite the relative complexity of analyzing their specificity.

Evolutionary Implications of the Patterns of Cross Reaction of Anti-HLA Antibodies

Bodmer (59,60) has proposed that each individual contains structural genes, arranged as a tandem series within the HLA region, for all the HLA-A,B,C products. Observed polymorphism would then result from selective expression of these genes, which would be inherited in a Mendelian fashion. This model stimulated many investigators to search for a malfunctioning of this control mechanism—hence, the generally abortive quest for alien histocompatability antigens on cancer cells.

The experimental basis for the model was that HLA-A,B polymorphisms were conserved among such widely divergent species as man and cows. Such polymorphisms would therefore have arisen before divergence of the species and would have been selectively maintained in both evolutionary lines. The model avoids the necessity for invoking strong selective forces on polymorphic differences. For in a tandem array of duplicated genes each HLA-A,B,C antigen is a product of a different gene, and differences perceived as allotypic are in fact akin to the isotypic differences found throughout evolution for the heavy and light chains of immunoglobulin. In interpreting the serological data no distincton was made between the two fundamentally different classes of polymorphic structures, those created by mutation and those revealed by mutation. However, the implication of Bodmer's arguments is that highly specific antigenic determinants, those created by mutation, were conserved between cows and men. Conserving of such determinants as A3 or B7 over long periods of evolutionary time would require some special explanation, unless the conserved polymorphic determinants represented structures of the ancestral gene products that remained in some allelic products and not in others. In this case the results would merely imply that the mutation rate of class 1 antigens was such that during the period since divergence neither cows nor man had accumulated new mutations in all alleles for all potential positions in the amino acid sequence.

Data from the original reports of species cross reactions indicated that the activities detected did not conform with known HLA types but were broad and similar to the activities of Bw4, Bw6 types. Monoclonal antibodies provided ideal reagents to reevaluate this question. We had accumulated some 30 anti-HLA-A,B,C reagents defining structures of both types and proceeded to screen them by indirect binding assay on cells from different species. We were able to confirm the previous findings that polymorphic cross reactions were common. In particular, cows were surprisingly cross-reactive compared to other non-primate species (48). In a total of 554 animals of 51 species there were no convincing reactions with monoclonal antibodies recognizing highly specific polymorphic determinants. By contrast, most of the monoclonal antibodies detecting broadly polymorphic determinants in humans defined polymorphisms in other species (43). These results show that the polymorphic structures conserved among species are the same structures that define broad polymorphisms within a species. There appears to be no selective conservation of highly specific antigenic determinants and thus no compelling reason for invoking Bodmer's model to explain HLA serology. All available information can be explained by the traditional model of multiple alleles coded for by a small number of loci, i.e. A,B, and C. These results also suggest a need to reconsider the raison d'etre of alien antigens.

Some Applications and Complications in the Use of Monoclonal HLA Antibodies

Our discussion has centered on describing the types and serological specificity of the anti-HLA antibodies we have obtained. It is apparent that a collection of such antibodies can be used to define different antigenic determinants of the HLA molecule. We were also interested in using these antibodies to investigate the role of HLA antigens in killing of virally infected target cells. In these experiments (61), different HLA antibodies were used to block T cell killing of influenza-infected target cells. Initial experiments showed that some antibodies blocked the killing response whereas others did not. We thought these different patterns might be identifying sites of the molecule that were differentially involved in cellular recognition. This hypothesis was shown to be false by a semiquantitative analysis of the blocking phenomenon. The property determining the extent of blocking was the avidity rather than the specificity of the antibody. Those antibodies that bound with sufficiently strong avidity to cover all HLA molecules under the conditions used caused blocking. The degree of blocking was inversely related to the proportionate covering of HLA sites.

In these experiments the effect of temperature was particularly important. The killing assays were performed at 37°C whereas the antibodies had been characterized mostly at 4°C. The avidity of antibodies often decreases with a change in temperature, and some antibodies that bind well at 4°C were shown to bind poorly at the higher temperature and to be poor blocking reagents. Garotta and Trucco have used temperature change as a method for elution of certain monoclonal antibody affinity columns (62). These considerations may be pertinent to assessing *in vivo* clinical use of monoclonal antibodies and their Fab fragments, in which a temperature higher than that normally used in the characterization of monoclonal antibodies is encountered.

These experiments showed that the HLA antigen of the virally infected target cell was a molecule directly involved in mediating the HLA-restricted cell interaction. Monomorphic and polymorphic HLA antibodies could be shown to block killing, and in the appropriate combinations polymorphic antibodies such as PA2.1 and MA2.1 would block only if their antigenic target were the restriction element. These studies demonstrated the potential use of anti-HLA antibodies in functional studies but highlighted the importance of understanding not only the specificity of the antibodies but also their affinity and avidity. Two other types of experiments confirmed this observation. An antibody, MRC OX3 against rat Ia antigens, was shown to bind significantly to human B cell lines of specificity DRw 1, 3, or 6 (4). It was subsequently shown that the antibody also had polymorphic reaction patterns in both rat and mouse and that in mouse the polymorphism was genetically mapped to the I-A region. Attempts to demonstrate binding of MRC OX3 to peripheral B cells of appropriate DRw specificity failed, as did attempts to inhibit binding to B cell lines with purified HLA-DR antigens. Two possible and very different interpretations of these results are that 1) MRC OX3 was directed against molecules genetically linked but different from those having DRw specificities, which were neither found on peripheral B cells nor present in preparations of DRw antigens; 2) MRC OX3 binds with very low affinity to HLA-DRw antigens so that binding is detected only with cells having a large amount of antigen, i.e., B cell lines. Even in the cases where binding is found, bivalent attachment is required to form a stable complex, and monovalent antigens, as found in solubilized preparations, cannot effectively inhibit this binding. It is also possible that a combination of these two interpretations may be correct, i.e., that MRC OX3 does bind weakly and is directed against molecules distinct from conventional DRw antigens. However, it is difficult to select the best working hypothesis without knowing the relative strength of binding of MRC OX3 to rat, mouse, and human cells and the relative strength of binding of monovalent Fab compound to divalent Fab'_2 or IgG.

A number of HLA antibodies were used to examine the distribution of HLA antigens on the epithelial cells of the thymus (63). These cells are thought to be involved in the establishment of MHC restriction; thus their own pattern of MHC antigenic expression is of some importance. Initial results with one monomorphic and one polymorphic antibody revealed two different patterns. The monomorphic antibody, W6/32, bound strongly to epithelial cells in both the medulla and cortex. In contrast the polymorphic antibody, PA2.1 (anti-A2), bound only to epithelial cells of the medulla in HLA-A2-positive thymuses. It was tempting to generalize differences in the expression of these two discrete classes of antigen-determinant in the thymus. However, it was also possible that differences in affinity could produce such differences, and W6/32 was known to be of higher affinity than PA2.1. Subsequent testing with a number of different polymorphic and polymorphic HLA antibodies showed both patterns of staining with different antibodies in both groups. The difference did not appear to correlate with affinity differences and is possibly due to allelic-specific patterns of antigen expression.

To avoid ambiguity in interpretation of experiments such as those described above we have begun to measure the binding properties of anti-HLA antibodies, using previously published methods (57,58,64). Two antibodies, W6/32 and BB7.2, exemplify the considerable variation possible in monoclonal antibodies directed against the same cell surface molecule.

BB7.2 is an IgG2a antibody with specificity for HLA-A2 and A28* (65). Staphylococcus Protein A binds, is cytotoxic, and provides a suitable reagent for HLA typing. The whole immunoglobulin has a binding or avidity constant for cells expressing HLA-A2 of 4.6×10^8 liters/mol. The binding to cells of other HLA types was not significantly greater than the binding to DAUDI, which expresses no HLA-A,B,C antigens. The binding constant of Fab' fragments of BB7.2 was almost two orders of magnitude less than that of IgG, which was entirely due to differences in the dissociation constant. Under normal conditions used in screening assays the binding of the Fab is undetectable due to its high rate of dissociation. In contrast, the bivalent IgG forms a readily detectable, stable complex. Thus the bivalency of the antibody combined with the polymeric nature of the antigen, i.e., cells, allows a weak affinity to give rise to relatively strong binding or avidity. The weak affinity of BB7.2 suggested that this antibody would not be useful in assays involving soluble, monomeric antigens where bivalency of the antibody would not enhance the strength of antigen-antibody binding. This supposition proved to be correct. BB7.2 immunoprecipitates HLA-A2 very inefficiently from solubilized extracts of biosynthetically radiolabeled cells, and solubilized HLA-A2 weakly inhibits the binding of BB7.2 to cells. The properties of BB7.2 are summarized in Fig. 2.

W6/32 is an IgG2a antibody specific for a monomorphic determinant of all HLA-A,B,C antigens (35,46). The binding constant or avidity of the IgG to cells is about 1×10^9 liter/mol^{-1}. In contrast to BB7.2 the binding constant of the Fab is a little greater than for the IgG, 3×10^9 liter/mol^{-1}, which was the result of a slightly greater rate of association. A similar two- to three-fold increase in the rate

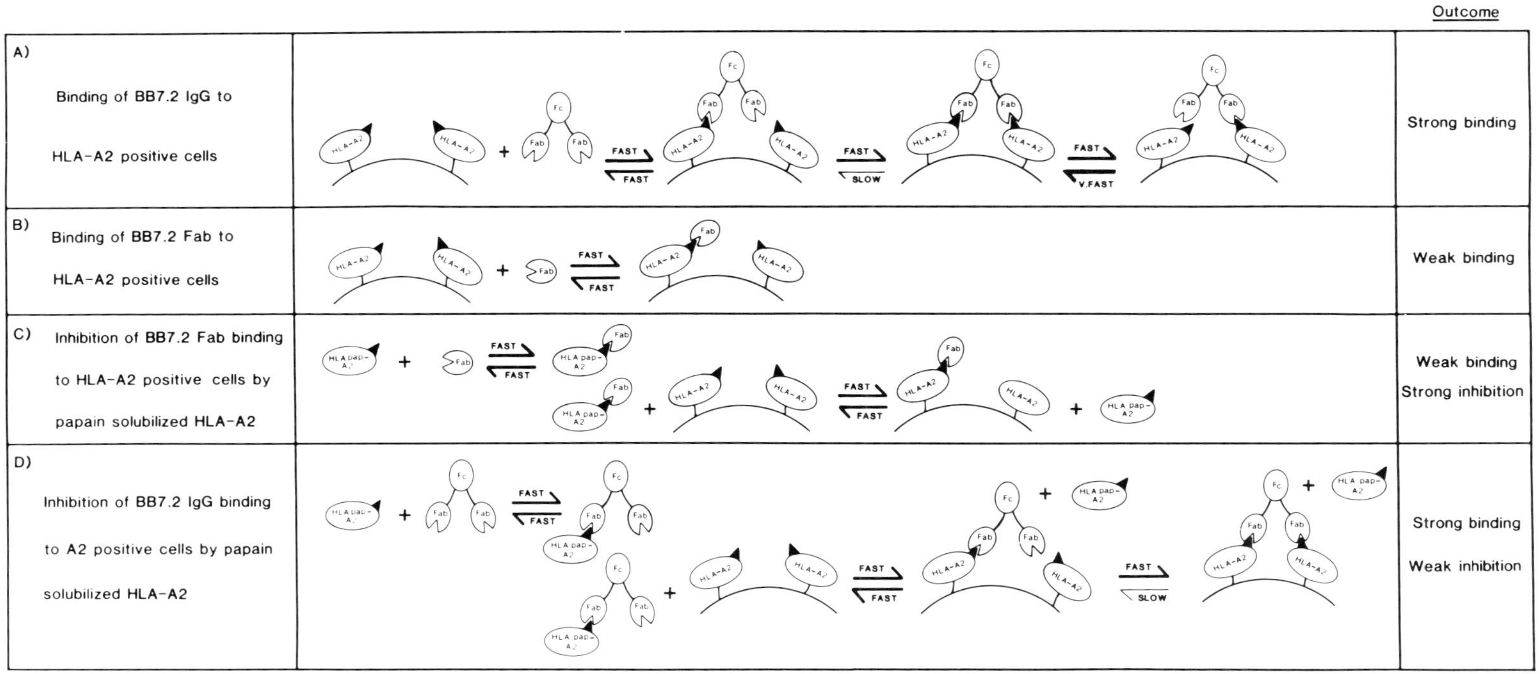

Fig. 2. The binding of BB7.2 antibody to cell surface and soluble HLA-A2. Papain-solubilized HLA-A2 is designated by HLA pap-A2. Surface HLA-A2 is designated HLA-A2 and is shown anchored into the cell membrane within which it can laterally move. Fab and Fc fragments of BB7.2 antibody are as designated, and the whole IgG is shown as a composite of two Fab's and one Fc. The scheme applies equally well for Fab' and Fab. The relative rates of reaction are as indicated and are emphasized by the breadth of the half arrow (65).

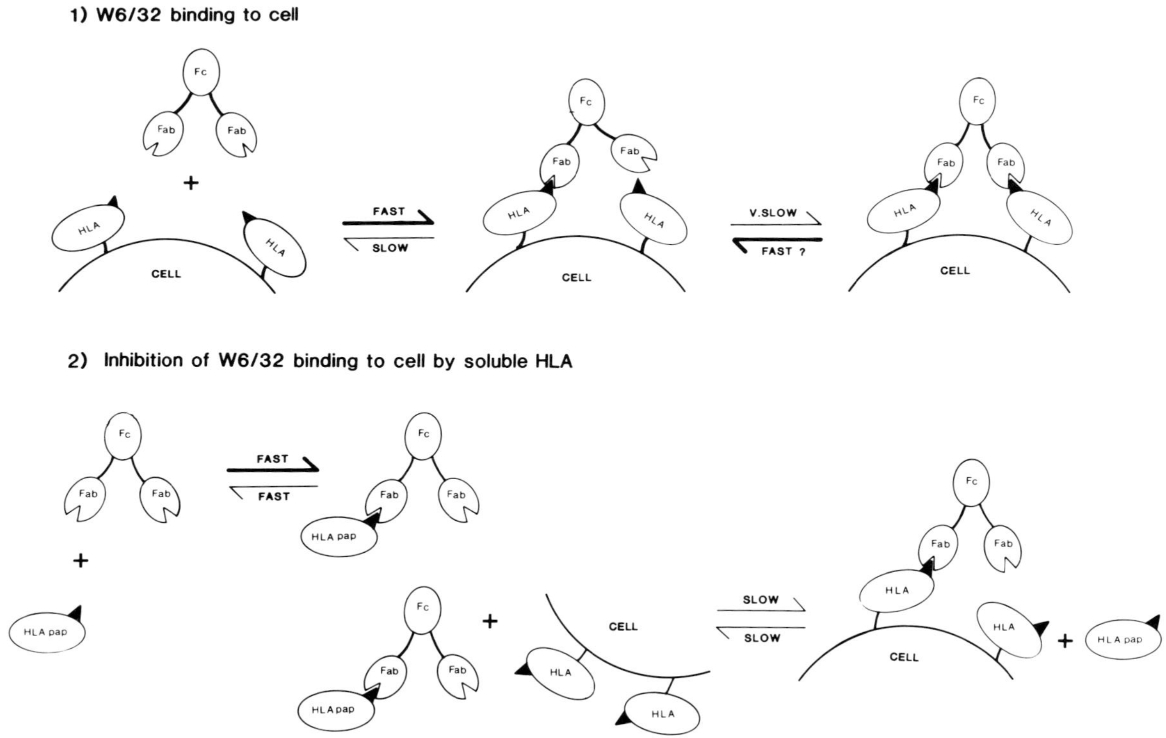

Fig. 3. The binding of W6/32 antibody to cell surface and soluble HLA antigens. The form of representation is as described in the legend to Fig. 2. The binding properties of Fab fragments made from W6/32 are similar to those of IgG, with the exception that bivalent binding is obviously not a possibility.

of association of Fab over IgG was observed for BB7.2 but was of little consequence to the difference between affinity and avidity due to the dramatic differences in the dissociation rates. These results and quantitation of the IgG molecules bound suggest that W6/32 binds to cells with a single combining site and does not relax to the extent that bivalent binding predominates. The interaction between W6/32 and either cells or solubilized antigen is comparable, as evidenced by its efficiency in immunoprecipitation and its stoichiometric inhibition by solubilized antigen. W6/32 may not bind bivalently to cells because of the presence of non-specific immunoglobulin chains producing only antibodies with a single active site or because bivalent binding is kinetically or thermodynamically unfavorable. These properties are summarized in Fig. 3.

Thus, although BB7.2 and W6/32 have avidity constants of comparable magnitude, their affinity constants are significantly different, because at equilibrium BB7.2 is all bound bivalently while W6/32 is bound monovalently to cells. These examples emphasize the need to characterize the binding of IgG and also of Fab fragments.

Coda

The monoclonal antibody method allows us to fully exploit the discriminatory potential of the mammalian immune system to make probes against a wide range of molecular structures. There is now considerable evidence that mouse monoclonal antibodies can be used for serologically dissecting the families of human histocompatibility antigens in a manner akin to that achieved with alloantisera. It is unlikely that each gene product will be defined in terms of combinations of a larger number of antigenic determinants. Quantitative comparisons will also be important. The picture obtained will not be identical due to intrinsic differences in using polyclonal versus monoclonal reagents. However, the level of understanding will be at least equivalent and most likely more accurate. There are already indications that structural interpretations of the serology of monoclonal antibodies correlate more closely with the chemical structure. The number of polymorphic monoclonal antibodies of different specificity that can be made against a single HLA gene product has been surprising. Whether these antibodies interact with distinct parts of the molecule or whether they bind with different geometry to the same basic piece of molecular structure is uncertain. Comprehensive blocking studies with Fab fragments have yet to be done; however, results with whole IgG indicate at least two polymorphic sites. Our own working hypothesis is that polymorphic residues are scattered throughout the surfaces of the HLA subunit not involved in β_2-m binding and that a continuum of overlapping polymorphic determinants exists.

Acknowledgments

The research described in this paper was supported under Grants 1R01AI17892 from the National Institutes of Health and Grant PCM80-17834 from the National Science Foundation. I would like to acknowledge my colleagues Frances Brodsky, Judy Ways, Rob McMaster, Andrew McMichael, and Bob Rouse for the enjoyable collaborations which generated the result and ideas. I thank Kathy Callahan for preparing the manuscript and Mike Graves for the drawings.

References

1. Parham, P, and WF Bodmer (1978). Monoclonal antibody to a human histocompatibility alloantigen, HLA-A2. Nature (Lond) **276**, 397-399.
2. Brodsky, FM, P Parham, CJ Barnstable, MJ Crumpton and WF Bodmer (1979). Monoclonal antibodies for analysis of the HLA system. Immunol Rev **47**, 3-61.
3. McKearn, TJ, FW Fitch, DE Smilek, M Sarmiento and FP Stuart (1979). Properties of rat anti-MHC antibodies produced by cloned rat-mouse hybridomas. Immunol Rev **47**, 91-115.
4. McMaster, WR, BC Winearls and P Parham (1979). A monoclonal mouse anti-rat Ia antibody which cross reacts with a human HLA-DRw determinant. Tissue Antigens **14**, 453.
5. Trucco, MM, G Garotta, JW Stocker and R Ceppellini (1979). Murine monoclonal antibodies against HLA structures. Immunol Rev **47**, 219-252.
6. Bono, R, F Hyafil, J Kalil, V Koblar, J Wiels, E Wollman, C Mawas and M Fellous (1979). Monoclonal antibodies against HLA-DRw antigens. Transplantation and Clinical Immunology 11, p 109. Excerpta Medica, Elsevier North-Holland.
7. Smilek, DE, HC Boyd, DB Wilson, CM Zmijewski, FW Fitch and TJ McKearn (1980). Monoclonal rat anti-major histocompatibility complex antibodies display specificity for rat, mouse and human target cells. J Exp Med **151**, 1139-1150.
8. Brodsky, FM, P Parham and WF Bodmer (1979). Monoclonal antibodies to HLA-DRw determinants. Tissue Antigens **16**, 30-48.
9. Zola, H, J Bradley, P Macardle, R McEvoy and M Thomas (1980). A hybridoma antibody which reacts with Human cells carrying the DRw4 tissue type. Transplantation (Baltimore) **29**, 72-73.
10. McMichael, AJ, P Parham, N Rust and F Brodsky (1980). A monoclonal antibody that recognizes an antigenic determinant shared by HLA-A2 and B17. Hum Immunol **1**, 121.
11. Parham, P, and J McLean (1980). Characterization, evolution and molecular basis of a polymorphic antigenic determinant shared by HLA-A and B products. Hum Immunol **1**, 131.
12. Ceppellini, R, G Garotta and MM Trucco (1980). Evaluation of xenogeneic monoclonal antibodies as HLA typing reagents. **In** Histocompatability Testing 1980, p 924. PI Terasaki, ed. UCLA Tissue Typing Laboratory, Los Angeles, California.
13. Boyd, HC, DE Smilek, RS Spielman, CM Zmijewski and TJ McKearn (1981). Monoclonal rat anti-MHC alloantibodies detect HLA-linked polymorphisms in humans. Immunogenetics **12**, 313-319.
14. Hansen, JA, PJ Martin, M Kamoun, B Nisperos and ED Thomas (1981). A supertypic HLA-DR specificity (DR 4 & 5) defined by murine monoclonal antibody. Hum Immunol **2**, 103-111.
15. Richiardi, P, A Amoroso, T Crepaldi, R Ceppellini and M Trucco (1981). A xenogeneic monoclonal antibody recognizing specificities controlled by HLA-A and B alleles. Immunogenetics **12**, 615-626.

16. Parham, P (1981). Monoclonal antibodies against two separate alloantigenic sites of HLA-B40. Immunogenetics **13**, 509-527.
17. Grumet, FC, BM Fendly and EG Engelman (1981). Monoclonal anti-HLA-B27 antibody (B27M[1]): production and lack of detectable typing difference between patients with Ankylosing Spondylitis, Reiters Syndrome and normal controls. Lancet **2**, 174-176.
18. Brodsky, FM (1979). Monoclonal antibodies for analysis of the HLA system. D Phil Thesis, Oxford University.
19. Parham, P, and FM Brodsky (1982). Mouse monoclonal antibodies against HLA-A,B,C antigens. **In** Monoclonal Antibodies and T Cell Hybridomas (Research Monographs in Immunology: Vol 3). GJ Hämmerling, U Hämmerling and JF Kearney, eds. Elsevier Publishing Co, Amsterdam.
20. Brodsky, FM, and P Parham (1982, in press). New aspects of HLA serology and biochemistry defined using monoclonal antibodies. **In** HLA Typing: Methodological Aspects and Relevance in Clinical Medicine. S Ferrone, BG Solheim, eds. CRC Press, Inc, Boca Raton, Florida.
21. Pappas, Synagoge, VIII 10xi, 1876-8. F Hultsch, ed. Berlin.
22. Svejgaard, A, M Hauge, C Jersild, P Platz, LP Ryder, L Staub Nielsen and M Thomsen (1979). The HLA system. **In** Monographs in Human Genetics **7**. L Beckman, U Hauge and M Hauge, eds. Karger, Basel.
23. Snell, GD, J Dausset and S Nathenson (1976). Histocompatibility. Academic Press, New York.
24. Klein, J (1975). Biology of the Mouse Histocompatibility-2 Complex, p 8. Springer-Verlag, New York.
25. Dorf, ME, ed (1981). The Role of the Major Histocompatibility Complex in Immunobiology. Garland STPM Press, New York, New York.
26. Coligan, JE, TJ Kindt, H Ueharn, J Martinko and SG Nathenson (1981). Primary structure of a murine transplantation antigen. Nature (Lond) **291**, 35-39.
27. Ploegh, HL, HT Orr and JL Strominger (1981). Major histocompatibility antigens: The human (HLA-A,B,C) and murine (H-2K,H-2D) class I molecules. Cell **24**, 287-299.
28. Klein, J (1979). The major histocompatibility complex of the mouse. Science **203**, 516-521.
29. Braun, WE (1979). HLA and disease: A comprehensive review. CRC Press, Inc, Boca Raton, Florida.
30. Dausset, J, and A Svejgaard, eds (1977). HLA and Disease. Williams and Wilkins, Baltimore, Maryland.
31. Lewontin, RC (1972). The Genetic Basis of Evolutionary Change. Columbia University Press, New York, New York.
32. Berggard, E, and AG Bearn (1968). Isolation and properties of a low molecular weight β_2-globulin occurring in human biological fluids. J Biol Chem **243**, 4095-4103.
33. Moller, G, ed (1974). β_2-microglobulin and HLA-A Antigen. Transplant Rev **21**.
34. Lancet, D, P Parham and JL Strominger (1979). Heavy chain of HLA-A and HLA-B antigens is conformationally labile: a possible role for beta 2-microglobulin. Proc Natl Acad Sci USA **76**, 3844-3848.
35. Parham, P, CJ Barnstable and WF Bodmer (1979). Use of a monoclonal antibody (W6/32) in structural studies of HLA-A,B,C antigens. J Immunol **123**, 342-349.
36. Brodsky, FM, and P Parham (1982,). Monomorphic anti-HLA-A,B,C monoclonal antibodies detecting molecular subunits and combinational determinants. J Immunol, in press.
37. Michaelson, J, E Rothenberg and EA Boyse (1980). Genetic polymorphism of murine β_2-microglobulin detected biochemically. Immunogenetics **11**, 93.
38. Gates, FT, JE Coligan and TJ Kindt (1981). Complete amino acid sequence of murine β_2-microglobulin: structural evidence for strain-related polymorphism. Proc Natl Acad Sci USA **78**, 554-558.
39. Krangel, MS, HT Orr and JL Strominger (1979). Assembly and maturation of HLA-A and HLA-B antigens *in vivo*. Cell **18**, 979-991.
40. Ivanyi, P (1981). Interspecies MHS relationships studied by serological and cellular cross-reactions. **In** Current Trends in Histocompatibility, p 133. RA

Reisfield, ed. Plenum Press, New York.

41. Trucco, MM, G Garotta, JW Stocker and R Ceppellini (1979). Murine monoclonal antibodies against HLA structures. Immunol Rev **47**, 219-252.
42. Brodsky, FM, WF Bodmer and P Parham (1979). Characterization of a monoclonal anti-β_2-microglobulin and its use in the genetic and biochemical analysis of major histocompatibility antigens. Eur J Immunol **9**, 536-545.
43. Brodsky, FM, and P Parham (1982). Evolution of HLA antigenic determinants: Species cross-reactions of monoclonal antibodies. Immunogenetics, in press.
44. Terhorst, C, A van Agthoven, K LeClair, P Snow, E Reinherz and S Schlossman (1981). Biochemical studies of the human thymocyte cell-surface antigens T6,T9,T10. Cell **23**, 771-780.
45. Cotner, T, H Mashimo, PC Kung, G Goldstein and JL Strominger (1981). Human T cell surface antigens bearing a structural relationship to HLA antigens. Proc Natl Acad Sci USA **78**, 3858-3862.
46. Barnstable, CJ, WF Bodmer, G Galfre, C Milstein, AF Williams and A Ziegler (1979). Production of monoclonal antibodies to Group A erythrocytes, HLA and other human cell surface antigens - new tools for genetic analysis. Cell **14**, 9-20.
47. Parham, P, PK Sehgal and FM Brodsky (1979). Anti-HLA-A,B,C monoclonal antibodies with no alloantigenic specificity in humans define polymorphisms in other primate species. Nature (Lond) **279**, 639-641.
48. Brodsky, FM, W Stone and P Parham (1981). Of cows and men: a comparative study of histocompatibility antigens. Hum Immunol **3**, 143-152.
49. Ma, NSF, TC Jones, AC Miller, AM Morgan and EA Adams (1976). Chromosome polymorphism and banding patterns in the owl monkey (Aotus). Lab Anim Sci **26**, 1022-1036.
50. Ma, NSF, RN Rossan, St T Kelley, JS Harper, MT Bedard and TC Jones (1978). Banding patterns of the chromosomes of two new karyotypes of the owl monkey, Aotus, captured in Panama. J Med Primatol **7**, 146-155.
51. Ma, NSF, T Simeone, J McLean and P Parham (1982). Chromosome localization and gene synteny of the major histocompatibility complex in the owl monkey, Aotus. Immunogenetics, in press.
52. Parham, P, and HL Ploegh (1980). Molecular characterization of HLA-A,B homologues in owl monkeys and other non-human primates. Immunogenetics **11**, 131.
53. Ma, NS (1981). Chromosome evolution in the owl monkey, Aotus. Am J Phys Anthropol **54**, 293-303.
54. Sanderson, AR (1977). HLA 'help' for human β_2-microglobulin across species barriers. Nature (Lond) **269**, 414-417.
55. Young, MD, DC Baerg and RN Rossan (1976). Studies with induced Malarias in Aotus monkeys. Lab Anim Sci **26**, 1131-1137.
56. Goulmy, E, A Termijtelen, BA Bradley and JJ van Rood (1977). Y-antigen killing by T cells of women restricted by HLA. Nature (Lond) **266**, 544-545.
57. Trucco, M, S DePetris, G Garotta and R Ceppellini (1980). Quantitative analysis of cell surface HLA structures by means of monoclonal antibodies. Hum Immunol **1**, 233.
58. Mason, DW, and AF Williams (1980). The kinetics of antibody binding to membrane antigens in solution and at the cell surface. Biochem J **187**, 1-20.
59. Bodmer, WF (1972). Evolutionary significance of the HLA system. Nature (Lond) **237**, 139-145.
60. Bodmer, WF (1973). A new genetic model for allelism at histocompatibility and other complex loci: polymorphism for control of gene expression. Transplant Proc **V**, 1471.
61. McMichael, AJ, P Parham, FM Brodsky and JR Pilch (1980). Influenza virus specific cytotoxic T lymphocytes recognize HLA molecules; blocking by monoclonal anti-HLA antibodies. J Exp Med **152**, 1955.
62. Garotta, G, and M Trucco (1981). HLA antigens temperature dependent elution from specific monoclonal antibody columns. Colloquium Protides of Biological Fluids **28**, p 463. H Peeters, ed.
63. Rouse, RV, P Parham, FC Grumet and IL Weissman (1982). Expression of HLA antigens by human thymic epithelial cells. Submitted to Hum Immunol.

64. Frankel, ME, and W Gerhard (1979). The rapid determination of binding constants for antiviral antibodies by a radioimmunoassay. An analysis of the interaction between hybridoma proteins and influenza virus. Immunochemistry **16**, 101-106.
65. Parham, P, and FM Brodsky (1981). Partial purification and some properties of BB7.2; a cytotoxic monoclonal antibody with specificity for HLA-A2 and a variant for HLA-A28. Hum Immunol **4**, 277-299.

III
Applications to Cancer

ANALYSIS OF CELL SURFACE MOLECULES ON HUMAN NEUROBLASTOMA CELLS AND LEUKEMIA CELLS

Roger H. Kennett and Zdenka L. Jonak
Department of Human Genetics
University of Pennsylvania School of Medicine

Mariko Momoi and Mary Catherine Glick
Department of Pediatrics
University of Pennsylvania School of Medicine
and
Children's Hospital of Philadelphia

Lois A. Lampson
Department of Anatomy
University of Pennsylvania School of Medicine
Philadelphia, Pennsylvania 19104

Investigators making antisera against human tumor cells to define tumor-associated antigens have viewed Köhler and Milstein's report (1) of monoclonal antibodies of predefined specificity with considerable enthusiasm. The ability to continually produce large amounts of a single antibody with a well-defined specificity suggested that many previously conceived methods for detection and therapy of tumors could now be applied.

Several investigators have reported monoclonal antibodies made against antigens on a variety of human tumors (2,3). Production of these antibodies involves attempts to define two types of antigens: 1) "tumor-specific antigens"--antigens that represent new molecules on the surface of tumor cells and thus directly reflect a molecular change involved in malignant transformation; 2) antigens that are operationally "tumor-specific"--antigens that, although not truly tumor-specific, can be used to discriminate tumor cells from most normal cells.

Antibodies to both of these classes of antigens may, in fact, be useful for identification and therapy of tumors. In the second case, special care will be needed to ensure that using the antibodies to lyse tumor cells or to deliver toxins or radiation specifically to the cells does not also selectively kill essential and irreplaceable normal cells, i.e., hematopoietic stem cells or neurons.

To define an antigen as being of class 1 involves comparing the structure of the gene for the antigen in normal and tumor cells, and it is in this respect that we can expect the new technologies of hybridomas and recombinant DNA to come together in important ways (3,4).

We will describe here our experiences in making monoclonal

antibodies against human neuroblastoma cells and human leukemia cells. We will attempt to evaluate progress in the production of monoclonal antibodies to human tumor antigens and will provide our perspective on future directions of such research.

Materials and Methods

The methods used in the work described here for production, characterization, and application of monoclonal antibodies have been reported previously (2,5,6-8).

Results and Discussion

For the past few years, work in our laboratories has been directed toward the production of monoclonal antibodies against human neuroblastoma cells and leukemia cells. Our intention was to define tumor-specific antigens or cell surface differentiation antigens and to use the antibodies to isolate molecules that could then be characterized biochemically and genetically. We have produced hundreds of antibodies against both types of human tumor cells and have concentrated on using human neuroblastoma cell lines and acute lymphoblastic leukemia cells as antigens or as a source of antigens. We will describe here our progress in defining tumor-specific antigens and will discuss future applications and approaches in the use of monoclonal antibodies to study malignant cells.

The monoclonal antibody that we have characterized and used to the fullest extent was made against the human neuroblastoma cell line IMR6 (5,6). This antibody, PI153/3, was originally characterized as reacting with neuroectoderm-derived tumors and fetal brain but as showing no detectable reactivity with adult brain or with any of the other human cell types in a panel including fibroblasts, lymphoid lines, peripheral blood cells, and various tumors with other tissue origins. While using this antibody to detect neuroblastomas metastasized to bone marrow, we noted that the antibody reacted with acute lymphoblastic leukemia cells from some patients (4). It was found, in fact, that PI153/3 reacts with B cell leukemias and non-T, non-B leukemias but not with T cell leukemias or myelongenous leukemia cells (9). Reaction with leukemia cells did make us consider the possibility that bone marrow lymphocytes were represented by the leukemia cells in a stage of differentiation and that in cases of regenerating marrow in neuroblastoma patients these cells would be detected by the antibody and mistaken for neuroblastoma cells. To avoid this misclassification, we have used a second antibody (P3B1C3) that reacts with lymphocytes and all the leukemias detected by

PI153/3 but not with neuroblastomas. Using these two antibodies together we could distinguish lymphoid cells (PI153/3+/P3B1C3+) from neuroblastomas (PI153/3+/P3B1C3-). These two antibodies make it possible to detect and define neuroblastoma in bone marrow, an important procedure for cases in which marrow may be removed, the patient treated, and the marrow returned to the patient after treatment.

Whether the same antibody can be used safely to remove neuroblastomas from the marrow depends on whether the lymphocytes expressing the antigen are replaceable by development from stem cell precursors.

This same antibody has been used to distinguish lymphoid tumors from neuroblastomas and can be used to distinguish stage IV (+) neuroblastoma from IVS (-), a special case of neuroblastoma that is usually left untreated and exhibits spontaneous regression. It can also, of course, be used to classify leukemias with regard to their cell of origin (9).

Other investigators have subsequently reported monoclonal antibodies that react with human neuroblastoma as well as with some other tumor types (10,11).

While characterizing the reactivity of this antibody and its use to detect metastasis, we continued to make monoclonal antibodies against neuroblastoma cells. We immunized mice with cells, cells coated with an antiserum made against another human cell type (6), membrane vesicles (12), KCL extracts (13), and NP-40 extracts.

Using each of these immunizing protocols, we have derived over 300 monoclonal antibodies that, on the basis of the first screening, appeared to be neuroblastoma-specific in that they did not react with the second cell type (fibroblast or lymphoblastoid line) used in the original assay. When tested against a panel of cells, all but two showed reactions with cells other than neuroblastomas. Figure 1 shows the reactions of these two antibodies, PI153/3, a control antibody, and other antibodies with characteristic patterns of binding. It could well be that, as in many other cases, the two antibodies that appear to be specific for neuroblastoma may react with determinants on other cell types. Similar results have been found in our production of antibodies against Reh (14), a non-B, non-T acute lymphoblastic leukemia cell line. Many antibodies that at first appear to be specific for Reh or ALL do in fact, after further screening, bind to other cells--both tumor cells and normal cells.

It is, in fact, interesting that more than 50% of the antibodies, similar to the PI153/3, react with both Reh and neuroblastomas. There are, of course, precedents for what could be described as tissue-specific antigens (e.g., mouse Thy-1 antigen) that are expressed both on neural and lymphoid tissues. What this implies about function or processes of differentiation or what it may have to do with the fact that some neural cells are in effect normally sequestered from the immune system remains to be defined.

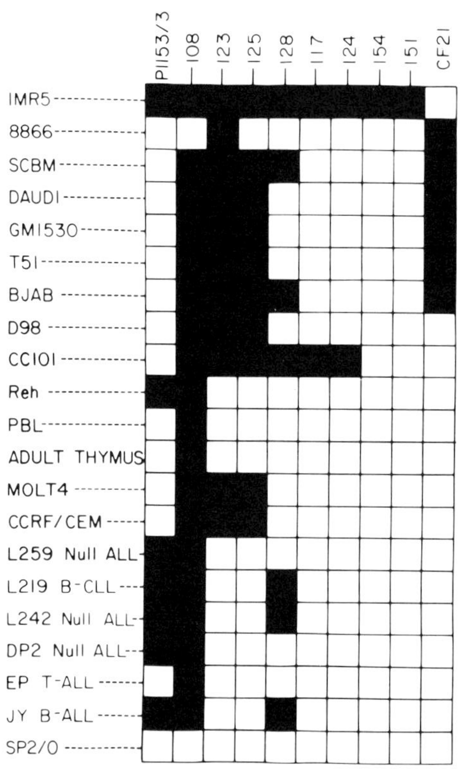

Fig. 1. Reactions of selected anti-neuroblastoma antibodies with a panel of human cell types. Antibodies were tested for binding to the indicated cell types using an enzyme-linked anti-immunoglobulin assay. ■ indicates a positive binding reaction. IMR5, neuroblastoma; 8866, SCBM, DAUDI, GM1530, T51 are B lymphoblastoid line; BJAB is an EBV-negative B lymphoblastoid line; D98 is a HeLa cell subline; CC101 is a fibroblast; Reh is a non-B, non-T ALL; MOLT 4 and CCRF/CEM are T-cell lines; the other cells are peripheral blood samples from the indicated type of leukemia, and SP2/0 is a mouse plasmacytoma used as a control. The antibody CF21 used as a control was made against the human B cell line, GM1530.

Monoclonal Antibody Specificity

It has become increasingly clear that even monoclonal antibodies exhibiting a very restricted pattern of reactivity often exhibit cross reactivity with other cell types. Since monoclonal antibodies, particularly those made in fusions with non-producer myeloma cells, have a single type of binding site reactive with a specific antigenic site, this cross reactivity may result because 1) the same molecule is present on the two cell types, 2) the same antigenic determinant is present on different molecules on the two cells, or 3) similar antigenic determinants are present on the two cell types.

Which of these statements accurately explains the cross reactivity can be determined only by isolating the molecules involved and comparing them by biochemical methods. The frequency with which explanations 2 and 3 represent the actual situation will affect the practicality of using monoclonal antibodies to deliver cytotoxic agents directly to cancer cells. If there is a significant amount of antigenic site cross reactivity with monoclonal antibodies, the possibility of using a single monoclonal antibody to define a truly tumor-specific antigen is reduced accordingly. Investigators have determined that the hemagglutin molecule of influenza virus, a protein with a molecular weight of 220,000, can be recognized on the order of 1000 different ways by monoclonal antibodies (15). If this is the case for most antigenic protein molecules, then the probability of antigenic site cross reactivity is a significant factor in defining specificity of monoclonal antibodies. In any case, defining antigens on different cell types as being the same antigen will require sufficient biochemical characterization to demonstrate their identity. With regard to specific therapeutic application, the reason for cross reactivity is not as important as whether the non-tumor cells that express the determinant are essential and irreplaceable.

A second observation we have made while screening monoclonal antibodies against human neuroblastomas is that cytolytic anti-β_2-microglobulin or anti-HLA antibodies do not lyse neuroblastoma cells (Table 1). Standard binding assays also do not indicate that these molecules are present on the surface of neuroblastoma cells, but such assays do detect the HLA molecules on a human glioma cell line (Fig. 2). Dr. Lampson has shown (16) that these molecules are present, but at a concentration at least an order of magnitude lower, by demonstrating that cell extracts can inhibit the binding of the same anti-HLA and anti-β_2-microglobulin antibodies to lymphoblastoid cells.

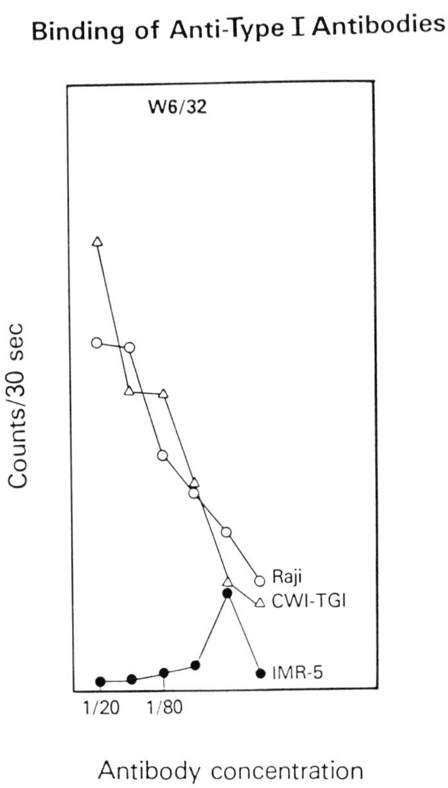

Fig. 2. Binding of anti-HLA monoclonal antibody W6/32 (17) to IMR-5, a human neuroblastoma; CW1-T61, a human oligodendroglioma; and Raji, a B-lymphoblastoid line. Binding of the antibody was detected using ^{125}I-labeled anti-Fab (18). Range of six background values: CW1-TG1, 392-580; Raji, 1032-1327; IMR-5, 195-396.

Table 1. Analysis of HLA and β_2 microglobulin expression by cytotoxicity

Values indicate the last dilution of supernatant or antiserum giving 50% lysis (mean of duplicate determinations).

Antibody/antiserum	Specificity	Neuroblastomas					B Cells	
		SKNSH	134A	IMR5	IMR32	NBM	RPMI-8866	DAUDI
PI153/3	Oncofetal antigen on neuroblastoma	64	16	32	8	16	0	0
L243	Ia	0	0	0	0	0	256	256
W6/32(10X)	HLA	0	0	0	0	0	256	0
Anti-β_2 serum (1/10)	β_2m	0	0	0	0	0	64	0

These observations illustrate again the difficulty of deciding purely on the basis of binding or cytotoxicity assays whether an antigen is present and the need to do biochemical analysis before concluding that an antigen is not present. Again, this suggests a need for caution in using monoclonal antibodies for therapy, because other cells that are not reactive under *in vitro* conditions may be affected when the antibody is administered to a patient or is used to test bone marrow.

The object of this discussion is not to be pessimistic about monoclonal antibodies as potential tools in tumor therapy but to indicate some possible pitfalls that should be considered and also to suggest alternative approaches that may complement those already available.

An Alternative Approach to the Definition of Tumor Cell Surface Antigens of Potential Therapeutic Significance

The search for a tumor-specific antigen is based on the assumption that a molecular change involves 1) the alteration of a cell surface molecule to produce an antigenic change or 2) the addition of a new molecule not expressed on the normal cell membrane. It is, of course, possible that the molecular changes coinciding with malignant transformation do not result in the appearance of new antigenic determinants on the tumor cell surface. Two alternative possibilities are diagramed in Fig. 3. The basic assumptions of these models are that 1) since a tumor, by definition, continues to divide when its normal counterpart would stop, there may be some molecular change limiting its ability to respond to a growth-control message (GCM) that would normally cause the cell to stop dividing and begin differentiating or performing a specific function and that 2) for the sake of simplicity, the receptor for the GCM is on the cell surface.

It is possible that, as depicted in Fig. 3A, the event leading to tumor cell formation is the loss of a receptor. This can be tested for by making antibodies against the normal cells and using them to find a molecule missing on the tumor cells. But this procedure is highly impractical for at least two reasons: 1) it is often difficult if not impossible to define the normal cell type that exactly corresponds to a given tumor and 2) if it were defined, it is unlikely that a large enough population of these cells could be obtained in a suspension pure enough to make the immunization and screening assays practical.

The second model, in Fig. 3B, represents a case in which the GCM receptor is not absent but is changed or has interacted with some other component so that it cannot receive the message. In this case, most if not all of the antigenic determinants on the tumor cell

A. LOSS OF RECEPTOR FOR GROWTH CONTROL MESSAGE (GCM)

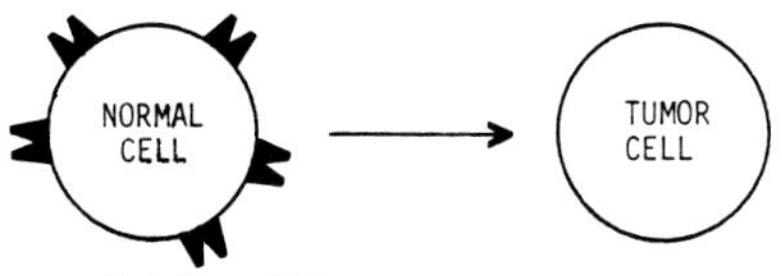

Tumor does not express receptor and cannot respond to GCM

Model predicts:

Antibodies to receptor on normal cell will not react with tumor cell.

Antibodies to receptors on normal cells may block GCM.

Antibodies may mimic effect of GCM on normal cells.

To test this model:

Find monoclonal antibodies that react with normal cells corresponding to differentiated state of the tumor, but do not react with the tumor cells

B. ALTERATION OF RECEPTOR FOR GROWTH CONTROL MESSAGE

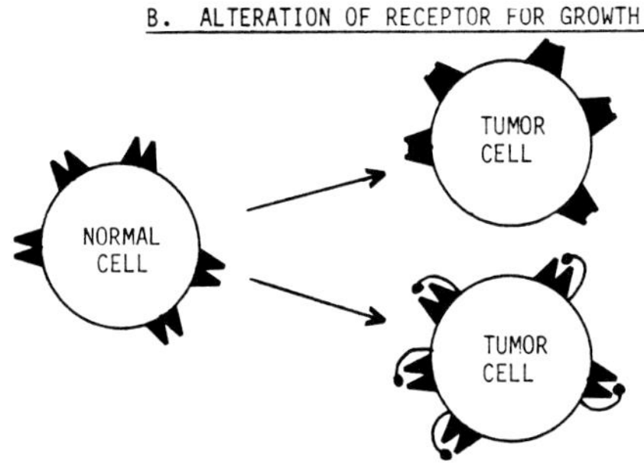

Receptor is modified so it cannot bind GCM

Other cell surface molecules interact with the receptor so it cannot bind GCM

Model predicts:

Antibodies may bind receptor on normal cells and on tumor cells.
Antibodies may mimic the effects of GCM.

To test this model:

Find monoclonal antibodies that react with tumor cells and see if they can mimic the effects of GCM.

Can they stop proliferation and induce differentiation?

Fig. 3. Two alternative mechanisms by which receptors for growth control messengers (GCM) may be involved in the primary alteration in malignancy. In both models, tumor cells continue to divide and/or fail to differentiate because they lack a functional receptor that would normally receive the message inducing the cell to stop dividing and to differentiate. The analysis of both possibilities has been made practical by the availability of monoclonal antibodies, reagents that are directed against single antigenic determinants and are available in large quantities. For the study of most human tumors, it may be more practical to test model B, because tumor cells are more likely to be available for immunization, assays, functional studies, and molecular analyses. Functional studies would also be easier because they could use tumor cells without identification of the GCM by looking for antibodies that by themselves or in combination inhibit cell proliferation and/or induce differentiation.

molecule will be present in the molecule as it is expressed in the corresponding normal cell. Because antibodies reacting with insulin receptors can mimic the effects of insulin (19)--"insulinomimetic" monoclonal antibodies have in fact been reported (20)—monoclonal antibodies binding to tumor cells should be reacted with these cells to test whether they can mimic the effect of the proposed GCM, stop the tumor cell from dividing, and perhaps even induce it to proceed to differentiate. This provides a way to identify antigens that may be involved in the control of cell division and/or growth.

On the basis of this model, we have tested 80 different antibodies to see if they inhibit the proliferation of the leukemia cell line Reh. Figure 4 shows the results of one of these experiments. In the antibodies tested, we have found that three inhibit Reh. This procedure allows us to pick from the many antibodies that bind to

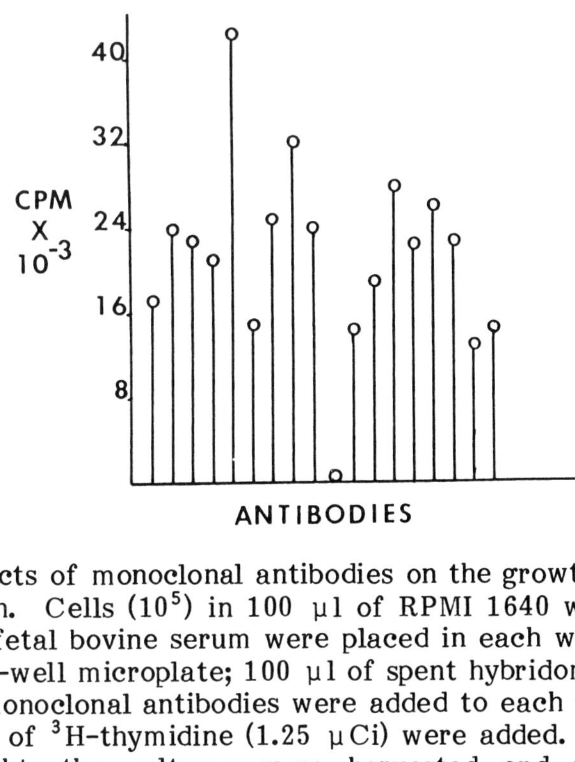

Fig. 4. Effects of monoclonal antibodies on the growth of leukemia cell line Reh. Cells (10^5) in 100 μl of RPMI 1640 with 20% heat-inactivated fetal bovine serum were placed in each well of a round-bottomed 96-well microplate; 100 μl of spent hybridoma supernatant containing monoclonal antibodies were added to each well. One day later, 50 μl of ^{3}H-thymidine (1.25 μCi) were added. After incubation overnight, the cultures were harvested and the extent of proliferation measured by the amount of ^{3}H-thymidine incorporated into TCA precipitable material. Samples were tested in quadruplicate. Results show that some of the hybridoma supernatants appear to inhibit Reh cell proliferation, and further tests of those are in progress. We have shown that the inhibiting activity titers out with the antibody-binding activity (21).

tumor cells the few that may be directed against molecules involved in growth regulation; these selected antibodies can be used to examine the cell surface molecules more closely. The molecules can then be isolated from tumor cells and normal cells and compared by other biochemical criteria for molecular alteration of the tumor cell molecule. This may be a way to pick out molecules that are present in relatively small numbers on the cell surface but perhaps play a significant role in cell division. It has even been suggested (22) that it may be useful to actually screen for monoclonal antibodies affecting such functions as growth control or division and in this way identify antigens that are very important functionally but that are present in too few molecules per cell to be picked up in standard binding assays.

Isolation of Minor Components from the Cell Surface

Detecting cell surface molecules by functional assays as suggested above will be useful only if the antibodies can be used to isolate and characterize the molecules identified. We will describe here the use of the antibody PI153/3 to isolate the corresponding neuroblastoma cell surface antigen. This work, which has been reported previously in detail (7), illustrates the possibility of using even a monoclonal antibody of the IgM class to isolate a cell surface molecule that constitutes a minor component (0.5%) of the total cell surface glycoprotein.

Assay of various cell fractions from IMR-5 neuroblastoma cells for their ability to inhibit cytolytic activity of PI153/3 on neuroblastoma cells indicated that there was no antigenic activity in glycolipid or ganglioside fractions but that the glycoprotein and pronase-digested glycopeptide fraction did show inhibiting activity and thus contained molecules bearing the PI153/3 antigenic determinant (Fig. 5).

Attempts to prepare an affinity column with this IgM antibody by binding it to cyanogen bromide-activated sepharose resulted in the loss of antibody-binding activity. Dr. Momoi circumvented this difficulty by preparing an affinity column of goat anti-mouse IgM and passing the PI153/3 ascites fluid over the column. Passage of NP-40 extracts labeled with D-(^{3}H)glucosamine over this column resulted in specific retention of a glycoprotein that could then be eluted with glycine buffer (Fig. 6 and 7). Analysis by inhibition of cytolytic activity demonstrated that the antigen present in the NP-40 extract was retained in the PI153/3 affinity column and was specifically eluted by the glycine buffer (Table 2).

Similar procedures carried out with other human neuroblastoma cells and other human and mouse cell types indicated that the antigen bound to and eluted from the PI153/3 column was detectable only on

Table 2. Purification of antigen from IMR-5 cells[a]

	Radioactivity[b]	Antigenic activity	
	cpm/10^8 cells	Units[c]/10^8 cells	Units/10^4 cpm
NP-40 extract	300,000	40	1
Pellet	130,000	0[d]	0
Immunoaffinity column			
Unadsorbed	300,000	0[e]	0
Eluted			
Glycine buffer	500	23	500
4 M urea	220	0	0

[a]Reproduced from (7) with permission.
[b]Glycoproteins were labeled with D-(^{3}H)glucosamine.
[c]A unit of activity was that amount of antigen inhibiting 50% of the complement-mediated cytolysis as measured by the activity of creatine phosphokinase in the cell pellet and was calculated to 10^8 cells as described in (7).

[d]After extraction, the pellet showed no inhibitory activity up to 5.5×10^6 cells.
[e]No inhibitory activity up to 6.6×10^6 cells.

the neuroblastoma cells and on the leukemia cell line Reh, which is known to express the antigen (Table 3). When the glycoprotein eluted from the affinity column was analyzed by SDS-PAGE electrophoresis, a specific peak with a molecular weight of approximately 20,000 could be identified (Fig. 8). The data to this point are consistent with the PI153/3 antibody reacting with the carbohydrate portion of a cell surface glycoprotein that on IMR-5 has a minimal molecular weight of 20,000. Whether the antigen detected on other cells such as Reh is the same molecule or simply a molecule with a similar antigenic determinant remains to be defined.

Work recently carried out in Dr. Glick's laboratory with Arthur Smith indicates that the antigen isolated from neuroblastoma cells (CHP-134) contains the antigenic determinant on a polypeptide larger than that of IMR-5 cells. This is, of course, consistent with the

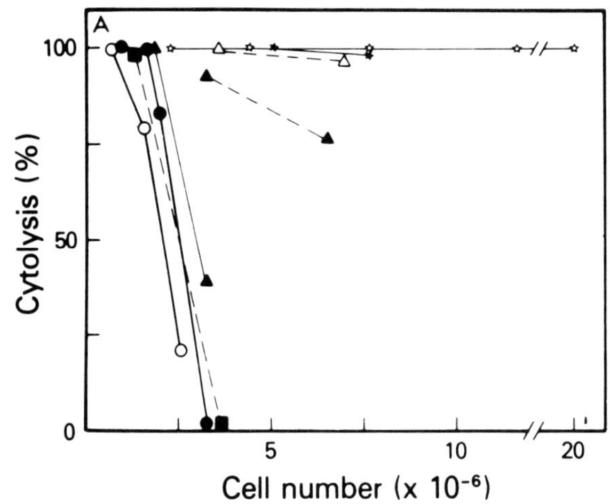

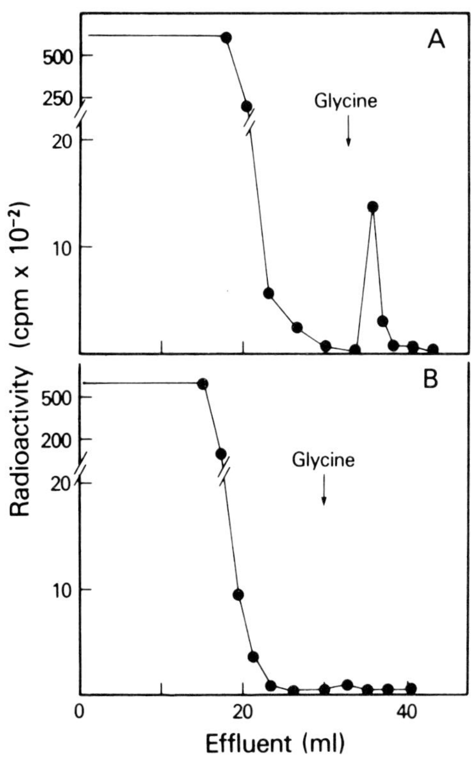

Fig. 6. Profiles of an NP-40 extract on immunoaffinity columns of two different monoclonal antibodies. Monoclonal antibodies PI153/3 (A) and P3B13C2 (B) were adsorbed to anti-IgM-Sepharose. An NP-40 extract (1.2×10^7 cpm) from IMR-5 cells labeled metabolically with D-(^{3}H)glucosamine was applied to each column and eluted with glycine buffer and 4 M urea. Reproduced from (7) with permission.

Fig. 5. Antigenic activity of cell fractions. The indicated fractions were examined for their ability to inhibit the lysis of IMR-5 cells by the antibody PI153/3. Lysis was measured by assaying the enzyme creatine phosphokinase in the cell pellet after treatment with antibody and complement. The fractions from IMR-5 cells were (closed circles, solid line), NP-40 extract; (open squares, broken line), trypsinate; (closed squares, broken line), pronase-digested trypsinate; (open stars, broken line), glycolipids; (closed stars, broken line), gangliosides; and an NP-40 fraction eluted from wheat germ agglutin-in-agarose with 0.1 M GlcNAc (closed triangles, solid line) followed by 0.3 M GlcNAc (closed triangles, broken line). (Open circles, broken line) indicates inhibition by an NP-40 extract from another neuroblastoma, CHP-134. Reproduced from (7) with permission.

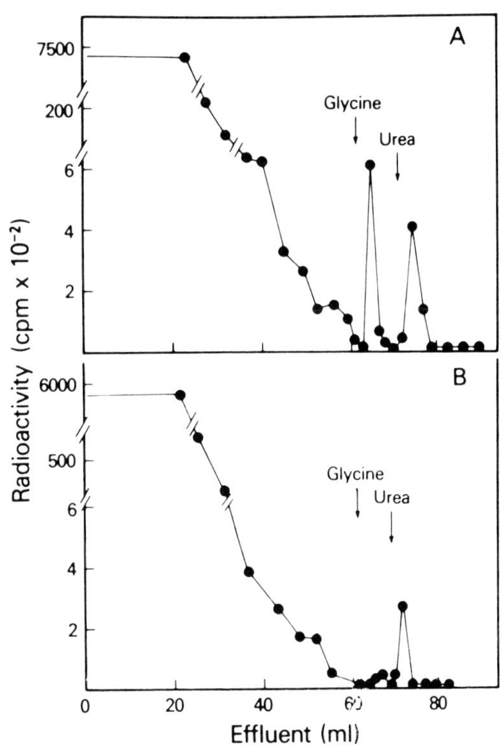

Fig. 7. Profile of radioactive trypsinates on immunoaffinity columns. Trypsinates (1.2 x 10^6 cpm) from IMR-5 cells (A) and hybrid (IMR-5 x IT-22) cells (B) labeled metabolically with L-(^{3}H)-fucose were adsorbed on immunoaffinity columns of monoclonal antibody PI153/3 and eluted with glycine buffer. Reproduced from (7) with permission.

Table 3. Selective elution from the immunoaffinity column and antigenic activity of various cell lines[a]

	Affinity column	Creatine phosphokinase assay[b]
NP-40 extract		
IMR-5	+	+
CHP-134	+	+
Reh	+	+
CHP-134-F	-	-
NIE-115	-	-
Trypsinate		
IMR-5	+	+
CHP-134	+	+
NIE-115	-	-
Hybrid[c]	-	NDF
Pronase-digested trypsinate		
IMR-5	+	+
CHP-134	+	+
CHP-134-F	ND[d]	-
NIE-115	-	-

[a]Reproduced from (7) with permission.
[b]Measured by the inhibition of complement-mediated cytolysis.
[c]IMR-5 x IT-22 (7).
[d]ND, not done.

antigen's being a carbohydrate and, in this case, being attached to a different protein. Thus, final conclusions concerning the reaction of a given monoclonal antibody with different cell types must await detailed biochemical analysis.

Table 4 summarizes the points made in the above discussion. Monoclonal antibodies are certainly useful for detection and classification of tumors, and even if they do not exhibit an absolute specificity for tumor cells, they will still be useful for delivery of drugs and other cytotoxic agents to these cells. It would not be surprising, though, if in the long run the most significant contribution to tumor therapy were a result of the increased understanding of cell structure and function derived from the application of monoclonal antibodies to the detection and characterization of molecules involved in growth regulation, cell division, and differentiation.

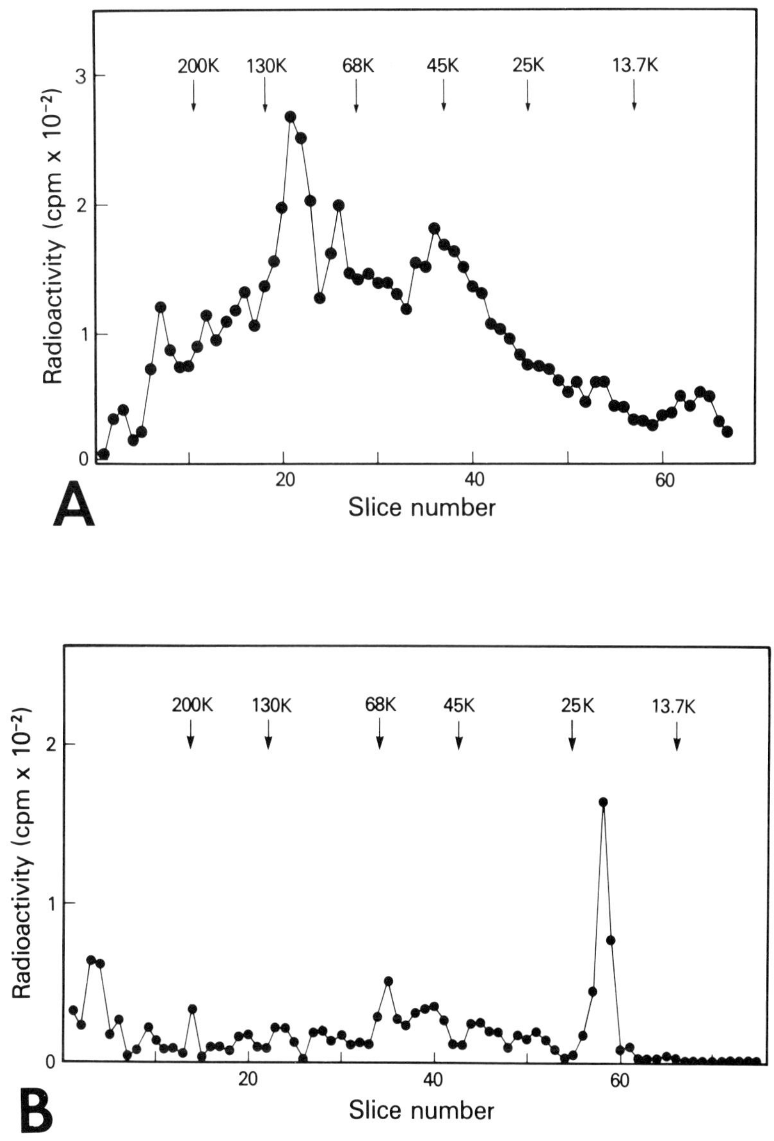

Fig. 8. Profiles of electrophoresis of radioactive glycoproteins from IMR-5 cells on a polyacrylamide slab gel under denaturing conditions. IMR-5 cells were labeled metabolically with D-(^{3}H)glucosamine and extracted with NP-40 in the presence of α-toluene/sulfonyl fluoride, included also in all subsequent procedures. The NP-40 extract was adsorbed to a column of wheat germ agglutinin-agarose or to the immunoaffinity column of monoclonal antibody PI153/3. Profiles of electrophoresis on polyacrylamide gels in 1% SDS under denaturing conditions of (A) total NP-40 extract, (B) eluate from immunoaffinity column. Reproduced from (7) with permission.

Table 4. Summary

1. Monoclonal antibodies against antigenic determinants on human neuroblastoma cells that have been reported are not "neuroblastoma-specific."
2. Even some of those that appear to have restricted patterns of reactivity often react with:
   Other tumors from neuroectoderm
   Human brain
   Lymphocyte subsets
   Fibroblasts
3. This may represent "cross-reacting" antigenic determinants on different molecules or differentiation antigens shared by nerve cells and cells of other tissues (Thy-1).
4. Even when not tumor-specific, monoclonal antibodies can be used in combinations to detect tumor metastasis and to classify tumor cells.
5. These same antibodies may be useful for immunotherapy if, when tested, they do not delete essential "stem cell" clones.
6. Monoclonal antibodies can detect differentiation antigens that are minor (<1%) components of the total antigen mixture in/on a cell.
7. Even monoclonal antibodies that do not readily immunoprecipitate these minor components can be used to isolate and characterize these molecules.
8. Monoclonal antibodies that react with both tumor and normal cells will be useful for characterizing differences between tumor/normal cell surfaces and for identifying molecules influencing cell growth and differentiation.

Acknowledgments

This work was supported by Grants CA24263 and P01 CA14489 from The National Institutes of Health and by grant PCM 79-26757 from The National Science Foundation.

References

1. Köhler, G, and C Milstein (1975). Continuous cultures of fused cells secreting antibody of predefined specificity. Nature (Lond) **256,** 495-497.
2. Kennett, RH, ZL Jonak, KB Bechtol and R Byrd (1981). Monoclonal antibodies as probes for cell surface changes in malignancy. In Fundamental Mechanisms in Human Cancer Immunology, pp 331-348. JP Saunders, JC Daniels, B Serrou, C

Rosenfeld and CB Denney, eds.
3. Kennett, RH, ZL Jonak and R Byrd (1981, in press). Cell surface changes in malignancy. In Methods in Cancer Research, Vol 19. H Busch, ed.
4. Kennett, RH, ZL Jonak and KB Bechtol (1980). Monoclonal antibodies to tumor associated antigens. In Monoclonal Antibodies, pp 155-168. RH Kennett, TJ McKearn and KB Bechtol, eds. Plenum Press, New York.
5. Kennett, RH, KA Denis, AS Tung and NR Klinman (1978). Hybrid plasmacytoma production: fusions with adult spleen cells, monoclonal spleen fragments, neonatal spleen cells, and human spleen cells. Curr Top Microbiol Immunol **81**, 77-91.
6. Kennett, RH, and F Gilbert (1979). Hybrid myelomas producing antibodies against a human neuroblastoma antigen present on fetal brain. Science **206**, 1120-1121.
7. Momoi, M, RH Kennett and MC Glick (1980). A membrane glycoprotein from human neuroblastoma cells isolated with the use of a monoclonal antibody. J Biol Chem **255**, 11914-11921.
8. Kennett, RH, TJ McKearn and KB Bechtol (1980). Appendix: Methods for production and characterization of monoclonal antibodies. In Monoclonal Antibodies, pp 361-419. RH Kennett, TJ McKearn and KB Bechtol, eds. Plenum Press, New York.
9. Greaves, MF, W Verbi, J Kemshead and R Kennett (1980). A monoclonal antibody identifying a cell surface antigen shared by common acute lymphoblastic leukemias and B lineage cells. Blood **56**, 1141-1144.
10. Cuttitta, F, S Rosen, AF Gazdar and JD Minna (1981). Monoclonal antibodies which demonstrate specificity for several types of human lung cancer. Proc Natl Acad Sci USA **78**, 4591-4595.
11. Kemshead, JT, F Walsh, J Pritchard and M Greaves (1981). Monoclonal antibody to ganglioside CQ discriminates between haemopoietic cells and infiltrating neuroblastoma tumor cells in bone marrow. Int J Cancer **27**, 447-452.
12. Scott, RE (1976). Plasma membrane vesiculation: a new technique for isolation of plasma membranes. Science **194**, 743-745.
13. Reisfeld, RA, MA Pelligrino and BD Kahan (1971). Salt extraction of soluble HLA antigens. Science **172**, 1134-1136.
14. Rosenfeld, C, A Goutner, C Choquet, AM Vinuati, B Kayibanda, JL Pico and MF Greaves (1977). Phenotypic characterization of a unique non-T, non-B acute lymphoblastic leukemia cell line. Nature (Lond) **267**, 841-843.
15. Klinman, NR, KA Denis and LA Sherman (1981). Defining the immune mechanism with monoclonal antibodies. In Vitro **17**, 1029-1035.
16. Lampson, L (1982). Expression of the major histocompatibility antigens in the human nervous system. In Monoclonal Antibodies to Neural Antigens. R McKay, MC Raff and LF Reichardt, eds. Cold Spring Harbor Laboratory, Cold Spring Harbor, New York.
17. Barnstable, CJ, WF Bodmer, G Brown, G Galfre, C Milstein, AF Williams and A Ziegler (1978). Production of monoclonal antibodies to group A erythrocytes, HLA and other human cell surface antigens - new tools for genetic analysis. Cell **14**, 9-20.
18. Lampson, L, I Royston and R Levy (1977). Homogeneous antibodies directed against human cell surface antigens: 1. The mouse spleen fragment culture response to T and B cell lines derived from the same individual. J Supramol Struct **6**, 441-448.
19. Kahn, CR, K Biard, JS Flier and DB Jarrett (1977). Effects of autoantibodies to the insulin receptor on isolated adipocytes. J Clin Invest **60**, 1094-1106.
20. Beachy, JC, and MP Czech (1980). Production of insulinomimetic antibodies against rat adipocyte membranes by hybridoma cells. J Supramol Struct **13**, 447-456.
21. Byrd, RL, ZL Jonak and RH Kennett (1981, in press). Monoclonal antibodies against human neuroblastomas and leukemias: detection of metastasis and of molecules involved in growth regulations. In Monoclonal Antibodies Workshop - Biol Response Modifiers NIH. Raven Press, New York.
22. Levy, R. Personal communication.

MONOCLONAL ANTI-IDIOTYPE ANTIBODIES AND THE BIOLOGY OF B CELL LYMPHOMA

Ronald Levy, David G. Maloney, Ada Hatzubai, Sheri Brown,
Jeanette Dilley and Richard A. Miller

Department of Medicine, Division of Oncology
Stanford University Medical Center
Stanford, California 94305

Considerable effort has been devoted to finding human tumor-specific antigens. Since the development of hybridoma technology (1), researchers have approached this problem by immunizing mice against human tumor cells and screening for monoclonal antibodies that can discriminate between tumor cells and normal cells (2). This effort has yielded several monoclonal antibodies that define tumor-associated antigens of two categories: those expressed on tumor cells in greater amounts than on normal cells (3) and those expressed on tumor cells but found only on rare populations of normal cells (4). The search continues for antibodies that will define antigens restricted exclusively to tumor cells.

Tumors of the B lymphocyte lineage offer a special opportunity for the production of antibodies to tumor-associated antigens (5,6). Each B cell tumor produces a different surface immunoglobulin molecule with a unique idiotype, composed of both a single light chain-variable and a single heavy chain-variable region (7-9). The cell surface immunoglobulin idiotype of a B cell tumor is an extreme example of a tumor-associated antigen found only on rare populations of normal cells. The frequency of any single idiotype in the normal population of B cells is about $1/10^6$ or less (10) except in certain exceptional cases (11).

In man, a large proportion of adult lymphomas are of the B cell type (12,13). Most of these have immunoglobulin in the cell membrane but do not secrete appreciable quantities (14). To produce anti-idiotype antibodies the idiotype protein is isolated and purified. Several approaches have been used to obtain idiotype from non-secreting B cell tumors (5,15,16); we have constructed hybridomas between the human malignant B cells and mouse myeloma cells (15). Once isolated and stabilized in their production of the human Ig, such cells can provide a continuing source of the idiotype protein. Anti-idiotype antisera as well as monoclonal antibodies have been prepared against the idiotype of a patient with nodular lymphoma. We have used these reagents, together with the idiotype, to study the biology and clinical parameters of the patient's disease (17).

Materials and Methods

The collection of malignant B cells from Patient Ka, their fusion with mouse myeloma cells, selection of human Ig-secreting hybridomas, and isolation and purification of the idiotype-bearing immunoglobulin have all been described previously (18).

Production of Anti-Id Antiserum

A New Zealand White rabbit was given repeated intradermal injections of 30 μg of the purified Ka protein in complete Freund's adjuvant and exsanguinated three weeks after the last injection.

The rabbit antiserum was rendered idiotype-specific by absorption on a series of sepharose columns containing covalently coupled (19) fetal calf serum proteins, mouse Ig, normal human Ig, and a human μλ myeloma protein. It was further absorbed on normal human peripheral blood lymphocytes (PBL). The anti-Id antibodies were then purified by absorption to a Ka protein sepharose column and eluted with 0.1 M acetic acid.

Monoclonal Antibodies

A BALB/c mouse was immunized intraperitoneally with Id-Ka (100 μg) in complete Freund's adjuvant at day 0. At day 7 the mouse was boosted intravenously with 100 μg Id-Ka in PBS. The mouse spleen was removed at day 10. The spleen cells were fused with P3/X63/Ag8.653 cells (20) according to Kennett's fusion protocol (21).

Clones were examined by radioimmunoassay (RIA) for secretion of antibodies specific for human μ or λ chain and for Id-Ka (see below). Subcloning of clones secreting these antibodies was performed by limiting dilutions into wells containing normal mouse spleen cells as feeders.

Radioimmunoassay

RIA to test for specificity of antibodies to human μ or κ chain and Id-Ka. A solid phase RIA was performed by using polyvinyl microtiter plates (Cooke Laboratory Products) coated by absorption with various human immunoglobulins at a concentration of 10 μg/ml. After coating, the plates were washed with PBS-5% FCS. To the coated wells, 25 μl of test culture fluid samples were added. The plates were then incubated overnight at 4°C and washed four times with PBS-5% FCS, after which ^{125}I-labeled goat anti-mouse κ was added. The plates were then incubated for at least another four h and washed. The wells were cut out with a hot wire device and counted in a gamma counter.

RIA for detecting Id-Ka or anti-Id-Ka antibodies in serum. Plates were coated with either Id-Ka or purified anti-Id-Ka antibodies. Binding of the complementary ^{125}I-labeled ligand (anti-Id-Ka in the first case and Id-Ka in the second case) was inhibited by test substances. The standard solutions, or the substances to be tested, were added to the coated wells. The plates were then incubated for at least two h at room temperature (longer incubation was carried out at 4°C) and washed four times; only when no free inhibitor was present was the ^{125}I-labeled ligand added. In this assay, Id-Ka and anti-Id-Ka could be distinguished from each other.

Production and Characterization of Monoclonal Anti-Id Antibody

Ka protein, a 19S IgM (λ) secreted by the mouse x Ka tumor cell hybridoma (K6H6), was isolated by affinity chromatography on a goat anti-human IgM protein sepharose column. This protein was used to immunize mice for the production of hybridomas with anti-idiotype specificity. These hybridizations produced three types of monoclonal antibodies (Table 1). Idiotype-specific antibodies bound only to the idiotype-bearing immunoglobulin and not to other isolated IgMs of either the κ or λ light chain type. Light chain-specific antibodies bound only to immunoglobulins containing the λ light chain, and IgM-specific antibodies bound to all IgM immunoglobulins regardless of their light chain type.

Table 1 shows the binding specificities of a series of such hybridomas. Clones DM1, 7B4, and 4D6 bound 20 to 50 times background to the Ka idiotype-bearing Ig and less than two times background to other human IgM proteins. These anti-idiotype reagents were of the IgM, IgGl and IgG2b isotypes. Clone DM1 was found to be specific for the λ light chain, while DM2 was specific for the IgM isotype.

Virtually unlimited quantities of the monoclonal antibodies were prepared from the ascites fluid of mice bearing the specific hybridoma. These antibodies were then used to investigate Patient Ka's malignancy.

Free Idiotype Protein in Serum of the Patient

Using a radioimmunoassay we found that the serum of Patient Ka contained material that could block the mutual binding of Id and anti-Id (18). Either free Id or anti-Id could have caused this blocking activity. Thus, the patient's serum might have contained Id, anti-Id antibody or complexes of Id-anti-Id.

Table 1. Binding of monoclonal antibodies to idiotype and other IgM immunoglobulins

Plates were coated with the IgMs at a concentration of 10 μg/ml. Coated plates were incubated with culture fluids. At the end of the incubation time the plates were washed, and ^{125}I-labeled goat anti-mouse κ was added. After additional incubation, the plates were washed, and the bound radioactivity in the wells was counted with a gamma counter. Data is expressed as ratio of counts bound/background counts (second stage only).

Clone	Description	Isotype	Idiotype[a] (IgMλ)	JHA[b] (IgMκ)	SATO (IgMκ)	RPR (IgMκ)	RSE (IgMλ)	AWA (IgMλ)	EBO (IgMκ)	FLA (IgMκ)
DM11	Anti-Id	IgM	20.4	1.0	1.0	1.0	1.3	1.1	1.5	1.1
7B4	Anti-Id	IgGl	27.1	1.0	1.2	ND	1.1	1.5	1.2	0.4
4D6	Anti-Id	IgG2B	51.9	1.1	1.1	ND	1.2	1.7	1.0	1.4
DM1	Anti-λ	IgM	20.9	1.1	2.0	1.9	22.8	47.0	4.6	2.0
DM2	Anti-μ	IgM	26.0	17.9	ND[c]	ND	48.0	89.4	ND	ND

[a]Idiotype bearing IgM was produced by human x mouse hybridoma K6H6.

[b]IgMs were isolated from sera of patients with Waldenstrom's macroglobulinemia by dialysis against low ionic strength buffer. They were found to be fairly pure by SDS-PAGE analysis.

[c]ND, not done.

To distinguish between Id and anti-Id, we used a site-consumption RIA (17). In this assay, the competitor is added first and washed away before the labeled ligand is added. When the plate was coated with anti-Id and the ligand was ^{125}I Id (17), unlabeled Id inhibited in this site-consumption RIA, but anti-Id did not. Conversely, when the plate was coated with Id and the ligand was ^{125}I monoclonal anti-Id (17), unlabeled anti-Id inhibited, but Id did not.

Analysis of Ka sera revealed that the blocking activity was present only in the assay for idiotype. Ka serum did not inhibit the assay for anti-idiotype. However, complexes of idiotype-anti-idiotype might still have been present.

This problem was further clarified when the patient's serum was fractionated on sephadex G-200 and assayed for blocking activity (Fig. 1). All of the activity was found in the 19S peak, once again ruling out the presence of free anti-idiotype antibody. When the 19S peak was radioiodinated and analyzed by immunoprecipitation with anti-idiotype antibody, it was found to contain only IgM and no IgG (17). From the absence of free anti-idiotype in serum according to the RIA and the absence of idiotype anti-idiotype immune complexes, we conclude that the patient made no anti-idiotype humoral immune response. Instead, the patient had free idiotype protein in his serum. From its size (19S rather than 7S), we conclude that the free Id represents low level secretion of the protein by the tumor cells rather than shedding of membrane protein.

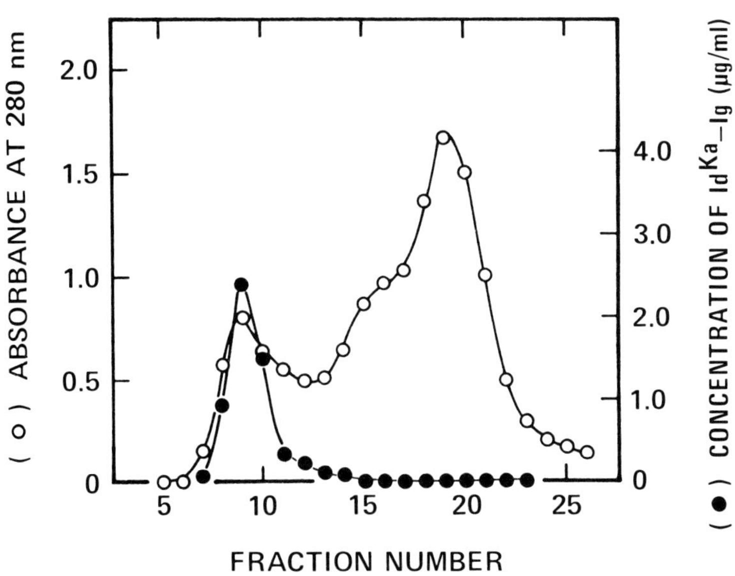

Fig. 1. Gel filtration of Ka serum. Ka serum was applied to a sephadex G-200 (150 ml) column equilibrated in PBS. Fraction size was 0.6 ml. Fractions were tested for the presence of Id by RIA.

Use of Monoclonal Anti-Id Antibody to Monitor the Patient's Malignancy

Using monoclonal anti-Id antibodies as a tumor-specific probe, we documented changes in the number of circulating Id-positive cells and in the amount of free Id as the patient's tumor burden varied. Biotinylated anti-Id was used as a first stage, and rhodamine or fluorescein-avidin as the second stage, to stain peripheral blood lymphocytes (PBLs) isolated from Patient Ka and from four normal donors. While PBLs isolated from normal donors did not stain with the anti-Id antibody, the percent of Patient Ka PBLs stained correlated with his clinical condition. Table 2 shows that the percent of Id-positive cells varied from a high of 75% of total mononuclear cells when his disease was progressing rapidly, to a low of 1-2% when he was in partial remission following chemotherapy.

Note in Table 2 that the concentration of circulating Id in the patient's sera also correlated well with the number of Id-positive cells and with the patient's clinical condition. Defined by RIA using a standard solution of purified Id as reference, the concentration of Id was lowest during apparent remissions and highest when his disease was most active and apparent.

Table 2. Percentage of Id-bearing cells and concentration of Id in peripheral blood

Date	% Id PBLs[a]	Concentration (μg/ml) of circulating Id[b]	Clinical condition
01/16/80	2	4	Remission
03/11/80	22	6	Remission
04/22/80	54	39	Disease progression
05/20/80	75	34	Active disease, chemotherapy begun
06/10/80	28	18	Partial response to chemotherapy
06/24/80	29	14	Continued response to chemotherapy
07/15/80	28	18	Dramatic response to chemotherapy
08/13/80	1	4	Stable partial remission

[a]Id+ refers to cells stained using biotinylated monoclonal anti-Id as first stage and rhodamine-avidin as second stage.

[b]Estimated from a standard curve by RIA.

Absence of T Cells Bearing Id or Anti-Id

To determine whether T cell response to the idiotype of the tumor occurred *in vivo*, Ka PBLs were double-stained for the presence on the same cell of T cell markers and Id. PBLs were incubated first with a mixture of biotinylated monoclonal anti-Id and fluoresceinated anti-Leu-1 (general marker for all peripheral T cells). After washing, rhodamine-avidin was added. In a typical sample taken during relapse, the anti-T cell antibody stained 30% of the cells, and anti-Id stained 55% of the cells. No double-stained cells were detected among several thousand examined, an indication that there were no Id-bearing T cells. Circulating Id in the Ka serum (Table 3) suggested that there were probably no T cells capable of binding Id. Any T cells with receptors for Id would have been detected as Leu-1- and Id-positive.

Elimination of Id-Positive Cells *In Vitro*

Using one monoclonal anti-Id antibody, we investigated two methods to eliminate the Id-positive cells *in vitro*. The first method, called "panning," selectively removed Id-positive cells from the total population of PBLs by binding them to a solid substrate coated with anti-Id. The second method, complement-mediated cytolysis, used the anti-Id antibody to fix complement and selectively kill the Id-positive cells.

Panning of the Id-positive cells was accomplished by incubating Ka PBLs in a petri plate coated previously with purified anti-Id anti-body. To monitor the method's efficiency, aliquots of the cells were stained with anti-Id antibodies before and after panning. Table 3 shows results of a typical experiment after one cycle of panning. More than 99% of the Id-positive cells were removed. The proportional increase in the percent of cells staining with the anti-peripheral T cell antibody indicates that the apparent depletion of Id-positive cells was real and not due to loss of membrane Id. Similarly, the κ bearing cells left after panning most likely represented normal B cells in the sample and further showed the specificity of the procedure.

Cytolysis of the Id-positive cells was accomplished with anti-Id antibody in the presence of rabbit complement. Cytolysis of Ka and normal PBLs by several monoclonal anti-human antibodies is compared in Table 4. The Id-positive cells were more susceptible to complement-mediated lysis than were normal PBLs. Anti-λ and anti-μ antibodies stained normal PBLs (2% and 5%, respectively) but did not lyse them, while both were able to lyse Id-positive cells. The anti-T cell antibody lysed approximately 70% of Ka PBLs (Id-negative) and normal PBLs; the anti-Id antibody stained and lysed only the Id-positive population of Ka PBLs, as determined by immunofluorescence following lysis. The anti-λ reagent behaved similarly. However, the anti-μ reagent failed to kill all the Id+ cells under the conditions employed here.

Table 3. Depletion of Id-bearing cells by panning

Antibodies used for staining	% cells stained	
	Before panning	After panning[a]
Anti-Id	55	0.7
Anti-T cell	30	82.0
Goat anti-μ	60	5.0

[a]In this experiment approximately 50% of the cells did not bind to the anti-Id coated plate. The results are typical of several experiments and represent a sample taken from the patient at a particular time. One thousand cells were counted and scored.

Table 4. Complement[a]-mediated cytolysis of Id-positive cells by monoclonal antibodies

Monoclonal antibodies	Class	% lysis[b]	
		Ka PBLs	Normal PBLs
DM11 (Anti-Id)	IgM	28	0
Anti-T cell	IgG2A	72	67
DM1 (Anti-λ)	IgM	30	0
DM2 (Anti-μ)	IgM	18	0

[a]Rabbit complement.

[b]Lysis determined by inability to exclude trypan blue dye. The results represent a typical experiment. In each case, 1000 cells were counted.

Discussion

The specificity and unlimited availability of the monoclonal anti-Id antibody enabled us to study a number of clinical issues. First, we monitored the patient's disease by following the percent of Id-positive cells in his blood. As we reported previously (18), this percent correlated well with the patient's clinical condition (Table 2). Circulating Id-positive cells increased when the patient's disease was relapsing but before this relapse became clinically apparent. After treatment with chemotherapy, the Id-bearing cells fell coincidentally with the clinical response. The anti-Id was used to detect Id protein in the serum. This Id-bearing immunoglobulin was 19S IgM and likely represented low-level secretion by the malignant cells rather than shedding of the 7S protein from the membrane. Like the number of Id+ cells, the concentration of Id protein changed in parallel with the patient's clinical status. Both parameters rose during relapse and fell during response to therapy.

In principal, every patient with B cell lymphoma can be monitored clinically in this manner. However, a specific anti-idiotype reagent will be needed by each individual—an effort that will be worth undertaking only if it enables more patients to survive. Improved monitoring of therapy or of remission status may improve current treatment regimens for B cell lymphoma, although this is by no means clear (22,23).

Alternatively, anti-idiotype reagents might be used to develop new approaches to therapy. Direct administration of anti-idiotype antibodies to patients (24) or elimination of idiotype-bearing cells from bone marrow prior to autologous bone marrow transplantation deserves consideration. In the first case, circulating idiotype protein in the serum of patients presents a problem requiring attention. Circulating Id would have to be removed if anti-idiotype antibodies were to reach the tumor cells *in vivo*. 19S IgM does not equilibrate rapidly between tissues and blood and would be difficult to remove. On the other hand, bone marrow purging of Id-bearing cells is less difficult technically. As we demonstrate here, panning or complement-dependent cytolysis are both extremely effective. The more difficult question posed by autologous bone marrow transplantation is whether more aggressive therapy will successfully eliminate residual tumor in the patient prior to the transplant.

In addition to purely clinical considerations, the anti-idiotype antibodies permit inquiry regarding the biology of B cell lymphoma. Studying humans rather than animal models is advantageous because the disease can be studied in the original tumor-bearing host. Our first question was whether evidence could be found for a host-immune response against the tumor clone, that is, for a host anti-idiotype response. By several criteria we concluded that the patient made no humoral anti-idiotype response. No free or complexed anti-idiotype could be found in the patient's serum at any point during his disease. We then attempted to look for T cells with anti-idiotype specificity. Total T cells were counted with a fluorescent anti-T cell hybridoma reagent, and cells bearing or binding Id were enumerated by a second color of fluorescence. No double-staining cells were detected, even though the T cells were bathed *in vivo* in an excess of Id protein. Of course, one cannot conclude from the absence of demonstrable Id-binding T cells that T cells with anti-Id specificity do not exist. They may have been below the limit of detection, they may have been sequestered in tissue compartments, or they may not bind antigen with sufficient avidity to be detectable by this method. One can conclude from the experiment that idiotype-bearing T cells do not exist in our patient with any detectable frequency. T cells bearing idiotype have been detected in patients with multiple myeloma or chronic lymphocytic leukemia by some (25-30), but not by other, investigators (31).

Does the host with B cell lymphoma allow the growth of a malignant clone because it fails to respond to the specific idiotype? This hypothesis might be tested by an attempt to induce an anti-idiotype response in the lymphoma-bearing host. Cooper and colleagues (31) have proposed that B cell malignancy actually represents the proliferation of pre-B cells, i.e., those cells that do not express surface Ig or even light chains. How could pre-B cells exist which give rise to a tumor population uniformly expressing a specific idiotype and therefore a specific light chain? Such pre-B cells would have to be committed to using a particular V_L gene even though they have not actually begun to express it. Ultimately, a test of the hypothesis will require the use of light chain nucleic acid probes to determine if the relevant pre-B cells have, indeed, already rearranged their light chain genes, therefore committing themselves to a specific V_L. If this is the case, it may still be possible to regulate the growth of the malignant clone through anti-idiotype mechanisms, since pre-B cells not expressing surface Id may ultimately be eliminated as they differentiate into B cells expressing Id.

Acknowledgments

This work was supported by American Cancer Society Grant IM-114. Dr. Levy is an Investigator of the Howard Hughes Medical Institute. D.G. Maloney is a Medical Scientist Trainee, Grant GM-07365, Public Health Service, from the National Institute of General Medical Sciences.

References

1. Köhler, G, and C Milstein (1975). Continuous cultures of fused cells secreting

antibody of predefined specificity. Nature (Lond) **256**, 495-497.

2. Levy, R, J Dilley and LA Lampson (1978). Human normal and leukemia cell surface antigens. Mouse monoclonal antibodies as probes. In Current Topics in Microbiology and Immunology, Vol 81, pp 164-169. F Melchers, M Potter and RN Warner, eds. Springer-Verlag, Berlin.
3. Levy, R, J Dilley, RI Fox and R Warnke (1979). A human thymus-leukemia antigen defined by hybridoma monoclonal antibodies. Proc Natl Acad Sci USA **76**, 6552-6556.
4. Ritz, J, TM Pesando, J Notis-McConarty, H Lazarus and SF Schlossman (1980). A monoclonal antibody to human acute lymphoblastic leukaemia antigen. Nature (Lond) **283**, 583-585.
5. Stevenson, GT, and FK Stevenson (1975). Antibody to a molecularly-defined antigen confined to a tumor cell surface. Nature (Lond) **254**, 714-716.
6. Lynch, RG, RJ Graff, S Sirisinha, ES Simms and HN Eisen (1972). Myeloma proteins as tumor-specific transplantation antigens. Proc Natl Acad Sci USA **69**, 1540-1544.
7. Frøland, SS, and JB Natvig (1972). Class, subclass, and allelic exclusion of membrane-bound Ig of human B lymphocytes. J Exp Med **136**, 409-414.
8. Schroer, K, DE Briles, JA vanBoxel and JJ Davie (1974). Idiotypic uniformity of cell surface immunoglobulin in chronic lymphocytic leukemia. Evidence for monoclonal proliferation. J Exp Med **140**, 1416-1420.
9. Fu, SM, RJ Winchester and HG Kunkel (1975). Similar idiotype specificity for the membrane IgD and IgM of human B lymphocytes. J Immunol **114**, 250-252.
10. Klinman, NR, and JL Press (1975). The B cell specificity repertoire: Its relationship to definable subpopulations. Transplant Rev **24**, 41-83.
11. Sigel, N (1977). Novel idiotype and antigen-binding characteristics in two anti-dinitrophenol monoclonal antibodies. J Exp Med **146**, 282-286.
12. Weissman, IL, R Warnke, E Butcher, R Rouse and R Levy (1978). The lymphoid system: Its normal architecture and the potential for understanding the system through the study of lymphoproliferative disease. Hum Pathol **9**, 25-45.
13. Filippa, DA, PH Lieberman, RA Erlandson, B Koziner, FP Siegal, A Turnball, A Zimring and RA Good (1978). A study of malignant lymphomas using light and ultramicroscopic, cytochemical and immunologic techniques. Am J Med **64**, 259-268.
14. Salmon, SE, and M Seligmann (1974). B cell neoplasia in man. Lancet **2**, 1230-1233.
15. Levy, R, and J Dilley (1978). Rescue of immunoglobulin secretion from human neoplastic lymphoid cells by somatic cell hybridization. Proc Natl Acad Sci USA **75**, 2411-2415.
16. Z Eshar, C Blatt, Y Bergman and J Haimovich (1979). Induction of IgM secretion from B cells by fusion. J Immunol **122**, 2430-2434.
17. Hatzubai, A, DG Maloney and R Levy (1981). The use of a monoclonal anti-idiotype antibody to study the biology of a human B cell lymphoma. J Immunol **126**, 2397-2402.
18. Brown, S, J Dilley and R Levy (1980). Immunoglobulin secretion by mouse x human hybridomas: An approach for the production of anti-idiotype reagents useful in monitoring patients with B cell lymphoma. J Immunol **125**, 1037-1043.
19. Axen, R, J Porath and S Ernback (1967). Chemical coupling of peptides and proteins to polysaccharides by means of cyanogen halides. Nature (Lond) **214**, 1302-1304.
20. Kearney, JF, A Radbruch, B Liesengange and K Rajewsky (1979). A new mouse myeloma cell line that has lost immunoglobulin expression but permits the construction of antibody-secreting hybrid cell lines. J Immunol **123**, 1548-1555.
21. Kennett, RH (1979). Cell fusion. In Methods in Enzymology, Vol 58, pp 345-357. WG Jacoby and IH Paston, eds. Academic Press, New York.
22. Jones, SE, Z Fuks, M Bull, ME Kaden, RF Dorfman, HS Kaplan, SA Rosenberg and H Kim (1973). Non-Hodgkins lymphoma. IV. Clinicopathologic correlation in 405 cases. Cancer **31**, 806-823.
23. Fisher, RI, VT DeVita, Jr, RL Johnson, R Simon and RC Young (1977). Prognostic factors for advanced diffuse histiocytic lymphoma following treat-

ment with combination chemotherapy. Am J Med **63,** 177-182.

24. Hamblin, TJ, AK Abdul-Ahad, J Gordon, K Stevenson and GT Stevenson (1980). Preliminary experience in treating lymphocytic leukemia with antibody to immunoglobulin idiotypes on the cell surface. Br J Cancer **42,** 495-502.
25. Preud'homme, J-L, M Klein, S Laboume and M Seligmann (1977). Idiotype-bearing and antigen-binding receptors produced by blood T lymphocytes in a case of human myeloma. Eur J Immunol **7,** 840-846.
26. Lea, T, ØT Førre, TE Michaelsen and JG Natvig (1979). Shared idiotypes on human peripheral blood B and T lymphocytes. J Immunol **122,** 2413-2417.
27. Binz, H, and H Wigzell (1977). Antigen-binding, idiotypic T lymphocyte receptors. Contemp Top Immunobiol **7,** 113-177.
28. Black, SJ, GH Hammerling, C Berck, K Rajewsky and K Eichman (1976). Idiotypic reactive with anti-idiotypic antibody. J Exp Med **143,** 846-860.
29. Eichmann, K, and K Rajewsky (1975). Induction of T and B cell immunity by anti-idiotypic antibody. Eur J Immunol **5,** 661-666.
30. Möller, G (1977). Idiotypes on T and B cells. Immunol Rev **34,** 1-164.
31. Kubagawa, H, LB Vogler, JD Capra, ME Conrad, AR Lawton and MD Cooper (1979). Studies on the clonal origin of multiple myeloma. Use of individually specific (idiotype) antibodies to trace the oncogenic event to its earliest point of expression in B cell differentiation. J Exp Med **150,** 792-807.

MONOCLONAL ANTIBODIES TO HUMAN MELANOMA

Joseph P. Brown, Karl Erik Hellström, and Ingegerd Hellström

Program in Tumor Immunology
Fred Hutchinson Cancer Research Center
Seattle, Washington 98104

Melanoma is an important model for studies of human tumor-associated antigens. It is a common, often fatal disease, and there is strong clinical evidence that melanoma patients can mount an immune response to their tumors (1). Melanoma cells can be grown relatively easily *in vitro*, and serological studies using melanoma patients' sera and cultured melanoma cells have demonstrated the existence of melanoma-associated antigens. Some of these antigens are restricted to the patients' own melanomas, while others are expressed by a number of melanomas (2). Melanoma-associated antigens have also been identified by heterologous antisera (3).

Köhler and Milstein (4) have shown that monoclonal antibodies can be obtained by fusing spleen cells from immunized mice with myeloma cells and growing antibody-producing hybrids in selective medium. This method clearly has great potential for identifying melanoma-associated antigens and has led to renewed interest in the serology of human melanoma. A number of groups have now described melanoma-associated antigens identified by monoclonal antibodies (5-9).

In the following pages we review our laboratory's progress toward obtaining monoclonal antibodies to human melanoma-associated antigens, using as an example p97, the antigen that we have characterized most thoroughly (5,10-14). We discuss the methods used to obtain the hybridomas and to determine the specificity of the antigens indentified. Structural and immunochemical studies of the antigens are described, and the application of the antibodies to the diagnosis and therapy of human melanoma is also discussed.

Generation of Hybridomas Producing Antibodies to Melanoma-associated Antigens

Fusion of mouse myeloma cells with spleen cells from a mouse immunized with human melanoma cells yields several hundred hybrids (15). These hybrids produce antibodies to a large number of melanoma cell surface antigens, including glycoproteins (15) and glycolipids (8). Selecting the few hybridomas producing antibodies to melanoma-associated antigens requires a screening procedure capable of testing hundreds of samples. We have used an autoradiographic binding assay (16) and immunoprecipitation (15) to obtain hybridomas producing antibodies to p97.

An attempt to obtain antibodies to the class 1 antigen of SK-MEL 28 melanoma yielded the first monoclonal antibody to p97 (2). BALB/c mice were immunized with the melanoma cells, and their spleen cells were fused with NS-1 myeloma cells (17). The resulting hybrids were grown in selective medium in microtest walls and tested two weeks after the fusion by the autoradiographic, indirect ^{125}I-labelled protein A binding assay (16). Samples of culture medium from the hybrids were replica-plated onto monolayers of melanoma cells in microtest wells. The samples were also tested on autologous fibroblasts. The cells were then incubated successively with rabbit anti-mouse immunoglobulin serum and ^{125}I-labelled *Staphylococcus aureus* protein A. Autoradiography revealed positive reactions. Many of the wells contained antibodies that bound to both cell types, but one well contained an antibody that appeared to be specific for the melanoma cells. Hybridoma 4.1, which produced an IgG1 antibody, was cloned from this well. Tests of a larger number of cell lines, using the indirect protein A binding assay, showed that the antigen recognized by monoclonal antibody 4.1 was expressed on a number of melanoma cell lines but was not present in detectable amounts on fibroblasts or B cell lines. Clearly, the antigen recognized by this antibody was not the AU antigen (2), which is present only on the SK-MEL 28 line used for immunization and screening, but it was of great interest to us.

For several reasons we felt that additional antibodies specific for the antigen recognized by antibody 4.1 would be useful, particularly antibodies of the IgG2 subclass, which have high affinity for protein A and are cytotoxic in the presence of complement. Antibodies to additional epitopes of the antigen molecule were also required so that we could develop an immunoradiometric assay to test tissues and serum for the antigen (see below). A subsequent fusion, in which spleen cells were fused with SP2/0 myeloma cells (18), was screened similarly and yielded a second hybridoma, 8.2 (13). Antibody 8.2, also IgG1, had a pattern of reactivity similar to that of antibody 4.1, and we subsequently confirmed that both antibodies recognized the same antigen molecule.

Preliminary biochemical characterization by immunoprecipitation and SDS-polyacrylamide gel electrophoresis (SDS-PAGE) showed that the antigen recognized by antibody 4.1 was a 97-kilodalton polypeptide. We then set out to obtain additional hybridomas producing antibodies to p97, using immunoprecipitation as a screening method (15). To reduce the work involved we first screened for wells containing antibodies of the IgG2 subclass, irrespective of their antigen specificity, using a rapid competition radioimmunoassay. Second, we pooled the samples before testing them. This enabled us to screen up to 500 wells with only 24 immunoprecipitation tests. The first fusion screened by immunoprecipitation yielded one hybridoma, 96.5, that produced an IgG2a antibody specific for p97 (15). Subsequent fusions screened by immunoprecipitation yielded four more hybridomas (118.1, 133.1, 133.2, and 133.3) that produced antibodies specific for p97 (10,13). We feel that immunoprecipitation is the method of choice for obtaining antibodies to cell surface antigens of known molecular weight, because the antibodies can be identified directly rather than by their pattern of reactivity on a panel of cells.

In addition to being a powerful screening method, immunoprecipitation gives useful information about the variety of protein antigens recognized by the mouse. We learned that, on varying either the immunizing melanoma cell line or the mouse strain immunized, a different set of proteins was immunoprecipitated. We also found that fibroblasts are a much better normal control cell type for screening than are B lymphoblastoid cell lines, since many more of the monoclonal antibodies produced by immunizing with melanoma cells bind to fibroblasts than bind to B cell lines. HLA-Dr antigens are in this respect an exception, being present on B cell lines and some melanomas, but not on fibroblasts (19).

When looking for antibodies to new melanoma-associated antigens, we use both the autoradiographic binding assay and immunoprecipitation. First we use the ^{125}I-labelled protein A binding assay to screen hybrids for antibodies that bind to the immunizing melanoma cell line. Then we test selected hybrids by immunoprecipitation of lysates of surface radioiodinated melanoma cells and fibroblasts. In this way we can identify hybridomas producing antibodies that bind to the melanoma cell surface, that recognize protein antigens, and that have a degree of specificity for melanoma.

Tissue Distribution of Antigens Identified by Monoclonal Antibodies

Whether an antigen is restricted to melanomas or whether it is also present on normal cells is clearly of great importance. A limited number of cell types such as fibroblasts, B cell lines, and carcinoma lines are generally tested during the screening phase, before the hybrids are cloned. However, the assays used for screening are designed primarily for speed, and they are not suitable for definitive determination of antigen distribution. Not only are they relatively insensitive, but they also cannot be used readily to assay tissues.

We have developed two assays to measure antigens in cultured cells and in tissue biopsy samples (10,12). The first is a binding assay using ^{125}I-labelled antibody. Monoclonal antibody is purified from ascites fluid by affinity chromatography on protein A-Sepharose (20) and labelled with ^{125}I to a specific radioactivity of about 30,000 cpm/ng. The test cells are incubated with the labelled antibody, washed, and counted for ^{125}I. The amount of antibody bound is proportional to the number of cells over a fairly wide range and can thus be calculated as molecules bound per cell. For assays of tissue specimens, a membrane preparation is tested, and results are calculated as nanograms of antibody bound per milligram of protein.

The sensitivity of the binding assay depends upon one's ability to determine precisely the amount of non-specific binding. One approach is to use as a negative control ^{125}I-labelled normal IgG of the same subclass as the specific antibody. However, because labelled IgG preparations differ considerably in the amount of non-specific binding, this approach is unreliable. A better solution is to use an excess of unlabelled antibody as competitor in a parallel incubation. Binding in the presence of the competitor is assumed to be non-specific and is subtracted from the amount bound in the absence of competitor. This assay can readily detect as few as 100 antigen molecules per cell.

The second approach uses a two-site immunoradiometric assay, which we refer to as the double-determinant immunoassay (DDIA) (10,12). The DDIA employs two monoclonal antibodies to two distinct epitopes of the target antigen. One antibody is coupled to a solid phase to form an immunoadsorbent, which is used to immobilize the antigen. The second antibody is labelled with ^{125}I and used to quantitate the bound antigen as in the binding assay described above. This assay is particularly suitable for antigens identified by monoclonal antibodies, both because purified antigen is not required and because the assay is more sensitive and specific than competition radioimmunoassay. The DDIA is more sensitive because the antigen can be concentrated on to the immunoadsorbent in the first incubation. Greater specificity results because an antigen must possess two epitopes to be detected by the DDIA, effectively eliminating any possibility of detecting an unrelated antigen that fortuitously cross-reacts with a single monoclonal antibody.

The binding assay and DDIA have both shown that although p97 is present in large amounts in many melanomas (about as much as HLA-A, B, C antigen), it is also present in small amounts in normal adult tissues, and in relatively large amounts in certain fetal tissues, particularly colon. We conclude that p97 is a melanoma-associated oncofetal antigen. Similar results were obtained by immunoprecipitation, except that this method was not sufficiently sensitive to detect p97 in normal adult tissues.

Structural and Immunochemical Analysis of Melanoma-associated Antigens

Structural studies of antigens identified by monoclonal antibodies are valuable for several reasons: they allow melanoma-associated antigens to be compared with one another and with other defined cell surface antigens; they may clarify the function of the antigens; and amino acid sequence data may facilitate structural gene isolation (21) and allow synthesis of oligopeptides for use as immunogens (see below).

Immunoprecipitation allows rapid isolation of radiolabelled antigen for analysis by SDS-PAGE. The molecular weights of protein antigens can be determined in this way; whether the proteins are glycosylated or phosphorylated can be determined by the use of different labelling procedures. In our hands the most sensitive labelling method is radioiodination, antigens being labelled either *in situ* by the lactoperoxidase method (22) or in solution in the presence of chloramine T (15). Radiolabelled cell lysates are incubated with monoclonal antibody. Immune complexes are isolated by adsorption to protein A-bearing *S. aureus* (23) and analyzed by SDS-PAGE and autoradiography. This method revealed that the antigen recognized by antibody 4.1 is a 97-kilodalton polypeptide. When melanoma cells were surface-labelled by periodate oxidation followed by reduction with tritiated borohydride, immunoprecipitation experiments showed that p97 became labelled. This evidence and the observation that neuraminidase digestion increased the electrophoretic mobility of ^{125}I-labelled p97 indicate that p97 is a sialoglycoprotein. Several other antigens, recognized by antibodies 3.1 (6) and 4.2 (Yeh et al., unpublished), could not be detected by immunoprecipitation. These antigens may be glycolipids.

To determine whether two antibodies recognize the same antigen, the technique of sequential immunoprecipitation is used. A radiolabelled cell lysate is incubated first with one antibody and *S. aureus*, and then is centrifuged. The antigen-depleted lysate is then tested by immunoprecipitation with the other antibody. We have used this method to show that four antibodies from our laboratory (4.1, 8.2, 96.5, 118.1) and six antibodies obtained from Dr. W. Dippold (M_{17}, L_1, L_{10}, R_{19}, I_{12}, K_5) all recognize the same molecule, and thus have established that p97 (5) and gp95 (8) are identical (13).

Epitope mapping experiments, in which unlabelled antibodies are tested for their ability to inhibit binding of radiolabelled antibodies to melanoma cells, have defined five distinct epitopes on the p97 molecule (13). Antibodies to three of these epitopes have been used to determine whether some cell types might express a protein related, but not identical, to p97. Carcinoma cells, T and B cell lines, and smooth muscle cells each bound the three antibodies in equimolar (though small) amounts. This suggests, but by no means proves, that these cell types express a molecule identical to the p97 on melanoma cells.

Immunodiagnosis and Immunotherapy

Monoclonal antibodies specific for melanoma-associated antigens offer several possibilities for immunodiagnosis of melanoma. One possible application is to screening sera for melanoma-associated antigens. However, the DDIA showed that normal human serum contained low levels of p97. Sera of a small minority of melanoma patients—those with advanced disease—contained concentrations two to three times greater, but most melanoma patients' sera did not have elevated levels. We conclude that screening sera for p97 is unlikely to be of diagnostic value. However, for other melanoma-associated antigens this approach may be of value and is certainly technically feasible if one uses the DDIA.

Localization of melanoma metastases by radionuclide imaging is promising both as a diagnostic technique and as a model system for the development of antibody-linked drug delivery systems (see below). Encouraging results have been reported for a mouse model system (24). Over the past year we have evaluated the usefulness of antibodies to p97 for radionuclide imaging both in nude mice bearing melanoma xenografts and in human melanoma patients.[1] By imaging experiments with ^{125}I-labelled antibody specific for p97, and by counting biopsy specimens from patients injected with ^{131}I-labelled anti-p97 antibody and ^{125}I-labelled normal immunoglobulin, we have found evidence that antibodies specific for p97 do, indeed, localize into melanoma metastases, although the degree of specific uptake is modest, only two- to three-fold over ^{125}I-labelled control antibodies. One of the key findings is that it is necessary to inoculate sufficient specific antibody, about 1 mg, to be in considerable excess over the circulating p97; otherwise a significant proportion of the radiolabel is complexed with antigen. Currently, we are investigating the use of Fab fragments, which are less immunogenic and are cleared more rapidly from the circulation. Radioisotopes such as ^{123}I and ^{111}In may allow tomographic scans to be obtained, greatly increasing the resolution and sensitivity of the method.

Another potential diagnostic application of monoclonal antibodies to melanoma-associated antigens is immunohistological typing of melanomas. Use of monoclonal antibody to diagnose an undifferentiated melanoma has already been reported (25). Also, for unknown reasons, many melanoma-associated antigens are not present in all melanomas. One explanation is that some melanoma-associated antigens may be differentiation antigens normally expressed at certain stages of the neural crest-melanoblast-melanocyte lineage (26). Antigenic characterization of melanomas may thus give insight into their origin, knowledge that should be of diagnostic and prognostic value.

Therapeutic application of monoclonal antibodies depends on their ability to localize to tumor metastases *in vivo* and to kill melanoma cells. As discussed above, we have evidence for the former. For the latter, several modes of action are possible. First, IgG2 monoclonal

---

[1] Larson, et al., unpublished observations.

antibodies to p97 can kill melanoma cells *in vitro* in the presence of rabbit complement, and cytoxicity is greatly enhanced by using two antibodies to two epitopes of p97 (14). Presumably, closely adjacent antibody molecules at the cell surface are particularly efficient at activating complement-mediated cytolysis. Secondly, we have observed antibody-dependent cellular cytotoxicity *in vitro*, using human effector cells. Monoclonal IgG2 antibodies have proven effective therapeutically in a mouse tumor model (27). However, several monoclonal antibodies that are cytotoxic to human tumor cells *in vitro* have been reported to be ineffective *in vivo* in nude mice bearing melanoma xenografts (28).

In collaboration with Dr. P. Casellas at Clin Midy (Montpellier) we have coupled a monoclonal antibody specific for p97 to the A chain of ricin. The resulting immunotoxin is cytotoxic to melanoma cells at concentrations at which free A chain and anti-dinitrophenol immunotoxin are completely ineffective. Similar results have been reported for monoclonal antibodies to colorectal carcinoma (29). Such immunotoxins hold promise as therapeutic agents, but their specificity and stability *in vivo* still have to be evaluated. A possible model system for initial evaluation of anti-p97 immunotoxins might be based on treatment of bone marrow that has been removed from melanoma patients to be used as an autologous graft (after high-dose chemotherapy of the patient) but that has been found to be contaminated with metastatic melanoma cells.

Discussion

Several groups have used monoclonal antibodies to identify antigens that are present in larger amounts in melanoma cells than in normal cells. However, none of these antigens has been shown to be absolutely restricted to melanomas; p97, for example, is present in certain fetal tissues and in small amounts in normal adult tissues. Some melanoma-associated antigens may, in fact, be differentiation antigens, normally present on melanoblasts, melanocytes or other cells of neural crest origin (25,26). Immunohistochemical methods should allow examination of normal melanoblasts and melanocytes *in situ* for binding of monoclonal antibodies. We have recently demonstrated the presence of p97 in cryostat sections of primary melanomas by the immunoperoxidase technique, and we are using this method to study normal and fetal tissues.

Lack of absolute specificity for melanoma may not preclude clinical application of monoclonal antibodies. A therapeutic protocol that kills both melanoma cells and, for instance, skin melanocytes may still be useful. Indeed, monoclonal antibody to Thy-1 antigen, which is present on a number of normal tissues, including brain, is useful in treating mouse leukemia (27). Also, conventional cancer therapies have severe side effects on certain normal cell populations.

The functions of melanoma-associated antigens, like those of many cell surface antigens, remain unknown. None of the identified melanoma-associated antigens have been shown to be directly involved in neoplastic transformation. Possibly, some are receptors for hormones, such as melanocyte-stimulating hormone, or for transport proteins, such as transferrin (30). However, there seems to be no simple way to determine the function of a particular melanoma-associated antigen.

Human monoclonal antibodies to melanoma-associated antigens would be of great clinical value; there are already reports of human monoclonal antibodies specific for a hapten and for a viral antigen (31,32). Fusing melanoma patients' lymphocytes with human myeloma cells might yield such antibodies, although antibodies to melanoma-associated antigens can be detected in only a few melanoma patients.

To obtain human monoclonal antibodies to melanoma-associated antigens already defined by mouse monoclonal antibodies, one could use purified antigen to immunize a human or to immunize human lymphocytes *in vitro*. However, it has been shown that synthetic oligopeptides, derived from the amino acid sequence of the antigen, can be used as immunogens. The antisera produced in response to the oligopeptides often recognize the native protein molecule (33). Amino acid sequence studies of p97, aimed at obtaining enough sequence data, are now in progress. Ultimately we hope to immunize human volunteers (melanoma patients) with the synthetic peptide and then to fuse their peripheral blood lymphocytes with human myeloma cells. The synthetic peptide could be used to assist in selecting hybridomas producing specific antibody by coupling to fluorescent microspheres and using the fluorescence-activited cell sorter (34).

Acknowledgments

We are grateful to Drs. Bill Dreyer, John Forstrom and David Teplow for helpful and stimulating discussions, and to Charles Hart and Cynthia Green for expert technical assistance. This work was supported by Grants CA 27841, CA 25558, CA 14135, and CA 19149 from the National Institutes of Health, and Grant IM 241 from the American Cancer Society.

References

1. Hellström, KE, and I Hellström (1972). Immunity to neuroblastomas and melanomas. Annu Rev Med **23**, 19-38.
2. Shiku, H, T Takahashi, HF Oettgen and LJ Old (1976). Cell surface antigens of human malignant melanoma. II. Serological typing with immune adherence

assays and definition of two new antigens. J Exp Med **144**, 871-873.

3. Galloway, DR, RP McCabe, MA Pellegrino, S Ferrone and R Reisfeld (1981). Tumor-associated antigens in spent medium of human melanoma cells; immunochemical characterization with xenoantisera. J Immunol **126**, 62-66.
4. Köhler, G, and C Milstein (1975). Continuous cultures of fused cells secreting antibody of predefined specificity. Nature (Lond) **256**, 495-497.
5. Woodbury, RG, JP Brown, M-Y Yeh, I Hellström and KE Hellström (1980). Identification of a cell surface protein, p97, in human melanoma and certain other neoplasms. Proc Natl Acad Sci USA **77**, 2183-2187.
6. Yeh, M-Y, I Hellström, JP Brown, GA Warner, JA Hansen and KE Hellström (1979). Cell surface antigens of human melanoma identified by monoclonal antibody. Proc Natl Acad Sci USA **76**, 2927-2931.
7. Carrel, S, RS Accolla, AL Carmagnola and JP Mach (1980). Common human melanoma-associated antigens detected by monoclonal antibodies. Cancer Res **40**, 2523-2528.
8. Dippold, WG, KO Lloyd, LT Li, H Ikeda, HF Oettgen and LJ Old (1980). Cell surface antigens of human malignant melanoma; definition of six antigenic systems with monoclonal antibodies. Proc Natl Acad Sci USA **77**, 6114-6118.
9. Koprowski, H, Z Steplewski, D Herlyn and M Herlyn (1978). Study of antibodies against human melanoma produced by somatic cell hybrids. Proc Natl Acad Sci USA **75**, 3405-3409.
10. Brown, JP, RG Woodbury, CE Hart, I Hellström and KE Hellström (1981). Quantitative analysis of melanoma-associated antigen p97 in normal and neoplastic tissues. Proc Natl Acad Sci USA **78**, 539-543.
11. Woodbury, RG, JP Brown, SM Loop, KE Hellström and I Hellström (1981). Analysis of normal and neoplastic human tissues for the tumor-associated protein p97. Int J Cancer **27**, 145-149.
12. Brown, JP, KE Hellström and I Hellström (1981). Use of monoclonal antibodies for quantitative analysis of antigens in normal and neoplastic tissues. Clin Chem **27**, 1592-1596.
13. Brown, JP, K Nishiyama, I Hellström and KE Hellström (1981). Structural characterization of human melanoma-associated antigen p97 using monoclonal antibodies. J Immunol **127**, 539-546.
14. Hellström, I, JP Brown and KE Hellström (1981). Monoclonal antibodies to two determinants of melanoma-associated antigen p97 act synergistically in complement-dependent cytotoxicity. J Immunol **127**, 159-160.
15. Brown, JP, PW Wright, CE Hart, RG Woodbury, KE Hellström and I Hellström (1980). Protein antigens of normal and malignant human cells identified by immunoprecipitation with monoclonal antibodies. J Biol Chem **255**, 4980-4983.
16. Brown, JP, JD Tamerius and I Hellström (1979). Indirect ^{125}I-labelled protein A assay for monoclonal antibodies to cell surface antigens. J Immunol Methods **31**, 201-209.
17. Köhler, G, CW Howe and C Milstein (1976). Fusion between immunoglobulin secreting and nonsecreting myeloma cell lines. Eur J Immunol **6**, 292-295.
18. Shulman, M, CD Wilde and G Köhler (1978). A better cell line for making hybridomas secreting specific antibodies. Nature (Lond) **276**, 169-270.
19. Winchester, RJ, C-Y Wang, A Crobotsky, HG Kunkel, KO Lloyd and LJ Old (1978). Expression of Ia-like antigens on cultured human malignant melanoma cell lines. Proc Natl Acad Sci USA **75**, 6235-6239.
20. Ey, PL, SJ Prowse and CR Jenkin (1978). Isolation of pure IgG1, IgG2a, and IgG2b immunoglobulins from mouse serum using protein A-Sepharose. Immunochemistry **15**, 429-436.
21. Houghton, M, AG Stewart, SM Doel, JS Emtage, MAW Eaton, JC Smith, TP Patel, HM Lewis, AG Porter, JR Birch, T Cartwright and NH Carey (1980). The amino-terminal sequence of human fibroblast interferon as deduced from reverse transcripts obtained using synthetic oligonucleotide primers. Nucleic Acids Res **8**, 1913-1931.
22. Gudjonsson, H, and S Johnsen (1978). HeLa cell plasma membrane. IV. "Iodination of membrane protein in synchronized cells." Exp Cell Res **112**, 289-295.

23. Kessler, S (1975). Rapid isolation of antigens from cells with a Staphylococcal protein A-antibody adsorbent: parameters of the interaction of antibody-antigen complexes with protein A. J Immunol **115**, 1617-1624.
24. Houston, LL, RC Nowinski and ID Bernstein (1980). Specific *in vivo* localization of monoclonal antibodies directed against the Thy 1.1 antigen. J Immunol **125**, 837-843.
25. Herlyn, M, WH Clark, Jr, MJ Mastrangelo, D Guerry, IV, DE Elder, D LaRossa, R Hamilton, E Bondi, R Tuthill, Z Steplewski and H Koprowski (1980). Specific immunoreactivity of hybridoma-secreted monoclonal anti-melanoma antibodies to cultured cells and freshly derived human cells. Cancer Res **40**, 3602-3609.
26. Quevedo, WC, Jr, and RD Fleischman (1980). Developmental biology of mammalian melanocytes. J Invest Dermatol **75**, 116-120.161.
27. Bernstein, ID, MR Tam and RC Nowinski (1980). Mouse leukemia: therapy with monoclonal antibodies against a thymus differentiation antigen. Science **207**, 68-71.
28. Herlyn, D, M Herlyn, Z Steplewski, JH Koprowski (1979). Monoclonal antibodies in cell-mediated cytotoxicity against human melanoma and colorectal carcinoma. Eur J Immunol **9**, 657-659.
29. Gilliland, DG, Z Steplewski, RJ Collier, KF Mitchell, TH Chang and H Koprowski (1980). Antibody-directed cytotoxic agents: Use of monoclonal antibody to direct the action of toxin A chains to colorectal carcinoma cells. Proc Natl Acad Sci USA **77**, 4539-4543.
30. Shindelman, JE, AE Ortmeyer and HH Sussman (1981). Demonstration of the transferrin receptor in human breast cancer tissue. Potential marker for identifying dividing cells. Int J Cancer **27**, 329-334.
31. Olsson, L, and HS Kaplan (1980). Human-human hybridomas producing monoclonal antibodies of predefined antigenic specificity. Proc Natl Acad Sci USA **77**, 5429-5431.
32. Croce, CM, A Linnenbach, W Hall, Z Steplewski and H Koprowski (1980). Production of human hybridomas secreting antibodies to measles virus. Nature (Lond) **288**, 488-489.
33. Sutcliffe, JG, TM Shinnick, N Green, F-T Liu, HL Niman and RA Lerner (1980). Chemical synthesis of a polypeptide predicted from nucleotide sequence allows detection of a new retroviral gene product. Nature (Lond) **287**, 801-805.
34. Parks, DR, VM Bryan, VT Oi and LA Herzenberg (1979). Antigen-specific indentification and cloning of hybridomas with a fluorescence-activated cell sorter. Proc Natl Acad Sci USA **76**, 1962-1966.

AS YOU SEE THEM
OR
HUMAN CANCER ANTIGENS VIEWED BY MONOCLONAL ANTIBODIES

Hilary Koprowski

The Wistar Institute of Anatomy and Biology
Philadelphia, Pennsylvania 19104

At present, the most successful approach to the analysis of human tumor antigens is through the study of antigens defined by monoclonal antibodies (1). The source of these antibodies is the hybridoma that is produced by the fusion of splenocytes from immunized mice and mouse myeloma cells (2). The human tumor material used to immunize the mice is freshly resected cancer or tumor cells maintained in tissue culture for long or short periods. Mice can be immunized with intact tumor cells that are either live or lightly fixed in gluteraldehyde, or with the tissue culture supernatant of tumors that secrete antigenic material into the medium (3). Finally, solubilized tumor cell membranes or 3M KCl extracts of tumor cells also produce an adequate immune response in mice to be used in producing antibody-secreting hybridomas.

Any one of the above preparations is injected intravenously into adult BALB/c mice, followed usually by an intravenous booster inoculation of the same material three to four weeks later. Spleens or lymph nodes are removed from these mice three to four days after the booster immunization, and the cells are processed for fusion with mouse myeloma cells and production of hybridomas (2).

When it is desirable to elicit an immune response to antigen produced by a growing tumor and then to use the mouse lymphocytes for fusion and production of hybridomas, human tumors can be given thymectomized, lethally irradiated mice that receive transplants of isologous bone marrow at the time of implantation of the tumor cells. In preliminary trials, however, hybridomas produced after immunization of mice with growing tumors secreted monoclonal antibodies that were cross-reactive with antigen(s) expressed by a variety of human tumors of origins different from that of the tumor growing in donor mice (4).

Making of hybridomas still remains a mystery, and the results of fusion experiments cannot be predicted. In parallel fusion experiments where mice are immunized with an apparently identical antigen preparation, one fusion experiment can result in an abundance of antibody-secreting hybridomas, whereas the other experiment results in none.

Monoclonal antibodies secreted by hybridomas produced after immunization of mice with either primary or metastatic melanoma can be divided into several classes, based on their reactivity or cross reactivity and on the identity of antigens immunoprecipitated and analyzed in gel diffusion (5). Only two monoclonal antibodies of several dozen investigated reacted with melanoma cells only. A larger number of monoclonal antibodies defined antigens expressed by melanomas and fetal tissue but not by other tumors or normal adult tissue. A still larger group of monoclonal antibodies reacted with a variety of tumor cells and also with some normal human cells. Finally, because most melanoma tumors express the DR antigen, the monoclonal antibodies produced quite often have DR specificity (6). Monoclonal antibodies that bind to melanoma cells and, then, only to fetal and adult melanocytes, immunoprecipitate polypeptides having the same molecular weight as polypeptides extracted from melanoma cells. However, monoclonal antibodies with specificity for melanoma cells and for other tumors of neural tumor origin immunoprecipitate antigens of three different molecular weights (5-7).

In parallel with the study of human melanoma, it is possible to investigate precursor lesions of the tumor, i.e., dysplastic nevi, which are readily observed and resected, in contrast with other human precancer lesions. Cells from dysplastic nevi and from a variety of other classes of nevi (common, compound, etc.) are relatively easy to grow in culture. Unlike the immortal melanoma cultures, nevi have a finite lifetime in culture, similar to normal human cells. Although cells of nevi are anchorage-independent in soft agar, progeny cells never spontaneously transform, and the cultures ultimately die out. Preliminary investigations show a normal karyotype for human nevi in contrast to the highly aberrant karyotype of melanoma cells (8).

Despite the behavioral similarity to normal human fibroblasts of cultures of nevi, including those recognized as premalignant lesions, nevi cells express almost all of the antigens expressed by melanoma cells and defined by a panel of monoclonal antibodies. Thus, the factors instrumental in the transformation of cells of nevi in the human organism are obviously inoperative in tissue culture.

Most, if not all, antigens of melanomas are proteins. The same is true of antigens defined by monoclonal antibodies secreted by hybridomas produced after immunization of mice with lung adenocarcinoma cells. All of the four monoclonal antibodies that bind to lung adenocarcinoma cells used for immunization of mice show cross reactivity with antigens expressed by other human tumor cells or even by normal cells (9). One of these antibodies also binds to cells of oat cell carcinoma, colorectal carcinoma, and breast carcinoma; it does not bind to melanomas and normal human fibroblasts, but it does react with human erythrocytes and peripheral blood lymphocytes. This antibody, of class Ig2a, mediates destruction, as will be mentioned below, of tumor cells to which it binds but conversely does not lyse erythrocytes or lymphocytes. Each of the four monoclonal antibodies immunoprecipitates a polypeptide of a different molecular weight (9).

Monoclonal antibodies secreted by hybridomas produced after immunization of mice with breast adenocarcinoma cells also immunoprecipitate polypeptides of a defined class. Of seven monoclonal antibodies reactive with breast carcinoma cells, three are cross-reactive with cells of other tumors and normal tissue, three seem to be restricted in their specificity to breast adenocarcinoma cells, and one binds only to cells used for immunization. Gel diffusion patterns of tumor extracts immunoprecipitated with these antibodies reveal six bands representing proteins of different molecular weights.

In contrast to the protein antigens of melanomas and of lung and breast adenocarcinomas, antigens defined by monoclonal antibodies secreted by hybridomas produced after immunization of mice with gastrointestinal tumors, are mostly glycolipids (10). Some of these monoclonal antibodies are directed against glycolipid constituents of normal human cells (11). These are Lewis B antigen, blood group B and lacto-N-fucosyl pentaose III-ceramide. The latter glycolipid seems to be identical with the stage-specific embryonic antigens (SSEA) (12). This antigen, first detected on blastomers of 8 cell mouse embryo (13), is expressed by mouse embryonic cells and is widely distributed in human tissues of different origin.

The glycolipid antigen defined by the gastrointestinal cancer monoclonal antibody is N-acetyl neuraminic acid-lacto-N-fucopentaosyl II-ceramide (14). This monosialoganglioside, referred to as GICA (gastrointestinal cancer antigen), was found only in cells of pancreatic, gastric, and colorectal carcinoma and in meconium but not in any other normal human tissue. It is also present on cell membranes as detected in an immunoperoxidase reaction in the presence of the specific monoclonal antibody (15). Using this technique, it was possible to demonstrate the presence of GICA on membranes of gastrointestinal carcinoma cells but not on normal tissue except for columnar epithelial cells of the secretory ducts in the pancreas and biliary tract. No normal cells of the colon or stomach seem to express GICA (15).

The only known biochemical pathway of synthesis of the terminal sugar portion of GICA is from lacto-N-fucopentaosyl II, the Lewis A antigen. A transferase thus far undetected in normal human tissue adds the N-acetyl-neuraminic acid determinant to the Lewis A compound. The availability of such a transferase might make possible the synthesis of GICA from the Lewis A compound, which is readily available. Another interesting aspect of the relationship between the Lewis A antigen and GICA is the possibility that Lewis A- and B-negative (Le a^-b^-) individuals may not be able to synthesize GICA. In preliminary assays, four colorectal carcinoma patients who were Le a^-b^- did not show the presence of GICA on their tumor cells or in their blood (see below). All other patients who expressed GICA secreted either Lewis A or Lewis B antigen. One must also consider the possibility that Le a^-b^- individuals may not be susceptible to cancers, the cells of which produce GICA (16), even though the role of glycolipids in malignant transformation is virtually unknown.

Gastrointestinal cancer antigen is secreted into the medium by cells of gastrointestinal cancer maintained in culture (3). Thus, it became of interest to analyze the sera of patients with gastrointestinal carcinoma for the presence of GICA secreted by the tumor tissue (17). The results of these bioassays showed that GICA was present in the sera of most patients with carcinoma of the pancreas or stomach and in about half of those with colorectal carcinoma (18). The absence of GICA in the blood does not necessarily indicate its absence in tumor tissue, as six out of eight patients with no detectable GICA in their sera showed the presence of GICA on the tumor cell surface (colorectal carcinomas) in the immunoperoxidase reaction (15).

Human tumors growing in nude mice were destroyed by one or more injections of tumor-specific monoclonal antibody (2,19), providing that the antibody was class Ig2a. Tumor-specific antibodies of different immunoglobulins displayed no antitumor effect, although they showed greater binding affinity for their target cells. Because tumor cells were not destroyed when exposed directly to the γ2a monoclonal antibody alone either in culture or prior to implantation in mice, it became clear that the antibody mediated a tumor-killing effect by interacting with effector cells in the organism. In nude mice, these would be either natural killer (NK) cells of the lymphoid series, or macrophages. The role of NK as a tumor-killing cell was shown to be highly unlikely since the tumor-suppressive effect was as pronounced in baby nude mice, in which the level of NK cells is low, as in adult nude mice. Furthermore, lowering the concentration of NK cells in adult nude mice by treatment with anti-interferon serum did not diminish the tumor-suppressive effect. These results pointed to macrophages as the most probable effector cells of monoclonal antibody-mediated tumor destruction. Moreover, because only Ig2a antibody mediated tumor destruction, only the fraction of macrophages displaying Fc receptors for Ig2a immunoglobulins would participate in the tumoricidal effect.

Evidence for the role of macrophages in tumor destruction was obtained in two types of experiments. In one, mice were treated with silica, which immobilizes macrophages, and the tumoricidal effect was abolished. In the second set of experiments, it was shown conclusively that mouse peritoneal macrophages mixed with Ig2a monoclonal antibody destroy the tumor cells that bind the antibody in cultures maintained for four to five days. Tumor cells were not destroyed if the tumor-specific monoclonal antibody was of an isotype other than Ig2a or if an Ig2a antibody with another specificity was used.

With the isolation and identification of antigens associated with human cancer and with the advent of new and unusual approaches to the diagnosis and eventual immunotherapy of human malignancies, monoclonal antibodies have moved from the software to the hardware category of goods. If wisdom prevails among scientists using this hardware, the era of monoclonal antibodies may bring results of far-reaching importance to biology and medicine such as those brought by recombinant DNA technology.

Acknowledgments

This investigation was supported by Public Health Service Grants CA-10815, CA-25874 and CA-21124, awarded by the National Cancer Institute, Department of Health and Human Services.

References

1. Koprowski, H (1980). Monoclonal hybridomas as a new tool in immunology. In Microbiology, pp 191-195. D Schlessinger, ed. American Society for Microbiology, Washington, DC.
2. Koprowski, H, Z Steplewski, D Herlyn and M Herlyn (1978). Study of antibodies against human melanoma produced by somatic cell hybrids. Proc Natl Acad Sci USA **75**, 3405-3409.
3. Chang, TH, Z Steplewski and H Koprowski (1980). Production of monoclonal antibodies in serum free medium. J Immunol Methods **39**, 369-375.
4. Herlyn, D, and H Koprowski (1982). Immune response in mice to growing human tumors. Submitted to J Immunol Methods.
5. Herlyn, M, Z Steplewski and H Koprowski (1982). Production and characterization of monoclonal antibodies against human malignant melanoma. Submitted to Cancer Investigation.
6. Mitchell, K, JP Fuhrer, Z Steplewski and H Koprowski (1980). Biochemical characterization of human melanoma cell surfaces: Dissection with monoclonal antibodies. Proc Natl Acad Sci USA **77**, 7287-7291.
7. Mitchell, KF, JP Fuhrer, Z Steplewski and H Koprowski (1981). Structural characterization of the melanoma-specific antigen detected by monoclonal antibody 691I5Nu-4-B. Mol Immunol **18**, 207-218.
8. Balaban, G, M Herlyn, D Guerry and P Nowell (1982). Karyotype stability in the primary tumor and multiple metastases of a human melanoma. AACR (abst), in press.
9. Mazauric, T, KF Mitchell, GJ Letchworth, III, H Koprowski and Z Steplewski (1982). Monoclonal antibody-defined human lung cell surface protein antigens. Cancer Res **42**, 150-154.
10. Magnani, JL, M Brockhaus, DF Smith, V Ginsburg, M Blaszczyk, KF Mitchell, Z Steplewski and H Koprowski (1981). A monosialo-ganglioside is a monoclonal antibody-defined antigen of colon carcinoma. Science **212**, 55-56.
11. Brockhaus, M, JL Magnani, M Blaszczyk, Z Steplewski, H Koprowski, KA Karlsson, G Larson and V Ginsburg (1981). Monoclonal antibodies directed against the human Le^b blood group antigen. J Biol Chem **256**, 13223-13225.
12. Hakomori, S, E Nudelman, S Levery, D Solter and BB Knowles (1981). The hapten structure of a developmentally regulated glycolipid antigen (SSEA-1) isolated from human erythrocytes and adenocarcinoma: a preliminary note. Biochem Biophys Res Commun **100**, 1578-1586.
13. Solter, D, and B Knowles (1978). Monoclonal antibody defining a stage-specific mouse embryonic antigen (SSEA-1). Proc Natl Acad Sci USA **75**, 5565-5569.
14. Magnani, J, B Nilsson, M Brockhaus, D Zopf, Z Steplewski, H Koprowski and V Ginsburg (1982). The antigen of a tumor-specific antibody is a ganglioside containing sialylated lacto-N-fucopentaose II. Fed Proc (abst), in press.
15. Atkinson, BF, CS Ernst, M Herlyn, Z Steplewski, HF Sears and H Koprowski. GI

tumor-associated antigen in immunoperoxidase assay. Submitted to Science.
16. Koprowski, H, M Blaszczyk, Z Steplewski, V Ginsburg, J Magnani and M Brockhaus (1982). Hypothesis: Lewis blood type may affect the incidence of gastrointestinal cancer (GIC). Submitted to Lancet.
17. Koprowski, H, M Herlyn, Z Steplewski and HF Sears (1981). Specific antigen in serum of patients with colon carcinoma. Science **212**, 53-55.
18. Herlyn, M, HF Sears, Z Steplewski and H Koprowski (1982). Monoclonal antibody detection of a circulating tumor-associated antigen: I. Presence of antigen in sera of patients with colorectal, gastric and pancreatic carcinoma. J Clin Immunol **2**, in press.
19. Herlyn, DM, Z Steplewski, M Herlyn and H Koprowski (1980). Inhibition of growth of colorectal carcinoma in nude mice by monoclonal antibody. Cancer Res **40**, 717-721.

IV
Applications to Drug Delivery Systems

HUMAN-HUMAN HYBRIDOMAS AND MONOCLONAL ANTIBODIES

Henry S. Kaplan and Lennart Olsson*

Cancer Biology Research Laboratory, Department of Radiology
Stanford University School of Medicine
Stanford, California 94305

A new era in immunology emerged when Köhler and Milstein (1,2) created a method for the fusion of mouse B lymphocytes to mouse myeloma cells to yield hybridomas able to secrete antibodies of predefined antigenic specificity. Clonal selection of these immortal hybridoma cell lines assured the monoclonality, monospecificity, and long term availability of their antibody products.

Although mouse and other rodent antibodies have been extraordinarily effective as reagents in laboratory investigations, their clinical use is limited because they are foreign proteins. Human immunoglobulin-producing cells have been fused to mouse myeloma cells to generate chimeric hybridomas (3-4). Although there have been rare instances in which long-term, stable production of human antibody has thus been achieved (5), most such hybrids have tended to be highly unstable due to the selective loss of human chromosomes.

An alternative approach to the creation of antibody-producing human lymphocyte cell lines has been to use human B lymphocytes transformed with Epstein-Barr virus (EBV) (6-8). This method appears to have limited practicality because the cultures often cease antibody production after a variable period (8). We have developed another alternative in the form of human-human hybridomas that secrete monoclonal antibodies of predefined antigenic specificity. They are obtained by the fusion of primed human lymphoid cells with HAT-sensitive human myeloma cells (9). This method should permit the generation of human monoclonal antibodies against a broad spectrum of predefined antigens.

Technical Considerations

Selection and Establishment of a HAT-sensitive Human Myeloma Cell Line

Murine myeloma cell lines usually are selected for 8-azaguanine-resistance in a single step procedure by cloning the myeloma cells in

*Present address: Department of Medicine A, State University Hospital, Copenhagen, Denmark.

soft agar in the presence of 8-azaguanine (usually 20 μg/ml). With mouse myeloma cell lines this procedure yields as many as 20 to 30 resistant clones/10^6 seeded myeloma cells. Thus, the more tedious selection procedures in liquid culture have not been necessary.

Nilsson et al. (10) established and characterized the human U-266 myeloma cell line. They reported that this IgE (λ)-secreting myeloma cell line grew slowly, required a feeder layer, and had a very poor cloning efficiency. In 1977, Kaplan requested and received samples of Nilsson's U-266 cell line to test it as a host for the replication of a C-type virus produced by the SU-DHL-1 human histiocytic lymphoma cell line (11,12). The initial passages of the U-266 cells had poor viability and growth rate. However, four to five months of painstaking selection of the healthiest miniwell cultures at each passage yielded a cell line with marked improvement in viability and growth rate; it no longer required the use of feeder layers. This line of myeloma cells also could be cloned in semi-solid agarose with an efficiency approaching 1%. A broth culture at that time was reportedly negative for mycoplasma.[1]

The U-266 cells were recovered from storage in liquid nitrogen and reestablished in culture. We tried initially, without success, to clone the cells in soft agar or agarose in the presence of 10, 15, or 20 μg/ml of 8-azaguanine. Colonies were rare and when harvested were not HAT-sensitive after expansion.

We had better results with liquid cultures and developed the following procedure to select for resistance to 8-azaguanine. A large inoculum of U-266 cells was grown in RPMI-1640 medium supplemented with 15% fetal calf serum (FCS) and 20 μg/ml of 8-azaguanine. After five days of cultivation, at least 99% of the cells were dead. The remaining viable cells were then separated from the dead cells on a Ficoll-Hypaque gradient (13) and cultivated for an additional two or three days in medium containing 20 μg/ml of 8-azaguanine. Viable cells remaining in the culture at this time were again isolated on a Ficoll-Hypaque gradient, washed, and seeded in a single microwell of a 96-well microtiter plate containing RPMI-1640 with 15% FCS and 5 μg/ml 8-azaguanine. Visible cell growth could be seen in this medium within about one week. As soon as growth was observed, the 8-azaguanine concentration was increased to 10 μg/ml. After approximately one additional week, as growth again resumed, the 8-azaguanine concentration was further increased to 15 μg/ml, and about one week later to 20 μg/ml, without any further inhibition of cell growth.

The cell culture was then expanded in RPMI-1640 with 15% FCS and 20 μg/ml 8-azaguanine, and cloned in microtiter plates by the

---

[1] The cells later were found to be contaminated with mycoplasma. The cell line has been freed of mycoplasma by treatment with heat, with or without antibiotics, followed by subcloning.

limiting dilution procedure. Growth curves were determined for five actively growing clones. The fastest growing clone, which had a cell population doubling time of about 18 to 20 h in exponential growth phase, was selected for use in human hybridoma production. This clone was initially designated U-266AR$_1$ and later identified as SKO-007 in the Stanford University Biological Organism Registry. These cells were found to be HAT-sensitive; 4 x 10^{-8}M was the lowest aminopterin concentration that assured the killing of all the myeloma cells. We consider it important to use a relatively low aminopterin concentration to obtain a maximum yield of hybridomas. However, variations in culture conditions may influence the HAT-sensitivity of the line, and so we recommend periodic titration of the minimum effective aminopterin concentration. The SKO-007 cell line was found to fuse readily with human lymphoid cells in the presence of polyethylene glycol (PEG). Dr. Rose Payne (Department of Medicine, Stanford University School of Medicine) determined the HL-A phenotype of the SKO-007 cell line as follows: HLA-A2, A3, B7, Bw60, Bw6, Cw3. Its karyotype, determined by Drs. Barbara Kaiser-McCaw and Frederick Hecht (Southwest Biomedical Research Institute, Tempe, Ariz.), is 44, X, -8, -17, -18, +2mar, +2min, t(1;1), t(2;?), t(3;?), t(11;?).

We attribute much of our success in the creation of the first human-human monoclonal antibody-producing hybridomas (9) to the use of the procedure (outlined above) to isolate a HAT-sensitive mutant of U-266. Use of a high 8-azaguanine concentration during the initial selection assured the killing of all cells with high or medium levels of HGPRT activity. Gradually increasing the 8-azaguanine concentration in surviving cultures permitted selection of variants with low HGPRT activity and the subsequent selection of mutants apparently devoid of the enzyme. Selection of the most rapidly growing clone is desirable, because such a clone is likely to confer high proliferation capacity on its fused hybridoma progeny, thus reducing the time required for cloning and growth of antibody-producing hybridomas. We have recently used this procedure to select HAT-sensitive mutants of two human malignant lymphoma cell lines.

Attempted Selection of a Non-producer Variant

Like its U-266 parent, the SKO-007 cell line produces IgE(λ) (Fig. 1). Thus, even after cloning, each hybridoma derived from SKO-007 is likely to produce several different immunoglobulin molecules as a result of the permuted assembly of the heavy and light chains encoded by the genes of the lymphoid and myeloma cell precursors. This permutation tends to reduce the yield of the desired monoclonal antibody produced by the hybridoma. Constructing hybridomas by the fusion of lymphoid cells with a non-producer myeloma cell line would therefore be advantageous, because the cloned progeny of such hybrids should produce only a single type of immunoglobulin molecule.

Earlier studies with mouse myeloma cell lines suggest that the loss of heavy chain production usually precedes the loss of light chain production (14). We have therefore used fluoresceinated anti-λ antibody to distinguish between myeloma cells with and without λ light chain secretion, and have used repeated sorting on a fluorescence-activated cell sorter (FACS III, Becton-Dickinson Co.). to isolate and clone non-secretory cells. Although such clones have appeared to be negative for the production of immunoglobulin products during the first three to four weeks of culture, they eventually have become positive for at least λ light chain secretion. Thus, we have not yet succeeded in selecting a non-producer variant of the SKO-007 human myeloma cell line but are trying other approaches to selecting such non-producers. In addition, we have selected, cloned, and grown the HAT-sensitive mutants of two human malignant lymphoma cell lines and have successfully fused them with human lymphoid cells. The resultant hybrids are currently being monitored for antibody production.

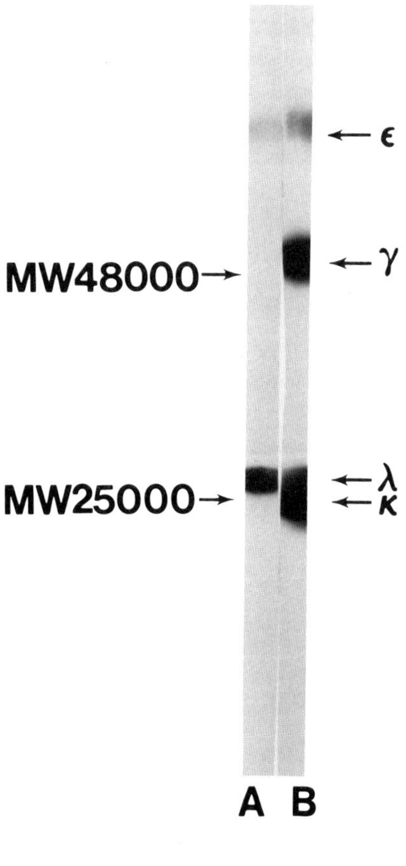

Fig. 1. SDS-PAGE of ^{14}C-leucine labeled supernatants immunoprecipitated with rabbit anti-human Ig. (A) Parental U-266AR$_1$ (SKO-007) myeloma cell line. (B) Cloned anti-CNP hybridoma cell line. κ, new kappa light chain; λ, lambda light chain of U-266AR$_1$ cells; γ, new gamma heavy chain; ε, epsilon heavy chain of U-266AR$_1$ cells.

Sensitization of Human Lymphoid Cells

In our initial experiments, we followed the Köhler-Milstein procedures as closely as possible by performing the immunization *in vivo*. Patients with previously untreated Hodgkin's disease were selected, since they are routinely submitted to a battery of immunologic tests, including sensitization and subsequent challenge with dinitrochlorobenzene (DNCB). About two weeks after initial testing, such patients undergo staging laparotomy and splenectomy (15). Spleens that, on pathological examination, appeared devoid of involvement by Hodgkin's disease, were used for hybridoma production. Single cell suspensions were prepared, freed of red blood cells and granulocytes by Ficoll-Hypaque gradient centrifugation, and enriched for lymphocytes by repeated brief incubation in plastic dishes and transfer of non-adherent cells. These lymphocyte-enriched mononuclear cell suspensions were then fused with the SKO-007 human myeloma cell line and incubated in HAT medium as described below. The spleen cells from two of three patients with Hodgkin's disease yielded a total of five HAT-resistant hybridoma clones producing IgG(κ) antibody with specific reactivity in radioimmunoassays for DNP-BSA (Table 1).

Table 1. Human-human hybridomas producing antibody to DNP

	Fusion no.		
	H - 1	H - 2	H - 3
Producer screen,[a] % positive wells	18	29	36
Specific assay,[b]			
No. positive wells	3	2	0
Cpm of positive wells	3814, 4072, 4301	3911, 4113	--
Cpm of negative wells, mean	1421	1262	1416
Ratio positive/negative pre-cloning	2.85	3.18	--
No. subcloned wells positive	24, 14, 23	19, 9	--
Cpm of positive subcloned wells, mean	12,318 ± 1743	14,162 ± 2936	--

[a] ^{125}I-Staphylococcus protein A binding.
[b] Binding to DNP-BSA.

Although this approach proved successful, it is clear that the spectrum of antigens for immunizing human subjects *in vivo* is severely limited, as is access to their spleen lymphocytes. Thus, development of a practical procedure for the production of human monoclonal antibodies will require techniques enabling human lymphoid cells to produce high titers of antibodies to a spectrum of antigens presented *in vitro*. In the murine hybridoma system the immunization schedule and the interval between the last antigen exposure and the harvest of spleen cells strongly influence the yield of specific hybridomas, suggesting that the state of differentiation of antigen-primed lymphocytes determines both the intensity of their antibody response and their susceptibility to fusion. The limited viability of human lymphoid cells *in vitro* severely restricts the immunization schedules that can be used in culture.

For our first *in vitro* sensitization experiments, we again used lymphoid cells from the uninvolved spleens of patients with Hodgkin's disease but incubated them with sheep red blood cells (SRBC) *in vitro*. Human spleen lymphoid cell suspensions, cleared of erythrocytes and granulocytes on a Ficoll-Hypaque gradient (13), were seeded in 30-mm petri dishes in RPMI-1640 with 15% fetal calf serum (FCS) and 2×10^{-5}M mercaptoethanol; SRBC were then added to a final concentration of 0.5%. The cells were incubated for five days at 37°C in air + 5% CO_2. Viable mononuclear cells were separated from dead cells on a Ficoll-Hypaque gradient, washed three times, and fused as above with U-266AR_1 myeloma cells. Initial screening with ^{125}I-labeled Staphylococcal protein A revealed several IgG-producing hybrids. However, none of these hybrids produced IgG antibody which was hemolytic for SRBC, in the presence of complement, in a Cunningham plaque-forming assay (16). When the remaining hybrids derived from this fusion were tested for anti-SRBC production in the plaque-forming assay, three cultures were positive. These cultures were incubated in 0.33% agarose in HAT medium with 15% FCS for one week and the emerging clones again tested for anti-SRBC production in a Jerne plaque-forming assay (17). Two clones with significant IgM antibody production were obtained. Thus, it is possible to generate human hybridomas producing antibody against an antigen to which lymphoid cells were primed *in vitro*.

Although the spleen is probably the optimal source of human lymphoid cells for *in vitro* immunizations, access to suitable spleen material is limited. Therefore, it is important to develop successful procedures for using the more readily available human peripheral blood lymphocytes (PBL). We have studied the influence of B cell mitogens on the yield of viable IgG- or IgM-producing hybrids following fusion of human PBL with SKO-007 cells. A low yield of immunoglobulin-producing hybrids was obtained by direct fusion of unstimulated PBL with SKO-007 cells (Table 2). However, stimulation of the cells with pokeweed mitogen (PWM) markedly increased the yield of immunoglobulin-producing hybrids to levels comparable

Table 2. Hybridoma Ig production by human lymphocytes fused with SKO-007 human myeloma cells

Source of lymphocytes	Wells seeded, total no.	Wells with viable hybrids		Wells with IgG production[a]		Wells with IgM production	
		no.	(%)	no. pos.	(%)	no. pos.	(%)
Spleen	288	176	61	107	37	64	22
PBL[b] unstimulated	288	94	33	45	16	37	13
PBL stimulated 7 days with LPS (50 μg/ml) prior to fusion	288	88	31	51	18	46	16
PBL stimulated 5 days with PWM (25 μg/ml) prior to fusion	288	242	84	146	51	134	47

[a]IgG and/or IgM production detected by radioimmunoassay 21 days after fusion.

[b]Peripheral blood mononuclear cells isolated from buffy coats on Ficoll-Hypaque gradients.

to those obtained with human spleen cells. Under these conditions lipopolysaccharide (LPS) failed to elicit any significant stimulation.

Further improvement of the *in vitro* immunization procedure is essential to the success of human hybridoma antibody production. The experimental difficulties are considerable, since complex interactions of multiple variables must be elucidated. Among various culture conditions we are currently evaluating are the relative merits of Iscove's medium (18) and RPMI-1640, and the advantages of the polyclonal activation system described by Hoffmann (19) compared to the standard PWM stimulation procedure. Methods of antigen presentation will require careful evaluation; different classes of antigens may require different methods of presentation. Antigens may be presented effectively by macrophages, when incorporated into liposomes, or when coupled to SRBC. When macrophages are used, the ratio of antigen-fed marcophages to lymphoid cells may be a significant variable. Presentation of human cell membrane antigens requires careful studies to determine whether co-cultivation of lymphoid cells with whole, intact human target cells (lethally irradiated, if necessary) yields responses as good as those provided by detergent-isolated cell membrane fractions presented by macrophages or in liposomes.

Fusion Procedure

It is not known whether the fusion procedures that have proven most successful in the production of mouse hybridomas will also be optimal for human hybridoma production. In our initial experiments, we used PEG with a molecular weight of 1500 successfully. However, it has recently been reported that the yield of mouse hybrids was optimal when a PEG with a molecular weight of 4000 was used (20). Other investigators have reported that the use of a slightly alkaline pH (approximately 8.0-8.1) (21) and/or of Ca^{2+} free medium during and immediately after fusion (22) can significantly increase the yield of viable hybrids.

An attractive alternative is the antigen-directed fusion procedure recently described by Bankert et al. (23). In this procedure, antigen was coupled to the myeloma cell line to increase the probability that antigen-primed B lymphocytes bearing specific antibody on their cell surfaces would bind and fuse preferentially and selectively to the antigen-coated myeloma cells. The procedure could be carried out successfully in the presence or absence of PEG. In one of the experiments reported by these investigators, the yield of specific antibody-producing clones was as high as 90%.

Parks et al. (24) described a highly efficient procedure for the selection of fused hybrids using the fluorescence-activated cell sorter and antigen coupled to fluorescent microspheres. This or similar procedures may be adapted to monitor the fusion step. Cell-sorter selection would be very useful in the selection of human hybridomas.

Cultivation and Cloning of Human Hybridomas

In our initial experiments, we observed that human hybrids require more time than mouse hybrids to grow out in HAT medium. The first viable HAT-resistant human hybrids were observed at 8 to 14 days, and additional hybrids emerged for three to four weeks during continued incubation. A variable still to be explored is the optimal time for adding HAT medium to the fused hybrid cultures. At present, we usually delay adding HAT medium until 24-48 h after fusion to permit the cells to recover from the toxic effects of PEG. However, the antigen-directed fusion procedure carried out in the absence of PEG would likely permit the immediate introduction of HAT medium. Alternatively, successful selection of fused hybrids with the cell sorter might obviate the need for HAT selection. We are now comparing the yield of viable hybrids in different culture media and in particular testing the relative merits of Iscove's medium vs. RPMI-1640. Earlier experiments (19) demonstrated the importance of optimal cell density in determining both the viability of hybrids and the yield of antibody-producing cultures (Table 3). Finally, we are evaluating the influence of feeder layers derived from human foreskin fibroblasts, human thymocytes, and human peripheral blood monocytes or spleen macrophages.

In vivo passage of mouse hybridomas in the peritoneal cavity results in a 100- to 1000-fold increase in production of antibody that can be harvested from ascites fluid. If the successful hetero-transplantation of human hybridomas into mice were feasible, similar increases in antibody production might be achieved, albeit at the price of admixture with murine serum proteins. Transplanting human

Table 3. Relationship between initial cell concentration and growth of functional hybrids

Data were obtained from three successive experiments with hybridized spleen cells of three patients with Hodgkin's disease.

No. of cells seeded/well on day 0	% wells with viable cells growing on day 10 after fusion	% wells producing IgG on day 21 after fusion
1×10^6	0, 0, 0	-- -- --
5×10^5	8, 3, 4	2, 0, 0
2×10^5	54, 64, 38	29, 36, 18
1×10^5	29, 32, 14	9, 11, 6
5×10^4	32, 17, 9	8, 3, 1

hybridomas into the peritoneal cavities of Pristane-primed nude athymic mice proved unsuccessful. We plan to do additional experiments using mice that have been immunosuppressed or rendered tolerant.

Human vs. Murine Monoclonal Hybridoma Antibodies

Monoclonal antibodies derived from murine hybridomas are highly effective analytic reagents for laboratory investigations of many problems in biology and medicine. Such monoclonal antibodies of high titer and high affinity are already available for a large number of antigens. In contrast, the production of monoclonal antibodies by human-human hybridomas is still in its infancy and must await the development of optimal techniques for antigen priming of human lymphocytes before a similar array of high titer human monoclonal antibodies can be made available. Thus it is now premature to attempt any detailed comparison of the potential of human vs. murine monoclonal antibodies. Nonetheless, a few general comments may be offered.

In general, it seems that murine and human monoclonal antibodies will be equally useful for *in vitro* diagnosis and analysis involving antigens that are not human gene products, although murine antibodies are likely to be preferred for practical and economic reasons. However, immunogeneticists have already observed that murine monoclonal antibodies have thus far failed to detect certain human major histocompatibility antigens readily detected by conventional anti-HLA antibodies. It has thus been suggested that intra-species lymphocyte responses to major histocompatibility antigens may yield human monoclonal antibodies whose range of antigenic specificity is broader than that of the murine antibodies. If so, human monoclonal antibodies will become useful *in vitro* reagents for HL-A histocompatibility testing.

However, it is clear that the major importance of human monoclonal antibodies stems from the expectation that they can be administered safely and repeatedly to human beings, and thus may well have significant applications in the prophylaxis, diagnosis and/or therapy of a broad spectrum of human diseases. This is not to suggest that murine monoclonal antibodies will have no role whatever in *in vivo* administration in man. It is quite conceivable that one or a few injections of murine antibodies may be well tolerated in human subjects. However, the highly significant differences in antigenicity of murine and human immunoglobulins make it probable that the repeated administration of a given murine antibody in therapeutic quantities will result in undesirable reactions. Since many types of treatment with monoclonal antibodies are likely to require repeated injections, it is clear that human monoclonal antibodies will be preferable in such situations. The fact that many thousands of humans have been safely and repeatedly injected with relatively large amounts of human immunoglobulin supports the expectation that human monoclonal antibodies will prove to be safe in clinical use. However, the fact that each such monoclonal antibody bears a single idiotype raises at least the theoretical possibility of a risk that human subjects may generate anti-idiotype antibodies in response to the administration of a human monoclonal antibody. In the murine disease models in which monoclonal antibodies have been used for therapeutic experiments to date, this appears not to have been a problem. Nonetheless, the possibility of complications stemming from anti-idiotype reactions must be carefully borne in mind in Phase I clinical trials with human monoclonal antibodies. Barring these and other as yet unforeseen difficulties, it seems likely that human monoclonal antibodies will achieve a major role in many aspects of clinical medicine during the next decade.

References

1. Köhler, G, and C Milstein (1975). Continuous cultures of fused cells secreting antibody of pre-defined specificity. Nature (Lond) **256**, 495-497.
2. Köhler, G, and C Milstein (1976). Derivation of specific antibody-producing tissue culture and tumor lines by cell fusion. Eur J Immunol **6**, 511-519.
3. Levy, R, and J Dilley (1978). Rescue of immunoglobulin secretion from human neoplastic lymphoid cells by somatic cell hybridization. Proc Natl Acad Sci USA **75**, 2411-2415.
4. Schwaber, J (1975). Immunoglobulin production by a human-mouse somatic cell hybrid. Exp Cell Res **93**, 343-354.
5. Schlom, J, D Wunderlich and YA Teramoto (1980). Generation of human monoclonal antibodies reactive with human mammary carcinoma cells. Proc Natl Acad Sci USA **77**, 6841-6845.
6. Koskimies, S (1979). Human lymphoblastoid cell line producing specific antibody against Rh-antigen. Scand J Immunol **10**, 371 (abst).
7. Steinitz, M, G Klein, S Koskimies and O Mäkela (1977). EB virus-induced B lymphocyte cell lines producing specific antibody. Nature (Lond) **269**, 420-422.
8. Zurawski, VR, Jr, E Haber and PH Black (1978). Production of antibody to tetanus toxoid by continuous human lymphoblastoid cell lines. Science **199**, 1439-1441.
9. Olsson, L, and HS Kaplan (1980). Human-human hybridomas producing monoclonal antibodies of predefined antigenic specificity. Proc Natl Acad Sci USA **77**, 5429-5431.
10. Nilsson, K, H Bennich, SGO Johansson and J Pontén (1970). Established immunoglobulin producing myeloma (IgE) and lymphoblastoid (IgG) cell lines from an IgE myeloma patient. Clin Exp Immunol **7**, 477-489.
11. Epstein, AL, and HS Kaplan (1974). Biology of the human malignant lymphomas: I. Establishment in continuous cell culture and heterotransplantation of diffuse histiocytic lymphomas. Cancer **34**, 1851-1872.
12. Kaplan, HS, RS Goodenow, AL Epstein, S Gartner, A Decève, and PN Rosenthal (1977). Isolation of a C-type RNA virus from an established human histiocytic lymphoma cell line. Proc Natl Acad Sci USA **74**, 2564-2568.
13. Böyum, A (1968). Separation of leucocytes from blood and bone marrow. Scand J Clin Lab Invest **21**, Suppl 97, 77-89.

14. Köhler, G (1980). Immunoglobulin chain loss in hybridoma lines. Proc Natl Acad Sci USA **77**, 2197-2199.
15. Glatstein, E, JM Guernsey, SA Rosenberg and HS Kaplan (1969). The value of laparotomy and splenectomy in the staging of Hodgkin's disease. Cancer **24**, 709-718.
16. Cunningham, AJ, and A Szenberg (1968). Further improvements in the plaque technique for detecting single antibody-forming cells. Immunology **14**, 599-601.
17. Jerne, NK, and AA Nordin (1963). Plaque formation in agar by single antibody-producing cells. Science **140**, 405-407.
18. Iscove, NN, and F Melchers (1978). Complete replacement of serum by albumin, transferrin and soybean lipid in cultures of lipopolysaccharide-reactive B lymphocytes. J Exp Med **147**, 923-933.
19. Hoffmann, MK (1980). Antigen-specific induction and regulation of antibody synthesis in cultures of human peripheral blood mononuclear cells. Proc Natl Acad Sci USA **77**, 1139-1143.
20. Fazekas de St. Groth, S, and D Scheidegger (1980). Production of monoclonal antibodies: strategy and tactics. J Immunol Methods **35**, 1-21.
21. Sharon, J, SL Morrison and EA Kabat (1980). Formation of hybridoma clones in soft agarose: effect of pH and of medium. Somatic Cell Genet **6**, 435-441.
22. Schneiderman, S, JL Farber and R Baserga (1979). A simple method for decreasing the toxicity of polyethylene glycol in mammalian cell hybridization. Somatic Cell Genet **5**, 263-269.
23. Bankert, RB, D DesSoye and L Powers (1980). Antigen-promoted cell fusion: antigen-coated myeloma cells fuse with antigen-reactive spleen cells. Transplant Proc **12**, 443-446.
24. Parks, DR, VM Bryan, VT Oi and LA Herzenberg (1979). Antigen-specific identification and cloning of hybridomas with a fluorescence-activated cell sorter. Proc Natl Acad Sci USA **76**, 1962-1966.

MONOCLONAL ANTIBODY THERAPY FOR MURINE LEUKEMIA

Christopher C. Badger and Irwin D. Bernstein

Medical Oncology and Pediatric Oncology Programs
Fred Hutchinson Cancer Research Center
1124 Columbia Street
Seattle, Washington 98104

and

Department of Pediatrics
University of Washington School of Medicine
Seattle, Washington 98195

We have used monoclonal antibodies against the Thy 1.1 differentiation antigen to successfully treat transplanted T cell leukemia (1-3). In these studies, a significant proportion of treated mice were cured by antibody after implantation of up to 3 x 10^5 SL2 leukemia cells. In those studies, the effectiveness of antibody therapy was found to be dependent on antibody isotype, with IgG_{2a} most effective, IgM ineffective, and IgG_3 of intermediate efficacy. We here briefly review our studies on the efficacy of monoclonal antibody therapy using IgG_{2a} anti-Thy 1.1 antibody. Included is a discussion of more recent efforts to identify factors that limit the anti-tumor effect of antibody.

Materials and Methods

Mice and leukemias. AKR/J mice were obtained from Jackson Laboratories. The transplantable AKR/J leukemia was derived from a spontaneous thymoma in an AKR mouse (2). The SL2 cells were maintained *in vitro* and *in vivo* by intraperitoneal inoculation of leukemic spleen cells. SL2 cells express high concentrations of Thy 1.1 both *in vivo* and *in vitro*. Tumors were implanted as single cell suspensions given subcutaneously in a volume of 0.1 ml in the flank.

Hybridomas and monoclonal antibodies. The generation and characterization of the IgG_{2a} monoclonal anti-Thy 1.1 antibody designated 19-E12 have been previously described (2). Hybrid cells secreting 19-E12 antibody were inoculated intraperitoneally into syngeneic (129 x BALB)F_1 mice for the production of hybridomas and ascites fluid that contained high concentrations (5-8 mg/ml) of monoclonal antibody. The concentration of monoclonal antibody in the ascites fluid was estimated by a competition binding assay. The ascites fluid was cytotoxic in the presence of rabbit serum as a source of complement. A titer of 10^{-6} (50% lysis endpoint) was observed against the Thy 1.1 AKR/J thymocytes and SL2 leukemic cells, but not against the Thy 1.2 AKR/Cu thymocytes and SL1 leukemia (titer < 10^{-2}).

Immunofluorescence studies. Cells for immunofluorescence studies were obtained from subcutaneous nodules, spleens, and lymph nodes. Tissue samples were minced in RPMI 1640 supplemented with 5% FCS (5% RPMI) and filtered through 40-μ nylon mesh. Viable cells were isolated on a Ficoll/Hypaque density gradient (Δ = 1.090) and used after being washed in 5% RPMI.

Cells were incubated for 30 min with antibody-containing ascites fluid (at a 1:1000 final dilution) or fluorescein-conjugated antibody in 5% RPMI 1640 at room temperature. The cells were then washed and, in indirect immunofluorescence studies, they were incubated with a 1:40 dilution of an affinity-purified fluorescein-labeled rabbit anti-mouse IgG or IgM serum (Litton Bionetics, Kensington, Md.) for 30 min on ice. We examined cells by flow microfluorometry using the FACS II system (Becton Dickinson) at a rate of 10^3 cells/s.

Effect of Antibody Dose on Therapeutic Effectiveness

Previous studies have demonstrated that IgG_{2a} anti-Thy 1.1 monoclonal antibody (19-E12) could delay the occurrence of systemic disease and prolong survival when up to 3 x 10^6 SL2 leukemia cells were implanted. Complete inhibition of tumor growth at the inoculum site was regularly achieved when mice were challenged with 10^5 but not with 10^6 cells (1-3). In these experiments, doses of 100 μl ascites fluid (containing approximately 0.5 mg antibody) were administered at three- to four-day intervals.

In more recent efforts, we determined the effectiveness of increased amounts of antibody given in a single dose, as well as in multiple doses over time. Animals implanted with 3 x 10^5 cells were treated with a single intravenous infusion of 19-E12 antibody of 100, 300, or 800 μl. The 800-μl dose was more effective than lower doses, curing 100% of animals. Single doses of 100 or 300 μl induced cure in only a portion of treated animals (Table 1).

Subsequently, we examined whether antibody could eliminate more than 3 x 10^5 cells. Animals were implanted with 3 x 10^5, 3 x 10^6, or 3 x 10^7 cells and treated with a relatively large single dose of 900 μl ascites fluid. Additional groups of mice were also treated with a multiple dose schedule consisting of either 100 or 900 μl followed by 50 or 450 μl, respectively, on days 3, 7, 11, and 14. The results demonstrated that treatment of mice challenged with 3 x 10^5 cells with a 900-μl dose with or without additional doses of 450 μl led to cure in 8/10 mice, while treatment with 100 μl cured

Table 1. Effect of antibody dose on 3 x 10^5 cells

AKR/J mice were implanted with 3 x 10^5 SL2 leukemia cells s.c. in the flank. One h later a dose of ascites fluid was infused via the retro-orbital venous plexus. The numerator is the number of animals cured, the denominator the number of animals treated.

Antibody dose	Experiment 1	Experiment 2	Total
0	0/5	0/5	0/10
100 μl	4/5	1/5	5/10
300 μl	2/5	0/5	2/10
800 μl	4/4	5/5	9/0

only 1/5 mice (Table 2). In contrast, when mice were challenged with higher doses of leukemic cells (3 x 10^6 or 3 x 10^7 cells) and treated with any of the antibody regimens, cures were not achieved. However, we did observe an increase in length of survival in the treated mice, and we noted that the increase in mean survival was approximately the same for mice treated with either the lower or the higher antibody dose regimens.

Thus, the maximum number of cells that could be consistently eliminated was 3 x 10^5 SL2 leukemia cells. We therefore asked whether this limitation was due to 1) failure of antibody to reach the subcutaneous implant of tumor, 2) failure of the host to reject antibody-coated tumor cells at the implant site, or 3) alteration in target antigen expression by the tumor cells.

Localization of Antibody *in vivo*

Antibody binding to the surfaces of tumor cells in a subcutaneous nodule was examined by quantitative immunofluorescence tests. Tumor cells (3 x 10^6) were implanted subcutaneously and allowed to grow for approximately two weeks, at which time a palpable subcutaneous nodule was present. A dose of antibody was then infused intravenously, the nodule excised, and viable cells isolated and examined for surface antibody by indirect immunofluorescence using the fluorescence-activated cell sorter. Cells from nodules were first examined at varying time intervals following antibody infusion to determine the time when maximal binding occurred. A typical result obtained from the FACS II is shown in Fig. 1. Binding was found to

Table 2. Effect of antibody therapy on increased cell doses

Animals were implanted with SL2 cells s.c. in the flank and antibody therapy started one h later. Treatment regimens were 100 μl i.v. day 0, then 50 μl i.p. days 3, 7, 11, and 14; 900 μl i.v. day 0; and 900 μl i.v. day 0, then 450 μl i.p. days 3, 7, 11, 14. Three surviving animals in each of the treated groups implanted with 3×10^6 cells were sacrificed on day 26, and two animals in the prolonged regimen groups challenged with 3×10^7 cells were sacrificed on day 20 for cell surface antigen studies. Survival in days (mean ± SD) was calculated from time to death or sacrifice.

	Cell dose					
	3×10^5		3×10^6		3×10^7	
Antibody dose	Cure	Survival	Cure	Survival	Cure	Survival
0	0/5	18 ± 3	0/5	16 ± 2	0/5	15 ± 1
100 then 50	1/5	29 ± 5	0/5	25 ± 3	0/5	22 ± 2
900	4/5	---	0/5	25 ± 3	0/5	25 ± 1
900 then 450	4/5	---	0/5	25 ± 3	0/5	21 ± 2

be maximal 24 h after antibody infusion. After infusion of 100 μl of antibody (approximately 0.5 mg) the mean fluorescence was 29% of that obtained by incubating the same cells with excess amounts of 19-E12 *in vitro*. The amount of antibody present on the cell surface was less at 12 and 48 h. Control tumors from animals infused with an irrelevant antibody did not show surface IgG at any time point.

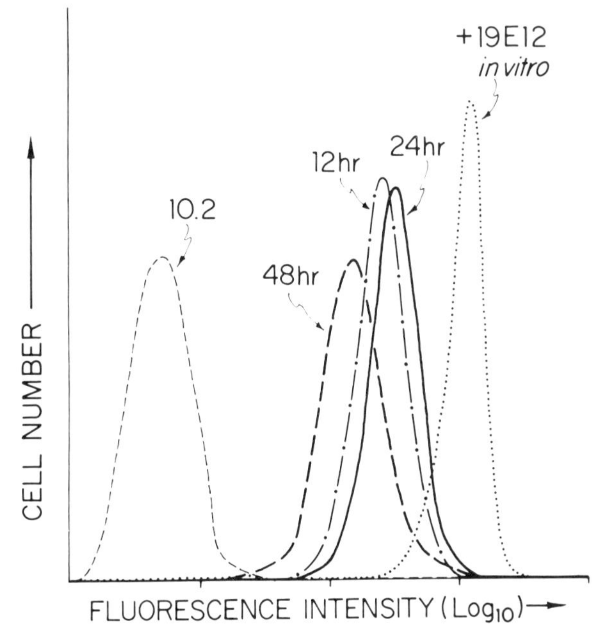

Fig. 1. Kinetics of *in vivo* antibody binding to tumor cell surfaces. Composite of representative FITC-anti-IgG fluorescence histograms from FACS II. AKR/J mice with palpable SL2 tumor nodules (0.5-1.0 cm diameter) given intravenous infusions of 100 μl 19-E12 or 10.2 (an IgG_{2a} antibody of irrelevant specificity) ascites fluid 12, 24, or 48 h prior to analysis. Excised nodules were minced and viable cells isolated on a Ficoll/Hypaque density gradient (Δ = 1.090). Cells were then tested by indirect immunofluorescence after incubation with 1) FITC-rabbit anti-mouse IgG (to determine antibody bound *in vivo*), or 2) 19-E12 ascites fluid (1:1000 dilution) and FITC-rabbit anti-mouse IgG (to determine the maximal amount of antibody that can bind to the cell surface), or 3) FITC-rabbit anti-IgM (to determine non-specific binding). Fluorescence was analyzed with the FACS II. Light scatter (size) patterns in each case demonstrated that a uniform cell population was being analyzed (data not shown). Location of control FITC anti-IgG fluorescence peaks with cells from untreated animals was always within 10% of FITC anti-IgM peaks and at least two orders of magnitude less than 19-E12 + FITC anti-IgG_1 peaks (data not shown).

With this approach, we were able to examine the relationship of the amount of antibody bound to tumor cell surfaces *in vivo* to the amount of antibody that was infused. Doses of 100 μl, 300 μl, or 800 μl of ascites fluid were infused into tumor-bearing mice, and the nodules were excised and examined at 24 h. Increased doses of antibody were associated with greater amounts of tumor cell surface antibody. Cells from the tumor nodule in animals given 100 μl showed that infused antibody coated 27% of available Thy 1.1 sites, 300 μl coated 51% of the sites, while 800 μl led to complete saturation of all Thy 1.1 sites. Thus, there appeared to be limited diffusion of antibody into the subcutaneous tumor, with very high doses of antibody required to achieve saturation of antigenic sites on the tumor cell surface.

Antigenic Nature of Cells Escaping Antibody Therapy

The probability that antigenic alterations limited the effectiveness of antibody has been previously discussed (3). In those experiments, animals were implanted with 3 x 10^6 SL2 cells and then treated with 100 μl on day zero followed by 50 μl every three-four days continuously. Animals were sacrificed when they developed enlarged spleens. Both spleen and subcutaneous nodule cells were isolated, and the expression of Thy 1.1, as well as of unrelated $H\text{-}2^k$ and gp70 antigens, was examined by immunofluorescence. Leukemic cells present in the spleen uniformly failed to express Thy 1.1, while $H\text{-}2^k$ and gp70 continued to be expressed at levels comparable to those in control tumors. The loss of Thy 1.1 appeared to have resulted from selection of metastatic variants as these cells failed to express Thy 1.1 after several *in vivo* passages in untreated mice. Thus, the metastatic disease in antibody-treated mice was due to antigen-negative variants.

When the tumor nodule at the implant site was similarly examined, a contrasting result was found, as the cells isolated from the nodule continued to express Thy 1.1 in levels comparable to those in control tumors. Indirect immunofluorescence demonstrated only small amounts of surface antibody, suggesting that the low dose, continuous antibody regimen did not produce high antibody levels in subcutaneous tissue.

Since a larger single dose of antibody had proven more effective in treating animals than the multiple lower doses used in the above experiments, it was possible that the persistence of antigen-positive cells in the nodule resulted from insufficient antibody at the site of implantation. Therefore, we repeated immunofluorescence studies in animals implanted with 3 x 10^6 cells and treated with either 100 or 900 μl ascites fluid followed by 50 or 450 μl, respectively, on days 3,

7, 11, and 14. Thirteen days after the last dose of antibody, when the animals had developed significant metastatic disease, the mice were sacrificed. An examination of the cell surface Thy 1.1 expression by the metastatic tumor cells in the spleens from treated mice demonstrated a failure of these cells to express the target antigen. This was true for mice treated with either the higher or lower dose regimen. Furthermore, tumor cells present in the subcutaneous nodule continued to express Thy 1.1 and had demonstrable surface antibody. In the animals treated with the higher dose regimen, 87% of the tumor cell surface Thy 1.1 sites were coated with antibody almost two weeks following the last dose of antibody. Thus, local failure resulted from persistence of antigen-positive cells even though high levels of antibody on the cell surface were maintained for prolonged periods. Antigen-bearing cells, however, were prevented from metastasizing by all the antibody regimens studied.

Discussion

To eliminate tumor cells, antibody must first bind to the tumor cell surface and then cooperate with host effector mechanisms, presumably effector cells (4-5). Thus, antibody might be expected to be more effective against intravascular tumor where the antibody-coated cells are exposed to Fc receptor-bearing cells in spleen, liver, and lymph nodes. In contrast, antibody might be expected to be less effective against extravascular tumor where smaller numbers of effector cells may have access to the tumor. Further, it can be expected that larger doses of antibody would be needed to coat antigenic sites on extravascular tumor cells rather than on metastasizing intravascular tumor cells. The results described in this report are consistent with these suggestions.

Achieving levels of antibody sufficient to saturate surface binding sites of subcutaneous tumor cells required infusion of approximately 5 mg antibody per animal, and this amount of antibody was needed to achieve maximum cure of mice challenged with 3 x 10^5 leukemic cells. Thus, it is important in antibody treatment to achieve high initial levels of antibody at the site of implantation.

Although amounts of antibody that would saturate the target antigen sites on the subcutaneous tumor cells could be achieved, only a maximum of 3 x 10^5 cells could be eliminated. This limitation presumably resulted from inadequate participation of host lytic mechanisms because cells growing locally were coated with antibody. Failure of cellular mechanisms may have been due to poor access to the subcutaneous site, insufficient total numbers of effector cells, or to a combination of both factors. These results are similar to those obtained using antiserum (4-6).

Antibody was very effective in preventing antigen-bearing cells from metastasizing even with relatively low doses of antibody. This presumably resulted from better access of effector mechanisms. Presumably, the emergence of antigen-negative variants can be reduced by treating mice with combinations of antibodies against different cell surface antigens expressed by the leukemic cells.

The collective results of these studies suggest that antibody therapy will be most useful in the treatment of small numbers of tumor cells that remain following conventional chemotherapy. Thus, it may provide a nontoxic method of eliminating the cells remaining after surgery and/or chemotherapy. In contrast, elimination of larger tumor burdens will require that antibody be used as a delivery system for toxic agents that will circumvent the requirement for participation of host effector mechanisms.

Acknowledgments

These studies were supported in part by Grants CA 09319 and CA 26386 from the National Institutes of Health.

References

1. Bernstein, ID, MR Tam and RC Nowinski (1980). Mouse leukemia: Therapy with monoclonal antibodies against a thymus differentiation antigen. Science **207**, 68-71.
2. Bernstein, ID, RC Nowinski, MR Tam, B McMaster, LL Houston and EA Clark (1980). Monoclonal antibody therapy of mouse leukemia. **In** Monoclonal Antibodies, pp 275-291. RH Kennett, TJ McKearn and KB Bechtol, eds. Plenum Press, New York.
3. Bernstein, ID, and RC Nowinski (in press). Monoclonal antibody treatment of transplanted and spontaneous murine leukemia. **In** Hybridomas in the Diagnosis and Treatment of Cancer. M Mitchell and H Oettgen, eds. Raven Press, New York.
4. Shin, HS, M Hayden, S Landley, N Kaliss and MR Smith (1975). Antibody-mediated suppression of grafted lymphoma. III. Evaluation of the role of thymic function, non-thymus-derived lymphocytes, macrophages, platelets, and polymorphonuclear leukocytes in syngeneic and allogeneic hosts. J Immunol **114**, 1255-1263.
5. Langlois, AJ, T Matthews, GJ Roloson, H-J Thiel, JJ Collins and DP Bolognes (1981). Immunologic control of the ascites form of murine adenocarcinoma 755. V. Antibody-directed macrophages mediate tumor cell destruction. J Immunol **126**, 2337-2341.
6. Shin, HS, JS Economou, GR Pasternack, RJ Johnson and ML Hayden (1976). Antibody-mediated suppression of grafted lymphoma. IV. Influence of time of tumor residency in vivo and tumor size upon the effectiveness of suppression by syngeneic antibody. J Exp Med **144**, 1274-1283.

TARGETING IN ERYTHROLEUKEMIC MICE: RADIOIODINATED AND CHELATED RADIOMETAL-CONJUGATED MONOCLONAL ANTIBODY

David A. Scheinberg and Mette Strand

Department of Pharmacology and Experimental Therapeutics
The Johns Hopkins University School of Medicine
Baltimore, Maryland 21205

and

Otto Gansow

Department of Chemistry
Michigan State University
East Lansing, Michigan 48824

In 1962, Frank Rauscher described an erythroblastic leukemia of mice characterized by a rapid and dramatic splenomegaly occurring within one to two weeks after the onset of the disease (1). The disease is caused by the Rauscher leukemia virus (RLV), an enveloped RNA tumor virus that buds from the surface of the infected, leukemic cells. The major envelope protein of the virion is a 70,000-dalton glycoprotein, gp70 (2), which is expressed in large amounts on the cell surface of the leukemic cells. A similar protein is expressed in small amounts on the surface of normal lymphoid and epithelial tissues of mice (3). Using the Rauscher leukemia as a model system and the Rauscher gp70 as the target antigen, we have investigated the potential diagnostic and therapeutic applications of a leukemic cell-specific monoclonal antibody.

The purified RLV gp70 (4) was used as an antigen for preparing a library of monoclonal antibodies. One of these hybridomas, 103A, produced an IgG-1 antibody specific for the Rauscher leukemia virus. The antibody also reacted with another largely homologous virus, the Friend leukemia virus. The IgG-1 immunoglobulin produced by the P3x63Ag8 myeloma cells was used as a control in all experiments.

Antibody Specificity

The specificity of the monoclonal antibodies was determined by direct and indirect binding to viruses using solid phase radioimmunoassays (5). The 103A demonstrated near maximal binding to the RLV and Friend leukemia viruses at dilutions in excess of 1:20,000 but did not bind to several other murine ecotropic or xenotropic viruses or to Feline leukemia virus even at low dilutions. The P3 immunoglobulin showed no binding to any of these viruses, at any dilution.

The cell specificity was determined by direct binding of ^{125}I-labeled 103A and P3 papain fragments to 2 x 10^6 live or glutaraldehyde-fixed cells (6) (Fig. 1). 103A bound to Rauscher leukemia cells, Friend leukemia cells and RLV-infected fibroblasts but did not bind to normal fibroblasts, splenocytes or thymocytes. The P3 immunoglobulin bound to none of the cells.

The binding of 103A to the virus-infected cells was specific and saturable as shown by competition assays (Fig. 2A). Unlabeled 103A completely competed for binding of the labeled 103 to leukemic cells, whereas P3 immunoglobulin showed no competition. Binding was also cell concentration-dependent (Fig. 2B).

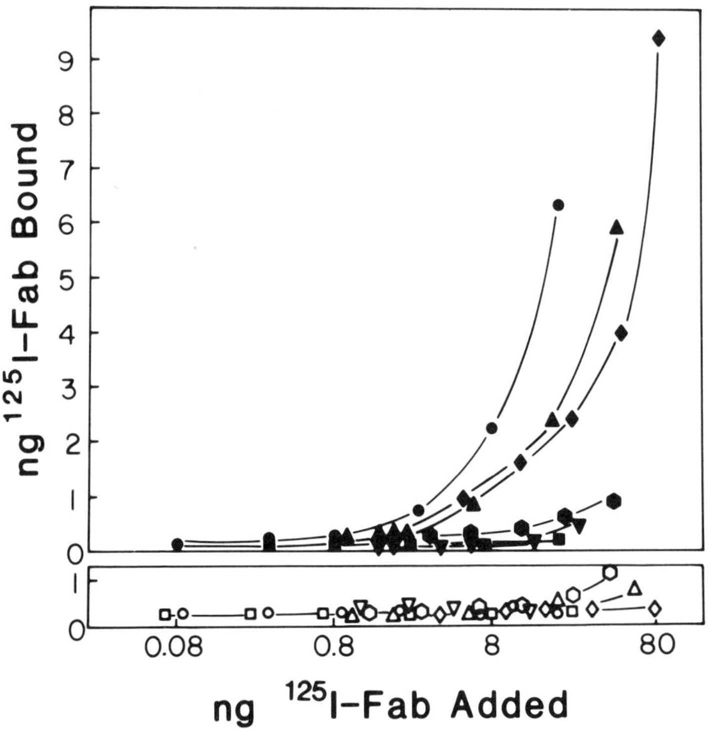

Fig. 1. Direct cell binding of ^{125}I-labeled papain fragments. Radioiodinated antibody fragments (5 μCi/μg) were incubated with 2 x 10^6 live or glutaraldehyde-fixed cells in 80 μl phosphate buffered saline (PBS) containing 0.1% bovine serum albumin (BSA). After 1 h at 4°C, cells were washed three times in the same buffer and the bound radiolabeled antibody was determined. Solid symbols: 103A; open symbols: P3. ● O, RLV-infected JLS-V9 cells; ▲ △, Friend erythroleukemia cells F4-6; ◆ ◇, Rauscher erythroleukemia cells; ■ □, BALB/3T3 cells; ▼ ▽, normal BALB/c spleen cells; ⬢ ⬡, normal BALB/c thymocytes. Details of all materials and methods in this paper are described elsewhere (11).

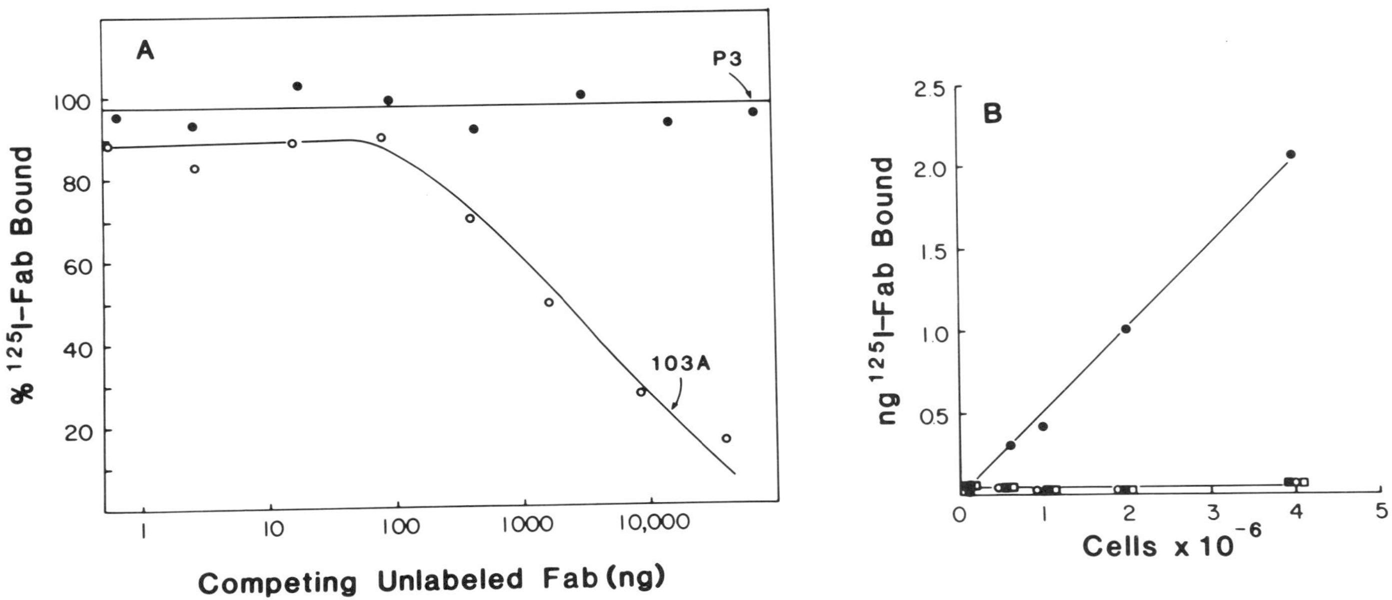

Fig. 2. Specificity of binding of ^{125}I-103A papain fragments to infected cells. (A) Specific competition by unlabeled 103A but not by unlabeled P3, for binding of 103A to RLV-infected JLS-V9 cells. Six ng of ^{125}I-103A (5 μCi/μg) was incubated with 2 x 10^6 RLV-infected JLS-V9 cells in the presence of a serial dilution of either unlabeled 103A O or unlabeled P3 ● as indicated. Binding was determined as in Fig. 1. (B) Cell concentration-dependence of binding. Binding of 9 ng of ^{125}I-103A or ^{125}I-P3 papain fragments to varying concentrations of cells as indicated. 103A ● and P3 O binding to RLV (JSL-V9) cells. 103A ■ and P3 □ binding to BALB/3T3 cells.

Targeting *In Vivo*

Since the binding of 103A showed complete specificity for leukemic cells *in vitro*, we investigated whether similar results could be obtained *in vivo*. Mice with advanced splenomegaly were injected intraperitoneally with ^{125}I-labeled IgG or papain fragments. Twenty to 24 h later these mice were sacrificed, their spleen cells isolated, and the amount of bound antibody per cell determined (Fig. 3).

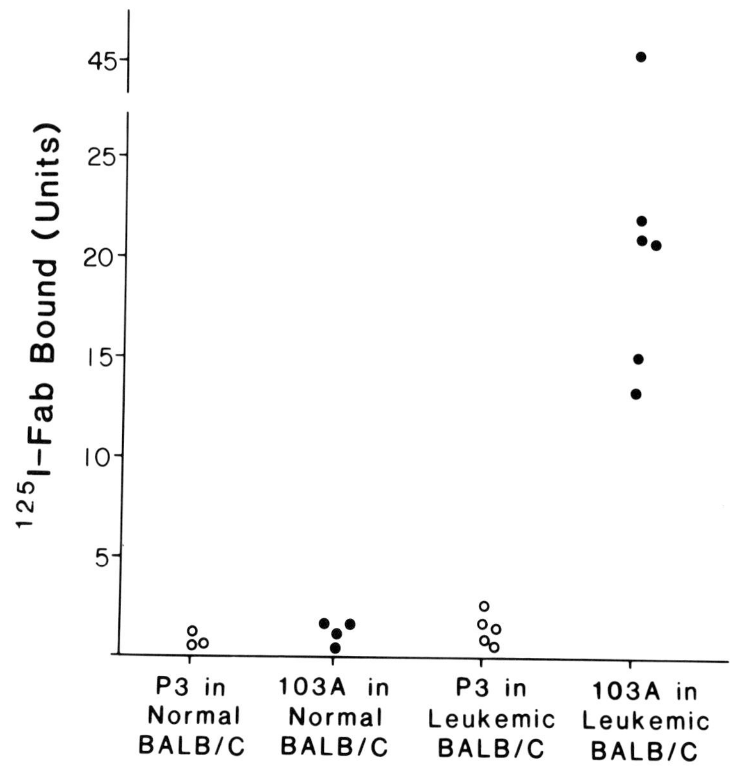

Fig. 3. Binding of ^{125}I-labeled papain fragments to spleen cells *in vivo* at 20 and 24 h after injection. P3 O, 103A ●. In order to compare results from different experiments, all data were normalized. One unit equals the mean of the binding of the P3 to 10^8 normal spleen cells, which ranged from 250–1000 cpm bound/10^8 cells. Normal spleens contained 10^8 cells and leukemic spleens 6–10 x 10^8 cells. Mice were injected with antibody intraperitoneally. Spleen cells were isolated from sacrificed mice and washed three times in PBS containing 0.1% BSA. The amount of ^{125}I-labeled antibody bound to 10^8 spleen cells was determined by counting the cells in a Coulter counter and measuring the radioactivity in an LKB γ counter.

There was no significant binding to normal spleen cells by either of the immunoglobulins, nor did P3 bind to leukemic spleen cells. In contrast, 103A showed significant binding to the leukemic spleen cells. We also isolated the thymocytes of these mice to examine the extent of binding of the antibodies to this organ. The 103A bound to thymocytes of leukemic mice, although the total amount bound was three times less than to the spleen cells. P3 did not bind to thymocytes of leukemic mice, and neither of the antibodies bound to thymocytes from uninfected mice.

The same data can be expressed as uptake ratios, that is, the binding of the antibody to leukemic cells in the live animals divided by the binding to analogous cells from uninfected animals (Table 1). At 20 to 24 h, the uptake ratios for both the papain fragments and the intact IgGs were about 20. Uptake ratios decreased greatly with time, ranging from 70 at 7 h after injection, to 20 at 24 h after injection, to less than 10 at 48 h after injection. The tumor specificity of this antibody indicated by such large uptake ratios suggested that diagnostic studies would be feasible in this model system, since polyclonal sera with uptake ratios as low as 4-5 have been reported to give reasonable scans of tumors in humans (8).

Table 1. Uptake ratios[a] of ^{125}I-labeled P3 and 103A in BALB/c mice[b]

	Papain fragments	Intact IgGs
P3	0.9 ± 0.4	1.9 ± 0.1
103A	23.2 ± 4.0	19.5 ± 1.5

[a]binding to leukemic cells/binding to normal cells.

[b]Data derived from experiments conducted as described in Fig. 3

[c]Mean ± SE in 4-8 mice.

Curative Monoclonal Antibody Therapy

Since the 103A bound only to infected cells expressing the target antigen, therapeutic treatments using this antibody should be expected to spare all normal cells. Therapy using antibody 103A was studied by treating leukemic mice with antibody. The course of the disease could be rapidly assayed by counting the 1-mm spleen tumor foci at 8 days after virus inoculation (9,10) or by weighing the spleens at 20 days. Spleen tumor foci represent clones of leukemic cells derived from a single virus infection on day 0. Foci are best visualized 7-9 days after infection following fixation in Bouin's solution. Normal mouse spleens weigh 100-150 mg, whereas the leukemic spleens weigh 1-1.5 g at 20 days. The experimental protocol was to inject mice intravenously at day 0 with approximately 20-30 focus-forming units of virus, which was enough to cause a 1000%-increase in spleen size at day 20. This virus inoculation was more than 100 times the dose necessary to cause leukemia in these mice. A single dose of antibody was injected at 72 h. This time span was selected to allow sufficient time for the onset of leukemia. Mice were sacrificed for assay at both day 8 and day 20.

The antibody was extremely potent. Animals were cured by a single dose of 5 μg or larger (Fig. 4). At these antibody concentrations, both the number of spleen foci on day 8 or the spleen weight on day 20 were reduced to normal levels. There is a sharp threshold of effectiveness at 1-2 μg. The 50%-effective dose was about 1.5 μg. The P3 IgG and the Fab'2 fragment of 103A (not shown) had no therapeutic effect. Therapeutic effects could be obtained at later times, although larger amounts of antibody were required.

What is most striking is that the monoclonal antibody behaved exactly like a drug: It has a defined chemical structure, and it had reproducible pharmacokinetics *in vivo*. The main advantage of this drug was its nearly absolute specificity; little was wasted on irrelevant tissues.

Antibody Conjugate Therapy: ^{131}I-103A IgG

The dose-response curve can be used as a baseline to investigate whether drugs, toxins, or cytotoxic radioisotopes conjugated to the antibody could enhance its therapeutic effects. In addition, the potency of each targetable agent could be compared quantitatively. As an antibody conjugate becomes more potent, the dose-response curve should shift to the left.

Antibody conjugated to beta particle-emitting radioisotopes was compared to unlabeled antibody for therapeutic potency. Iodine-131 was chosen because it is readily coupled to IgG. In addition, ^{131}I-labeled polyclonal antisera have been reported by Bale, Order, and others to have therapeutic effects against solid tumors (11,12). We investigated whether similar results could be obtained against the Rauscher leukemia using antibody 103A. Leukemic mice were injected with ^{131}I-labeled 103A IgG as described above. As a control, equal amounts of unlabeled antibody were injected into additional mice. Doses of antibody were in the ascending linear part of the dose-response curve. The ^{131}I-labeled antibody was no more potent than the unlabeled antibody as measured by both spleen foci and spleen size. It is possible that in this model system, unlike the

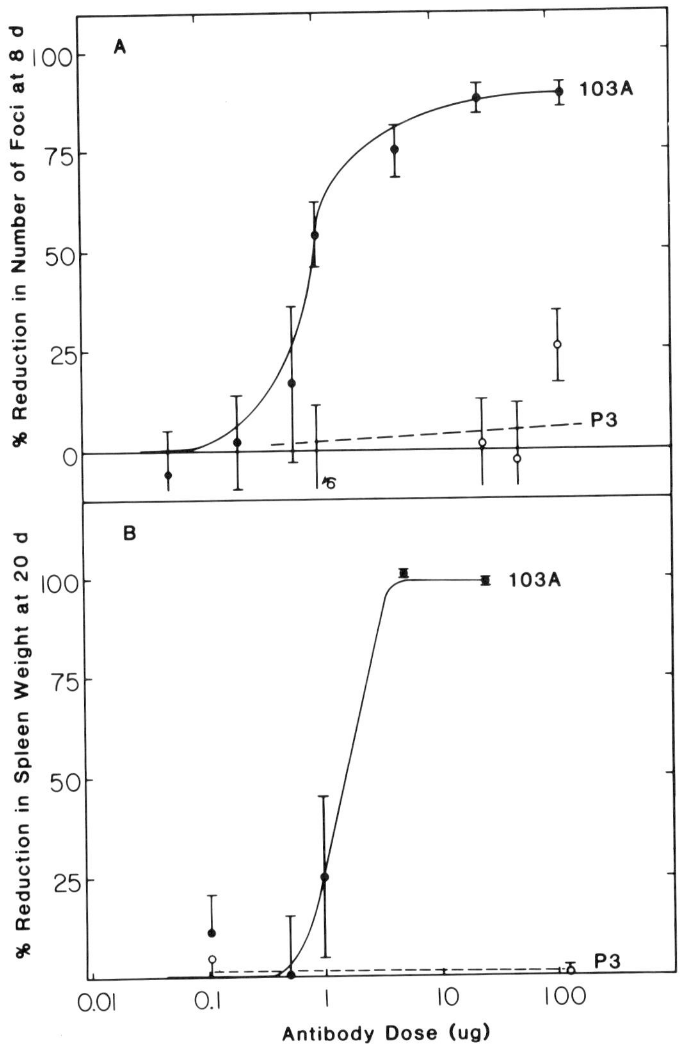

Fig. 4. Dose-response curve for immunotherapy of Rauscher erythroleukemia in BALB/c mice. Experiments were conducted as described in the text using a single dose of antibody intraperitoneally 72 h after RLV infection. P3 IgG (O----O) and 103A IgG (●——●) are shown. Each point represents the mean ± SE of 6-9 mice. Infected but untreated mice were used in each experiment as controls. (A) Therapeutic response was measured as the percent reduction from control spleen foci: 100% reduction was no foci; 0% reduction was 20-30 foci depending on the experimental group. (B) Therapeutic response was measured as the percent reduction from control spleen weight: 100% reduction was a normal spleen 100-150 mg; 0% reduction was a 1-1.5 g spleen, depending on the experimental group. Experiments were conducted as described in the text using a single dose of antibody intraperitoneally 72 h after RLV infection.

situation with large solid tumors, ^{131}I was not effective. Beta particles emitted from this isotope may have effects only in large tumors where a sufficient concentration of emission can be obtained.

Bifunctional Radiometal Chelates

Some of the most versatile alternatives for labeling antibodies include the bifunctional metal chelates (Fig. 5) that are covalently attached to the antibody by a sidearm. The substituted cryptates, recently described by Otto Gansow et al. (13), are the most complicated chemically but can potentially carry the most lethal radioisotopes, including metals of the lanthanide and actinide series. Targeted, chelated isotopes of this class could emit extremely high-energy alpha particles or even undergo nuclear fission on the tumor cell surface. A simpler bifunctional chelate based on EDTA would allow the targeting of somewhat more benign isotopes, including the group III A and the transition metals. The diethylene triamine pentaacetic acid (DPTA) class, based on pentaacetic acid, is similar to the EDTA group. Edgar Haber and coworkers have investigated this group of agents coupled to polyclonal antibodies (14).

The chelatable radiometals that have suitable characteristics include gallium-67 and -68, scandium-47, technetium-99m, and indium-111. All have short half lives, from 68 min to 3.2 days, that spare the patient large doses of radiation, and all are bound to EDTA with stability constants of 10^{-24} or more. ^{67}Ga, ^{68}Ga, ^{99m}Tc, and ^{111}In are ideal for scanning because they emit low energy gamma radiation or positrons. Scandium-47, which emits beta particles, is possibly useful for therapy.

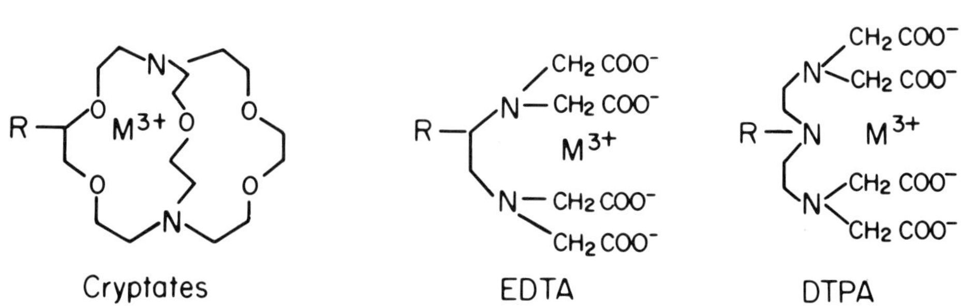

Fig. 5. Three bifunctional metal chelates: substituted cryptates (13); bifunctional EDTA (15) and diethylenetriamine pentaacetic acid (14).

Typical alpha emitters that might be bound by the chelates are radium-224, lead-212, bismuth-212, and actinium-225. In comparing beta emitters such as ^{47}Sc and ^{131}I, with an alpha particle emitter, two points are important. First, the energy released is 10 times higher with an alpha emitter, and second, the pathlengths of the alpha particles are 50 times shorter. The distance a beta particle travels is 1-2 mm in tissues, whereas an alpha particle will travel only 20-60 microns. Thus, the effect of the released energy of these larger particles is many hundreds of times greater and is restricted to the area of the targeted tumor cell. Beta particles may damage normal tissue surrounding a targeted tumor. ^{224}Ra is especially useful because it decays through four additional daughter nuclides of relatively short half life, each of which emits a high-energy alpha particle. Thus, the delivery of a single radium atom to a tumor cell mass may kill more than one cell.

Targeting of Radioiometal Chelate-Conjugated Monoclonal Antibody

For initial studies of radiometal-conjugated monoclonal antibody we have attached an EDTA-based chelate to antibody 103A for use in the Rauscher leukemia model system. The synthesis of the bifunctional EDTA chelate was based on the method of Meares and his coworkers (15). This chelate was attached to the 103A antibody as follows: The chelate containing iron, trace labeled with ^{59}Fe, was coupled to the antibody, using carbodiimide to yield a molar ratio of approximately one chelate per antibody. The iron was then removed by ascorbate reduction and dialysis in the presence of EDTA. The conjugate was labeled with high specific-activity ^{67}Ga or ^{111}In and tested for binding activity *in vitro* and *in vivo*.

In solid phase radioimmunoassays ^{111}In-labeled 103A bound specifically with high titer to the RLV, as had the ^{125}I-labeled 103A. ^{111}In-labeled P3 showed no binding. The specificity to leukemia cells also remained intact (Fig. 6). The 103A bound to the erythroleukemia cells but not to control leukemia cells, and the P3 bound to none of the cells. The effect of the chelate on the biological activity of the antibodies *in vivo* was tested by directly comparing the spleen targeting of chelate-conjugated and -unconjugated antibodies that had been labeled with ^{125}I. No difference in uptake ratio was observed between chelate-conjugated and underivatized antibodies. Therefore, the conjugation protocol did not alter the biological activity and specificity of the antibodies *in vitro* or *in vivo*. Finally, ^{111}In-labeled 103A showed specific targeting to the leukemic spleens, as had the ^{125}I-labeled 103A.

We have begun preliminary experiments to examine the diagnostic potential of these radiometal chelate-conjugated antibodies. Normal and leukemic mice were injected intravenously with ^{111}In-labeled

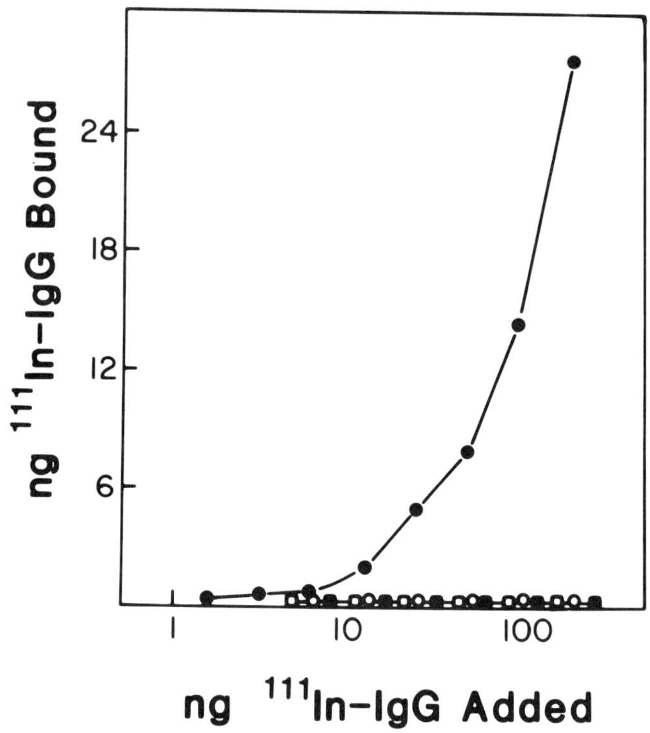

Fig. 6. Direct cell binding of ^{111}In-labeled 103A and P3; analysis was conducted as described in Fig. 1. The specific activity of the ^{111}chelate-conjugated monoclonal antibody 103A was 0.25 μCi/μg, closed symbols; and P3, 0.13 μCi/μg, open symbols. Binding to Friend erythroleukemia cells, ● O; binding to P3653 myeloma cells, ■ □.

103A IgG. At 1, 3, and 5 h after the injections of the labeled antibody, gamma-camera images were made of the animals. All exposures were identical and are photographs of the actual images without subtraction or enhancement (Fig. 7). In the normal mouse the labeled antibody initially showed a distribution similar to that in the blood. The lungs, heart, liver, spleen, and bladder were visible. With increasing time, the distribution of label became more diffuse, and no specific organ appeared to be labeled. The spleen of this mouse was isolated, and the specific activity was determined. The spleen weighed 150 mg or 0.7% of the mouse weight; 66,000 cpm, or 0.7% of the injected labeled antibody, was recovered in the spleen. Therefore, the distribution of the antibody in the normal mouse was random.

In the leukemic mice, the infected spleens were visible at 60 min and became even more distinct with time. The true anatomical locations as well as the radioactivity per gram of all of the spleens were verified upon autopsy. As indicated in the images, the 8-day spleen was located laterally, and the 20-day spleen filled most of the abdomen. The spleen of the 8-day leukemic animal weighed 350 mg or 1.7% of total body weight; 1.1 x 10^6 cpm or 11% of the injected dose was recovered in this spleen. This was a remarkable finding since such imaging *in vivo* is complicated by shed antigen in the form of virus particles, viral antigen on other infected tissues such as the thymus and liver, and the continuous metabolism and clearance of the antibodies. The P3 immunoglobulin labeled with ^{67}Ga showed only diffuse labeling similar to the normal mouse injected with 103A (data

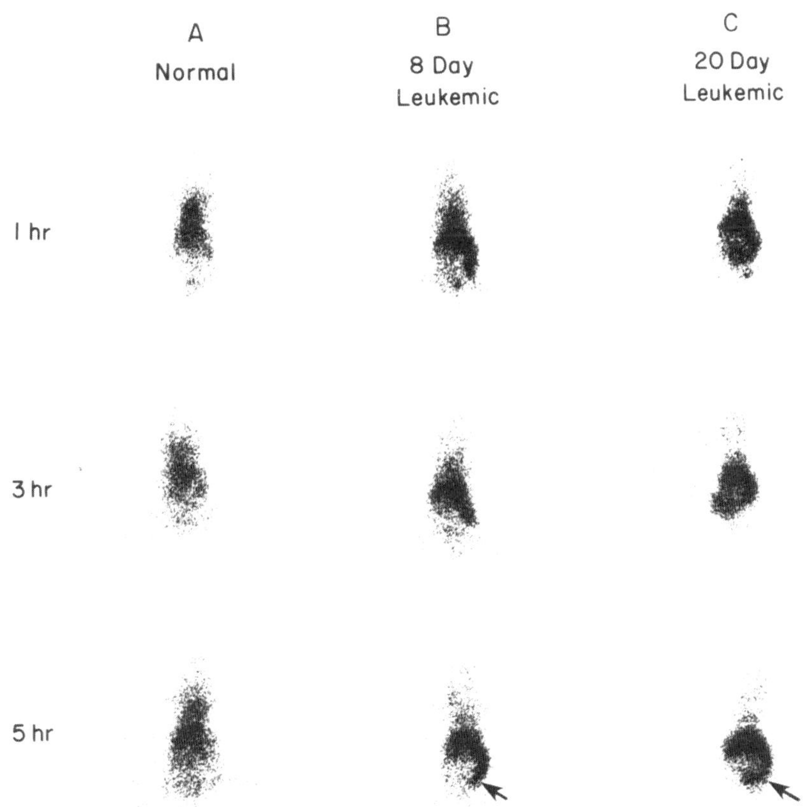

Fig. 7. Photographs of gamma-camera scans of normal and leukemic BALB/c mice injected with ^{111}In-103A. Mice are shown lying on their backs, their heads at the top, their spleens on the right. All scans contain 1.5 x 10^4 recorded disintegrations. Column A is a normal mouse; B, a mouse with leukemia for 8 days; C, a mouse with leukemia for 20 days. Rows 1, 2, and 3 are scans made at 1, 3, and 5 h after injection of the labeled antibody. Arrows point to spleens.

not shown). When injected alone, ^{111}In was taken up in small amounts in several organs, but there was no specific uptake in leukemic as compared to normal spleens. As expected, ^{111}In-chelate was very rapidly cleared following injection and was not detected in any organ. In summary, these results showed high resolution imaging, capable of distinguishing tumor masses as small as 350 mgs, without subtraction or enhancement using radiometal-chelated conjugated monoclonal antibodies. Moreover, this technique may allow conjugation of lethal radioisotopes, perhaps with better than single-hit cytotoxicity, to a targetable antibody and thus is a potentially powerful new therapeutic tool.

Acknowledgments

We thank A. George for excellent technical assistance, J. Gobel, National Institutes of Health, for help with the nuclear images, Dr. J. Klein for iodine-131, and L. Cumor for typing of the manuscript. This research was supported by National Cancer Institute contract NO181052. D.A. Scheinberg was supported by National Institutes of Health Medical Scientists Training Grant GM07309.

References

1. Rauscher, FJ (1962). A virus-induced disease of mice characterized by erythrocytopoiesis and lymphoid leukemia. J Natl Cancer Inst **29**, 515-543.
2. Strand, M, and JT August (1973). Structural proteins of oncogenic ribonucleic acid viruses. J Biol Chem **248**, 5627-5633.
3. Lerner, RA, CB Wilson, BC Del Villani, PJ McConahey and FJ Dixon (1976). Endogenous oncornaviral gene expression in adult and fetal mice: Quantitative, histologic, and physiologic studies of the major viral glycoprotein, gp70. J Exp Med **143**, 151-166.
4. Strand, M, and JT August (1976). Structural proteins of ribonucleic acid tumor viruses. Purification of envelope core and internal components. J Biol Chem **251**, 559-564.
5. Mariuzza, R, and M Strand (1981). Chemical basis for diversity in antibody specificity analyzed by hapten binding to monoclonal anti-4-hydroxy-3-nitrophenacetyl (NP) immunoglobulins. Mol Immunol **40**, 847-855.
6. Strand, M (1980). Transformation-related antigens identified by monoclonal antibodies. Proc Natl Acad Sci USA **77**, 3234-3238.
7. Scheinberg, DA, and M Strand (1982). Leukemic cell targeting and therapy by monoclonal antibody. Cancer Res **42.**
8. Mach, J-P, S Carrel, M Forni, J Ritschard, A Donath and P Alberto (1980). Tumor localization of radiolabeled antibodies against carcinoembryonic antigen in patients with carcinoma. N Engl J Med **303**, 5-10.
9. Axelrad, AA, and RA Steeves (1964). Assay for Friend leukemia virus: Rapid quantitative method based on enumeration of macroscopic spleen foci in mice. Virology **24**, 513-518.

10. Pluznik, DH, and L Sachs (1964). Quantitation of a murine leukemia virus with a spleen colony assay. J Natl Cancer Inst **33**, 535-546.
11. Bale, WF, MA Countreras and ED Grady (1980). Factors influencing localization of labeled antibodies in tumors. Cancer Res **40**, 2965-2972.
12. Order, SE, JL Klein, P Alderson, S Siegelman and P Leichner (1980). Use of isotopic immunoglobulin in therapy. Cancer Res **40**, 3001-3007.
13. Gansow, OA, AR Kausar and K Triplett (1981). Synthesis and characterization of some bifunctional 2β:2:1 cryptands. J Heterocycl Chem **18**, 297-303.
14. Khaw, BA, JT Fallon, HW Strauss and E Haber (1980). Myocardial infarct imaging of antibodies to canine cardiac myosin with indium-111-diethylenetriamine pentaacetic acid. Science **209**, 295-296.
15. Yeh, SM, DG Sherman and CF Meares (1979). A new route to "bifunctional" chelating agents: conversion of amino acids to analogs of ethylenedinitrilotetraacetic acid. Anal Biochem **100**, 152-159.

SELECTIVE KILLING OF LEUKEMIA CELLS BY ANTIBODY-TOXIN CONJUGATES

Jonathan W. Uhr, Keith A. Krolick, and
Ellen S. Vitetta

Department of Microbiology
University of Texas Southwestern Medical School
Dallas, Texas 75235

We have exploited the demonstration that the idiotype (Id) of a cell surface Ig of a B cell tumor represents a clonally-expressed tumor-specific marker (1). We have conjugated the A chain of the plant toxin, Ricin, to affinity-purified anti-Id and have attempted to kill murine neoplastic B lymphocytes with such conjugates. These studies have utilized the BCL_1 tumor, which resembles the prolymphocytic variant of human chronic lymphocytic leukemia (CLL) (2-5). The malignant cells are of B cell origin and bear immunoglobulin (Ig) on their surface. The tumor grows primarily in the spleen and blood of recipients, and invasion of the bone marrow occurs late in the course of the disease (2). Depending on the number of tumor cells injected, recipient mice survive for three to five months.

In the first series of experiments, tumor cells were treated *in vitro* with an anti-Id covalently coupled to A chain (anti-Id-A chain). The preservation of antibody activity and the presence of A chain in these conjugates were established by a solid-phase radioimmunoassay (RIA). Antibody-A chain conjugates were reacted with antigen (BCL_1 Ig or OVA), and the presence of antibody or A chain was subsequently demonstrated by binding of radiolabeled antibodies against the rabbit Ig or the ricin A chain. The results of treating BCL_1 cells and normal splenocytes with such conjugates are shown in Fig. 1. Protein synthesis was irreversibly inhibited in the BCL_1 cells that were killed (6). The specificity of the inhibition was firmly established by the lack of effect of the control conjugates on BCL_1 cells and the lack of effect of anti-Id-A chain conjugates on normal splenocytes. Hence, *in vitro*, anti-Id-A chain conjugates can kill neoplastic B cells that bear the corresponding Id specificity.

In the above experiments, the inhibition of protein synthesis correlated well with the percentage of tumor cells in the treated population. However, since injection of only 10 BCL_1 cells into normal BALB/c mice will cause tumor (2), the adoptive transfer assay represents a more sensitive measurement of the number of residual viable tumor cells in a treated cell population. For such experiments, an affinity-purified polyvalent rabbit anti-mouse Ig (RAMIg) that binds to both the BCL_1 tumor cells and to normal B cells (7) was used. Spleen cells from BCL_1-bearing mice were treated with an optimal concentration of the specific (RAMIg-A) or control (RαOVA-A) antibody conjugate (8). Approximately 80% of the spleen cells were tumor cells as judged by morphology and by immunofluorescent analysis following staining with anti-BCL_1 Id. After treatment, 10^4 cells were injected into normal BALB/c mice. A group of mice also received untreated cells. At 6 and 12 weeks after adoptive transfer, recipient mice were sacrificed and examined for tumor cells in the spleen and for leukemia. Untreated cells, or cells treated with the control conjugate, caused significant tumor. Animals receiving the cells treated with RAMIg-A chain had a concentration of Id^+ cells just above the level of control staining, and the number of Id^+ cells did not increase between 6 and 12 weeks. Furthermore, WBC in the blood of RAMIg-A chain-treated mice never exceeded levels observed in normal mice (5-10 x 10^6/ml). Therefore, it is probable that

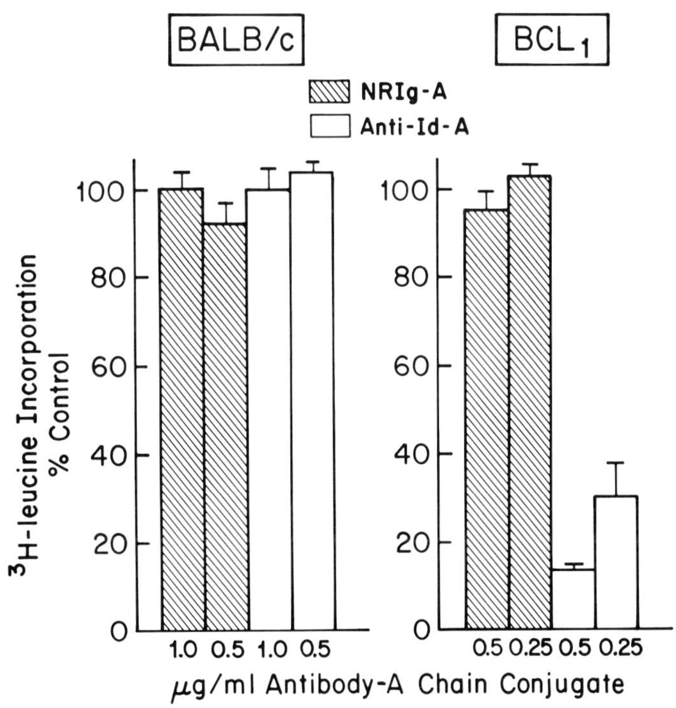

Fig. 1. Inhibition of protein synthesis in BCL_1 tumor cells by affinity-purified anti-Id-A chain. BALB/c spleen cells (2 x 10^5) were pulsed for 15-30 min with various concentrations of anti-Id-A chain at 4°C, washed, and then cultured in triplicate for two days in the presence of LPS at 50 μg/ml. Cultures received 1 μCi of ^3H leucine, were incubated an additional 14-16 h, and were then harvested and analyzed for incorporation of leucine into protein. Hatched bars, NRIg-A; empty bars, anti-Id-A (6).

treated animals contained no viable tumor cells, although the possibility exists that growth of a small number of tumor cells was inhibited by an immune response transferred with the treated splenocytes. Adoptive transfer experiments using *untreated* tumor cells have shown that, 12 weeks after transfer of tumor cells, all the animals receiving 10 tumor cells and 20% of the animals receiving 1 tumor cell have overt tumor. Based on these results, we estimate that the animals injected with spleen cells treated with RAMIg-A chain received less than 10 viable tumor cells. Thus, when an inoculum of 10^4 tumor cells was used, at least 99.9% of the cells were eliminated.

One approach (9) to management of patients with disseminated neoplasia involves removal of bone marrow before the patient is treated with supralethal doses of chemotherapy and/or radiotherapy to kill all tumor cells, followed by administration of the autologous bone marrow to reconstitute the hemopoietic system. One major problem with this approach is that the bone marrow may contain tumor cells. To surmount this problem, we have applied the antibody-A chain technique to treat marrow cells from BCL_1-bearing mice in order to eliminate tumor cells. The marrow from animals with advanced tumors contains about 10-20% tumor cells (1). As shown in Fig. 2, the transfer of untreated or RαOVA-A chain-treated marrow cells into normal mice causes tumor at six weeks. Marrow treated with RAMIg-A chain did not cause detectable tumor at this time. Thus, as with BCL_1 cells in the spleen, RAMIg-A chain is highly effective in killing BCL_1 tumor cells in the marrow (8).

The markedly potent effect of the antibody-A chain conjugates is contrasted with the results of similar experiments using RAMIg and C' to kill BCL_1 cells in bone marrow. In such experiments, hepatosplenomegaly was readily apparent three to four weeks after adoptive transfer, and the spleens and blood of the recipient mice contained large numbers of tumor cells (data not shown). It is estimated from the length of time needed to achieve the observed level of splenomegaly and from the fact that the injected bone marrow contained 10-20% tumor cells, that 10% of the original 10^5 tumor cells injected had escaped being killed by antibody and C'. In fact, a killing of 90-95% for antibody and C' is considered to be very effective cytotoxicity. The above results emphasize the advantage of using antibody-A chain compared to C'-mediated cytotoxicity.

To demonstrate that marrow cells treated with antibody-A chain contain functional stem cells, treated cells were transferred into lethally irradiated mice (8). Preliminary experiments had established that a dose of 750r was 100% lethal for normal BALB/c mice but that all of these mice could be rescued with an intravenous injection of 10^6 (but not 10^5) normal bone marrow cells. Thus, mice given 750r were injected with 10^6 untreated or RAMIg-A chain-treated marrow cells from a BCL_1-bearing mouse. Although both groups were rescued by this dose of marrow cells, the mice given untreated

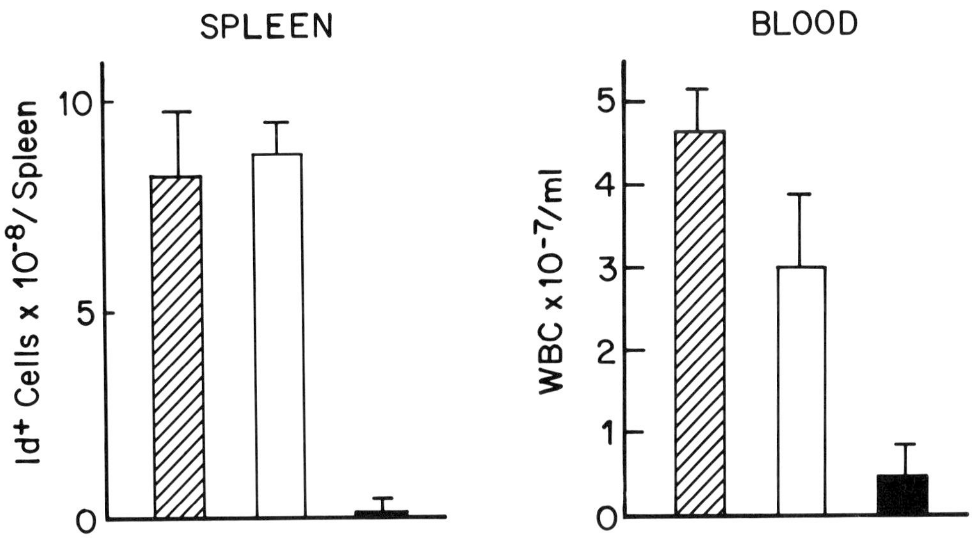

Fig. 2. Adoptive transfer of bone marrow cells treated with RAMIg-A chain from BCL_1-bearing mice into normal recipients. Bone marrow cells (10^6) containing 1-2 x 10^5 tumor cells were treated for 15 min at 4° with 1 μg/ml/10^7 cells with either RAMIg-A chain (solid bars) or RαOVA-A chain (empty bars). The treated cells, as well as untreated cells (hatched bars), were washed and injected intravenously into groups of five normal BALB/c mice (10^6 cells/mouse). At six weeks following adoptive transfer, mice were sacrificed and examined for Id^+ (tumor) cells in the spleen and for leukemia (8).

marrow cells had tumor cells in their spleens six weeks later. In contrast, the mice given bone marrow cells treated with RAMIg-A chain had no detectable tumor and exhibited normal numbers of T and B cells in their spleens.

These results indicate that 1) virtually all (>99.9%) BCL_1 tumor cells bear sIg, i.e., the BCL_1 tumor does not have a major pre-B cell component; 2) treatment with RAMIg-A chain eliminates Ig^+ tumor cells from the marrow but leaves sufficient numbers of stem cells intact; 3) neoplastic B cells can be destroyed by a conjugate using an antibody that is *not* tumor specific. Thus, for the above approach to autologous bone marrow transplantation, a tumor-*reactive*, stem-cell-*non-reactive* antibody is all that is required.

Further experiments will be required to determine if all the BCL_1 tumor cells have been killed by the above approach. In addition, it should be emphasized that spontaneous B cell leukemias in man could have malignant pre-B cells (10), i.e., surface Ig^- in addition to surface Ig^+ leukemic cells. Elimination of Ig^- leukemic cells would require treatment with a monoclonal antibody to a differentiation antigen that is expressed on pre-B cells and not on stem cells.

Acknowledgments

This work was supported by Grants AI-11851, AI-12789, CA-28149 and CA-23115 from the National Institutes of Health.

References

1. Fu, SM, RJ Winchester and HG Kunkel (1975). Similar idiotypic specificity for the membrane IgD and IgM of human B lymphocytes. J Immunol **114**, 250-252.
2. Slavin, S, and S Strober (1977). Spontaneous murine B-cell leukaemia. Nature (Lond) **272**, 624-626.
3. Krolick, KA, PC Isakson, JW Uhr and ES Vitetta (1979). BCL_1, a murine model for chronic lymphocytic leukemia: use of the surface immunoglobulin idiotype for the detection and treatment of tumor. Immunol Rev **48**, 81-106.
4. Muirhead, MJ, JM Holbert, Jr, JW Uhr and ES Vitetta (1981). BLC_1, a murine model of prolymphocytic leukemia: I. Effect of splenectomy on growth kinetics and organ distribution. Am J Pathol **105**, 306-315.
5. Galton, DAG, JM Goldman, E Wiltshaw, D Catovsky, K Kenry and GJ Goldberg (1974). Prolymphocytic leukaemia. Br J Haematol **27**, 7-23.
6. Krolick, KA, C Villemez, P Isakson, JW Uhr and ES Vitetta (1980). Selective killing of normal or neoplastic B cells by antibodies coupled to the A chain of ricin. Proc Natl Acad Sci USA **77**, 5419-5423.
7. Pure, E, and E Vitetta (1980). The murine B cell response to TNP-polyacrylamide beads: the relationship between the epitope density of the antigen and the requirements for T cell help and surface IgD. J Immunol 125, 1240-1242.
8. Krolick, KA, JW Uhr and ES Vitetta (1982). Selective killing of leukaemia cells by antibody-toxin conjugates: implications for autologous bone marrow transplantation. Nature (Lond) **295**, 604-605.
9. Gale, RP (1980). Autologous bone marrow transplantation in patients with cancer. J Am Med Assoc **243**, 540-542.
10. Vogler, LB, J-L Preud'homme, M Seligmann, WE Gathings, WM Crist, MD Cooper and FJ Bollum (1981). Diversity of immunoglobulin expression in leukaemic cells resembling B-lymphocyte precursors. Nature (Lond) **290**, 339-341.

GLYCOLIPID TUMOR CELL MARKERS AND THEIR MONOCLONAL ANTIBODIES: DRUG TARGETING AND IMMUNOSUPPRESSION

Sen-itiroh Hakomori, William W. Young, Jr.,* and David Urdal

Fred Hutchinson Cancer Research Center
Seattle, Washington 98104
and
University of Washington
Seattle, Washington 98195

Glycosphingolipids are ubiquitous components of plasma membrane (1), representing a large variety of cell surface antigens as listed in Table 1. The list increases as the use of monoclonal antibody becomes more widespread. Although the real function of glycosphingolipids is not known, remarkable changes in glycolipid composition and metabolism have been associated with the process of malignancy (1). Often the blocked synthesis of complex glycolipids in transformed cells is accompanied by an accumulation of a certain type of glycolipid. In some cases such accumulation or the appearance of new glycolipids may result from activation of a new glycolipid synthesis that is virtually absent in progenitor cells. A few examples of the accumulation of specific glycolipid haptens in experimental tumors and in human cancer are listed in Table 2. Some of them may be recognized as tumor-associated antigens.

Two approaches have been taken to identify the tumor-associated glycolipid antigen. In the first approach, chemical identification of glycolipid antigen followed by production of antibodies is used to characterize the tumor antigen's distribution and quantity, as well as the effect of antibodies on tumor growth. The second approach depends on the identification of glycolipid antigens recognized by established tumor-specific antibodies, an approach made possible only by the development of tumor-specific monoclonal antibodies (41,42). In this article we describe a systematic development of the first approach, which has been described in a series of papers from our laboratory (33,34,52-55).

Identification of Ganglio-N-triosylceramide ($GgOs_3Cer$) as the Tumor-associated Cell Surface Marker for Mouse KiMSV Sarcoma and L5178Y Lymphoma

A glycolipid was found to accumulate in BALBc/3T3 cells transformed by the non-productive Kirsten strain of murine sarcoma virus

*Present address: Department of Pathology, University of Virginia School of Medicine, Charlottesville, Virginia 22901.

Table 1. Glycolipid cell surface markers and antigens

1. Blood group antigens:
   ABH (2); Le^a, Le^b (3); Ii (4-6); P, P_1, P^k (7).
2. Heterophile antigens:
   Forssman (8); Hanganutziu-Deicher (9,10).
3. Lymphoid subpopulation markers:
   GM_1, $GgOs_4Cer$ for T cell subpopulation (11,12); $LcnOs_4Cer$ for unknown B/T (13); $GgOs_4Cer$ for NK (14,15); Thy-1 ganglioside (16).
4. Differentiation antigens:
   Forssman (17,18); Ii (19); F9 (20,21); TerC (22); SSEA-1 (23,50).
5. Glycolipids reacting with "auto-antibodies," or anti-glycolipid antibodies present in sera of patients with autoimmune diseases:
   Ii-active glycolipid (4-6); sialosylparagloboside (7); "experimental ganglioside syndrome" and neuritis (24); sulfatide and cerebroside in experimental encephalomyelitis (25,26); globoside and Forssman in paroxysmal hemoglobinuria (27); multiple sclerosis (28,29); experimental allergic neuritis (30); systematic *Lupus* erythmatosus (31).
6. Glycolipid tumor-cell-surface markers or antigen:
   $LcnOs_4Cer$ in NILpy tumor (32); $GgOs_3Cer$ in KiMSV tumor (33); lymphoma L5178Y (34); $GgOs_4Cer$ in human acute lymphoblastic leukemia (35); Forssman antigen in human gastrointestinal tumor (36); A-like antigen in human O or B tumor (37-39); P, P_1 antigen in human p tumor (40); a monosialo ganglioside (structure unidentified) in human colonic carcinoma (41); unknown glycolipid in human melanoma defined by monoclonal antibody (42).

(3T3KiMSV cells) (33), and in mouse lymphoma L5178Y (34). The accumulated glycolipid was identified as asialo GM_2 (ganglio-N-triosylceramide; GalNAcβ1→4Galβ1→4Glcβ1→1Ceramide; $GgOs_3$ Cer). Coupled with this chemical change are immunologic alterations indicating that $GgOs_3Cer$ could function as a tumor-associated marker in these tumor cells. The chemical level of $GgOs_3Cer$ was approximately 20-fold greater in 3T3KiMSV cells than in 3T3 cells. When intact cells were treated sequentially with galactose oxidase followed by (^{3}H)-borohydride, the labeling of $GgOs_3Cer$ was more than 30-fold greater in 3T3KiMSV cells than in non-transformed cells (33). Chemical analysis of this glycolipid in various tissues and organs indicated its virtual absence in various tissues, except for a trace quantity detected in erythrocytes and spleen. No organs or tissues had such a high level of $GgOs_3Cer$ as was found in KiMSV tumors (Table 3) (33). The rabbit antibodies directed to $GgOs_3Cer$ reacted strongly by indirect immunofluorescence with 3T3KiMSV cells. A small population of unidentified cells in testicles and seminal vesicles showed weak immunofluorescence (Table 4, Halfpap and Hakomori, unpublished observation). Therefore, $GgOs_3Cer$ is not an absolutely specific product of KiMSV tumors, but its presence in very high concentration at the tumor cell surface is unique and was subsequently found to be a useful target for immunotherapy and immunochemotherapy (see subsequent sections and Discussion).

This glycolipid was expressed not only in KiMSV tumor cells but also in various clones of lymphoma L5178Y (34). Some clones contain a high level while others contain a low level of this glycolipid, and its expression at the cell surface varied significantly (34, see Fig. 1). It is possible that 3T3KiMSV cells may also have such a clonal variation in the expression of $GgOs_3Cer$ (see Discussion). Examination by thin-layer chromatography of lymphoma L5178Y glycolipids revealed the presence of these analogues of $GgOs_3Cer$, showing three clearly separate bands. These have been identified as three components having different ceramides, the first containing C20-24 fatty acids, the second C16 fatty acid, and the third C16-α-hydroxy fatty acid (D. Urdal, Thesis, University of Washington).

Table 2. Accumulation of specific glycolipids in experimental tumors and in human cancer

1. *In vitro* transformants and experimental tumors:

    Lactosylceramide accumulation in BHKpy cells (43)
    Paragloboside ($LcnOs_4Cer$) in NILpy cells (32,44)
    Asialo GM_2 ($GgOs_3Cer$) in 3T3KiMSV cells (33) and tumors in lymphoma L5178Y (34)
    Unidentified neutral fucolipids and fucoganglioside (fucosyl GM_1) in rat hepatoma (45)
    Fucolipid accumulation in precancerous liver (46)

2. Human cancer:

    Le^X glycolipid in human colonic adenocarcinoma (47)
    Lactosylceramide in human gastric cancer (48)
    Fucosylceramide in human colonic cancer (49)
    Polyvalent and polyfucosylated Le^X structure in human colonic cancer (50)
    Forssman glycolipid in human cancer (51,52)

Table 3. Distribution of neutral glycolipids in normal BALB/c tissues and cultured cells

Expressed as μg glycolipid/100 mg dry residue. The glycolipid fraction was prepared, and the quantity of glycolipids present in the fraction was determined by the "comparative dilution method" (56).

	CMH[a]	CDH-sulfatide[b]	CTH	Asialo GM_2	CTT	CP[c]
3T3 cells	136	34	ND[d]	3.4	11.3	16
3T3KiMSV cells	115	46	ND	69	35	10
Brain	100	39	ND	ND	ND	ND
Thymus	87	ND	44	ND	ND	ND
Lung	5	ND	10	ND	40	ND
Liver	3	1	0.2	ND	2	ND
Kidney	8	40	2	ND	24	8
Spleen	20	4	2	e	10	16
Erythrocytes	15	3	ND	e	2	ND

[a]The abbreviations used are CMH, ceramide monohexoside; CDH, ceramide dihexoside; CTH, ceramide trihexoside; CTT, ceramide tetrasaccharide; CP, ceramide pentasaccharide.

[b]CDH and sulfatide did not separate under the conditions used.

[c]CP data include more complex neutral glycolipids as well as CP.

[d]ND, no detectable spot.

[e]As acetylated derivatives, a spot of glycolipid was detected on TLC which migrated slightly more slowly than asialo GM_2; the quantity was estimated for spleen and erythrocytes as 2.0 and 0.6 μg/100 mg dry residue, respectively.

Table 4. Distribution of glycolipid markers in various tissues in BALB/c Mouse (♂) (Halfpap and Hakomori, unpublished observation)

Anti-sera	Kidney	Spleen	Stomach	Liver	Testicle	Seminal vesicle	KIMSV tumor (K-234)
Pre-immune	-	-	-	-	±	-	-
Anti-$GgOs_3Cer$	-	a	-	-	±	±	+++
Anti-$GgOs_4Cer$	++ (some unidentified area)	a	+	-	+	±	±
Anti-$GbOs_4Cer$	-	a	+	-	±	+	±
Anti-$GbOs_5Cer$	++	a	++ (some layers)	-	++	++	+++ (patchy area)[b]

[a]Non-specific staining due to the presence of T cells with Fc receptors.

[b]Strongly positive in some patchy areas, which may represent inflammatory cellular elements.

$GgOs_3Cer$: ganglio-N-triosylceramide (asialo GM_2); $GgOs_4Cer$: ganglio-N-tetraosylceramide (asialo GM_1); $GbOs_4Cer$: globoside; $GbOs_5Cer$: Forssman glycolipid.

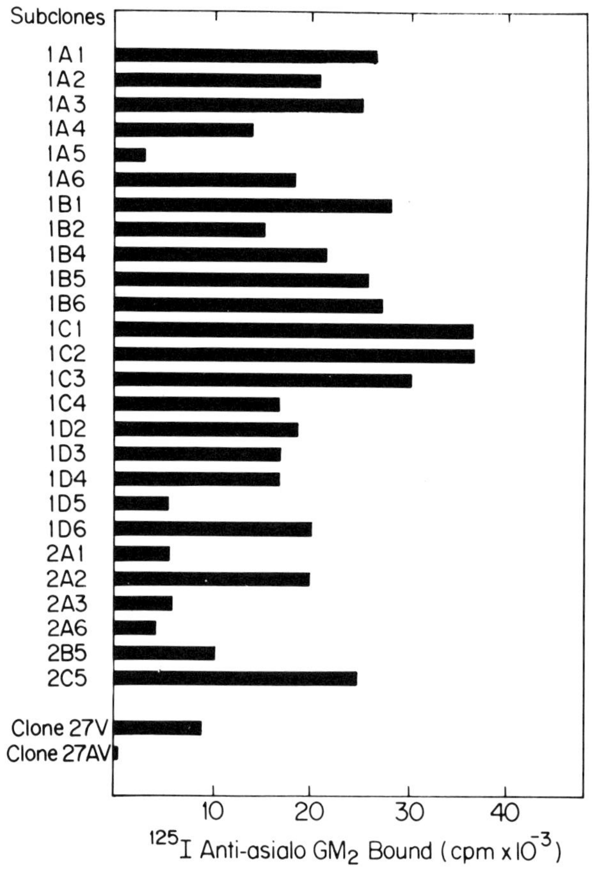

Fig. 1. Clonal variation of mouse lymphoma L5178Y in their expression of ganglio-N-triosylceramide. Binding of ^{125}I-anti-GgOs$_3$Cer to clones is indicated. These clones were derived from clone 27V (second from the bottom). In contrast, non-expressor clone 27AV did not contain this glycolipid (bottom line).

The Production of Polyclonal and Monoclonal Antibodies Directed to GgOs$_3$Cer

Polyclonal antibodies. Rabbit antibody was prepared directed to GgOs$_3$Cer by immunization with an emulsion containing bovine serum albumin and the glycolipid, and was subsequently purified on an affinity column to remove anti-bovine serum albumin antibody. The anti-glycolipid antibody was found to be specific for GgOs$_3$Cer by immunodiffusion and complement fixation and did not react with other glycolipids, including GM$_2$-ganglioside (33). With these antibodies a strong, membrane-associated fluorescence of the transformed cells could be demonstrated, and the immunofluorescence was completely abolished by absorption of the rabbit antibody with $GgOs_3Cer$ liposomes. Rabbit antisera with a similar immunological specificity directed to $GgOs_3Cer$ can be prepared by repeated intravenous injection of 3T3KiMSV cells; however, a similar immunization with normal 3T3 cells resulted in no production of antibodies directed to $GgOs_3Cer$ (33).

Monoclonal antibodies. Using the hybridoma technique introduced by Köhler and Milstein (57), we have tried to develop monoclonal antibodies directed to $GgOs_3Cer$ (53). Two hybridoma cell lines producing two antibodies, one identified as IgM and the other as IgG_3, have been successfully isolated. The IgM antibody was found to be directed to one side of the carbohydrate residue, while the IgG_3 antibody was directed to the other side of the same carbohydrate chain as shown in Fig. 2. This conclusion was based on the fact that the reactivity of IgM antibody was not inhibited by modifying the N-acetyl group of the terminal N-acetylhexosamine residue, whereas it was greatly inhibited by modifying the C6 primary hydroxyl group of the terminal N-acetylhexosamine residue. In contrast, IgG_3 antibody was inhibited strongly by modifying the N-acetyl group of the terminal N-acetylhexosamine residue but was not influenced by changing the C6 primary hydroxyl group of the terminal N-acetylhexosamine residue (see Table 5).

The effect of antibodies and complement and the effect with K-cells *in vitro* on 3T3 and 3T3KiMSV cells were studied first. KiMSV tumor cells were lysed effectively in the presence of complement and anti-$GgOs_3Cer$ antibodies but not in the absence of complement (Fig. 3). The antibody-dependent killing of 3T3KiMSV cells in the absence of complement but in the presence of human K-lymphocytes (ADCC) (Fig. 4) was remarkable.

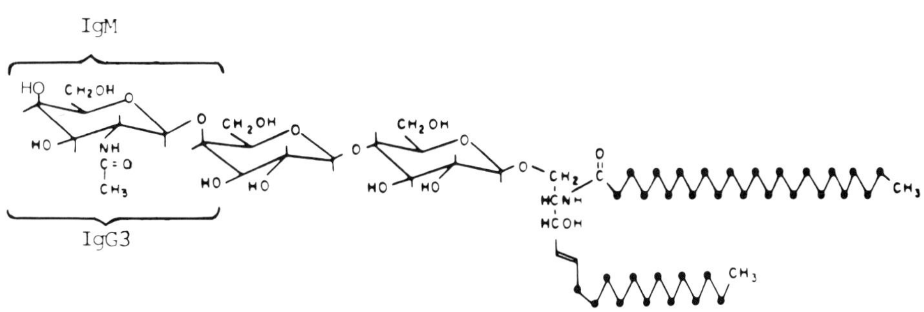

Fig. 2. Structure of ganglio-N-triosylceramide and two regions recognized by two monoclonal antibodies. IgG3 recognizes the site of the terminal N-acetyl group of N-acetylgalactosamine, and IgM recognizes the opposite site of the molecule (53).

Table 5. Inhibition by glycolipid of guinea pig erythrocyte hemagglutination caused by anti-asialo GM_2 antibodies

Glycolipid inhibitor	Concentrated hybridoma supernate		Rabbit anti-asialo GM_2	
	2D4 (IgM)	D11G10 (IgG_3)	IgM	IgG
Asialo GM_2	3.1[a]	3.1	1.6	12.5
Asialo GM_2-NH_2	> 100	> 100	nd[b]	nd
Asialo GM_2-re-N-acetylated	1.6	6.3	1.6	12.5
Asialo GM_2-N-propionylated	1.6	3.1	3.2	12.5[c]
Asialo GM_2-N-butyrylated	0.8	> 100	6.4[c]	>100
Asialo GM_2-C6 aldehyde	>100	6.2	12.5[c]	100
Glucosylceramide Ceramide dihexoside GM_2, GM_2 methyl ester GM_1, asialo GM_1, globoside Ceramide trihexoside Lacto-N-triosylceramide	>100	>100	nd	nd

[a] Minimum dose of glycolipid in μg/ml that inhibits three hemagglutination doses of antibody. Glycolipids were tested in the presence of auxiliary lipids.

[b] nd, not determined.

[c] Inhibition even at the highest glycolipid concentrations was not complete.

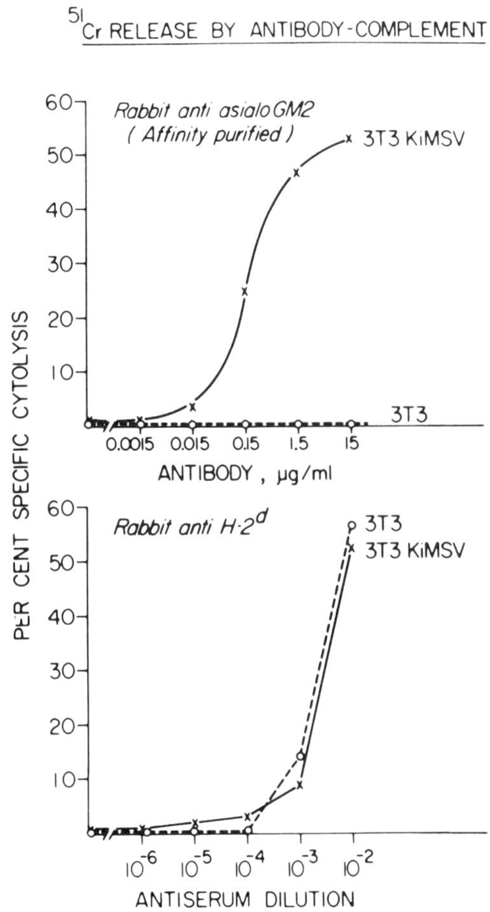

Fig. 3. Cytotoxicity of BALB/c 3T3 and 3T3-KiMSV cells by antibody-complement. The cytotoxicity assay was performed in V-bottom microtiter plates, and all dilutions were made with MEM plus 10% fetal calf serum. Each well received the appropriate antibody dilution plus 5 x 10^3 labeled target cells in a total volume of 0.15 ml. Following incubation at room temperature for 30 min, and at 37°C for 45 min, the plates were centrifuged at 300 x *g* for 1 min, and 0.1 ml of the cell-free supernatant was assayed for ^{51}Cr content.

Immunotherapy of Mouse Lymphoma L5178Y by Monoclonal Antibodies Directed to Tumor-associated $GgOs_3Cer$ (53,54)

Subsequently, we studied the effect of passive immunization on tumor growth *in vivo* with monoclonal antibodies directed to $GgOs_3Cer$. Two monoclonal antibodies were directed to two distinct portions of the non-reducing terminus of the glycolipid (53; see previous section).

Pooled ascites fluids from mice bearing each of these hybridomas contained 15 mg/ml of the IgM antibody produced by clone 2D4 (53) and 4 mg/ml of the IgG3 antibody produced by clone D11G10 (53). A nonspecific control ascites fluid contained 10 mg/ml of the monoclonal IgG3 antibody produced by clone 3. Because mice of the DBA/2 strain are known to have low concentrations of complement component C5, certain groups of mice received injections of native guinea pig serum as a complement source.

In the initial experiment mice received on day 0 intraperitoneal

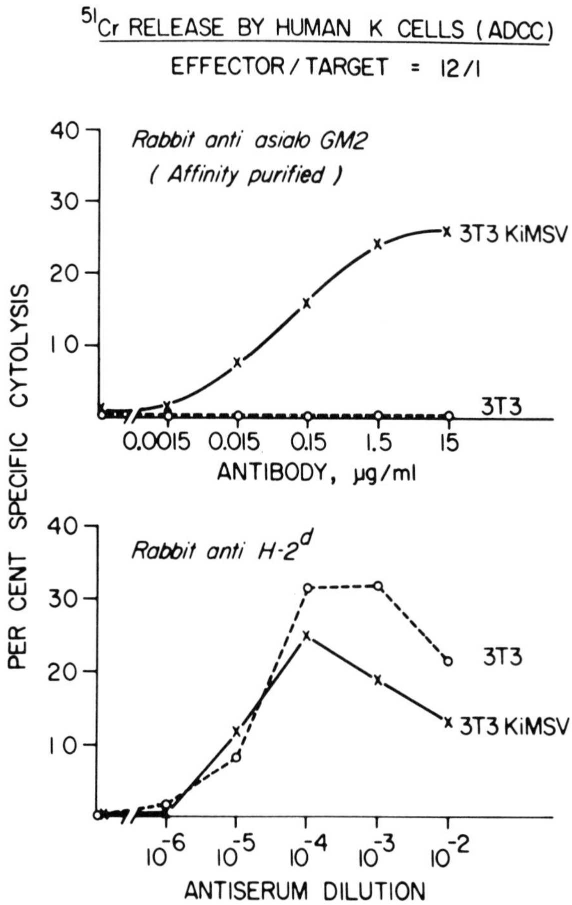

Fig. 4. Antibody-dependent cell-mediated cytotoxicity of BALB/c 3T3 and 3T3KiMSV cells. Human peripheral blood lymphocytes were purified by Ficoll-Hypaque separation followed by incubation at 37°C for 1 h to remove adherent cells. The cytotoxicity assay was performed in a microtiter plate, each well containing 6×10^4 lymphocytes, 5×10^3 ^{51}Cr-labeled 3T3 or 3T3KiMSV cells, and appropriate dilutions of antibody in a final volume of 0.2 ml. The plates were centrifuged at 300 x *g* for 1 min, then incubated at 37°C for 4 h. After incubation 0.1 ml of the cell-free supernatant was assayed for ^{51}Cr content.

inoculations of 10^6 L5178Y-subclone 1A1 cells (a dose at least 2 logs greater than the 100% lethal dose). Therapy began on day 1 and consisted of intraperitoneal injections of hybridoma ascites fluids with or without guinea pig serum (Fig. 5A). The median survival time of untreated mice was 34 days; treatment with guinea pig serum alone or with IgM antibody to $GgOs_3Cer$ alone did not significantly improve survival. Only one of three mice treated with the IgM antibody to $GgOs_3Cer$ plus complement was a long-term survivor. In contrast, the mice treated with the IgG3 antibody to $GgOs_3Cer$, either with or without complement, showed prolonged survival. In fact, five of these seven mice were apparently cured as judged by their survival 120 days after they were inoculated with the tumor cells.

In the second experiment this protective effect of the IgG3 antibody to $GgOs_3Cer$ was reproduced (Fig. 5B). To rule out nonspecific effects of IgG3 antibodies, we treated one group of mice with ascites fluid containing the nonspecific monoclonal IgG3 antibodies produced by hybridoma clone 3, which did not show reactivity with the subclone 1A1 lymphoma cells by immunofluorescence (data not shown). This antibody failed to protect mice against challenge with the subclone 1A1 cells; the median length of survival for this group was 31 days compared to 30 days for the untreated group. In this experiment the IgM antibody to $GgOs_3Cer$ had a slightly protective effect. However, therapy with the ascites fluid containing IgG3 antibody to $GgOs_3Cer$, either with or without complement, was most effective. Of the 12 mice treated with intraperitoneal injections of the IgG3 antibody, 9 survived at least 120 days after they were injected with tumor cells. In addition, intravenous therapy with IgG3 antibody to $GgOs_3Cer$ provided significant protection in three of six mice, indicating that the IgG3 antibody was effective not only locally after injection into the peritoneal cavity but also systemically.

In two control experiments we tested whether this protection was due to a specific effect of the antibody to $GgOs_3Cer$, or to a nonspecific anti-tumor activity in the hybridoma ascites fluid. First, IgG3 antibody to $GgOs_3Cer$ was purified from ascites fluid on a Protein A-Sepharose column (Pharmacia). Treatment with doses (0.31 mg of protein) of the purified antibody equivalent to the concentration in the ascites fluid effectively protected mice against growth of subclone 1A1 tumor cells (Fig. 5B). Figure 5C shows that the antibody to $GgOs_3Cer$ was ineffective in protecting mice against challenge with the lymphoma-cell-variant clone 27AV that did not display $GgOs_3Cer$. Neither the IgM antibody plus complement nor the IgG3 antibody altered the survival of mice inoculated intraperitoneally with 10^5 clone 27AV cells.

Immunotherapy of Mouse KIMSV Sarcoma by Polyclonal Antibodies to $GgOs_3Cer$: Polyclonal Antibodies Are More Effective than Monoclonal Antibody

The effect of polyclonal antibodies to $GgOs_3Cer$ raised in rabbit, passively immunized intravenously to mice, is shown in Fig. 5D. In this experiment KiMSV sarcoma cells were inoculated intraperitoneally, and tumor growth was significantly inhibited by intravenous administration of the polyclonal antibodies. As compared to monoclonal antibodies, the effective doses were found to be much lower, possibly because of a strong induction of ADCC mechanisms. Similar doses directed to $GgOs_4Cer$ (asialo GM_1) did not inhibit tumor growth.

A Crucial Problem Basic to Specific Immunotherapy

A crucial problem basic to specific immunotherapy is the potential escape of antigen-deficient variants from immune control. To determine if the tumor cells that survived treatment with the IgG3 antibody to $GgOs_3Cer$ contained altered amounts of $GgOs_3Cer$, we compared ascites cells from a treated mouse that survived 76 days with those from an untreated mouse (Table 6). The cells were cultured *in vitro* for one month prior to glycolipid analysis to eliminate host cells. In addition, to detect any possible variation in the amounts of $GgOs_3Cer$ among these cells resistant to IgG3 immunotherapy, we determined the glycolipid pattern of a few clones derived from 1A1G3 (Table 6). The $GgOs_3Cer$ in cells from the untreated mouse was about half that of the 1A1 cells used for challenge. In contrast, the cells from the treated mouse (1A1G3) contained only 10% of the $GgOs_3Cer$ present in the 1A1 cells.

Table 6. Concentrations of $GgOs_3Cer$ in L5178Y lymphoma cells (from Ref. 54)

The 1A1-tu cells were harvested from the peritoneal cavity of an untreated mouse 71 days after it was challenged with 10^5 1A1 cells. The 1A1-G3 cells were harvested from a mouse 76 days after it was challenged with 10^6 1A1 cells; this mouse was treated with ascites fluid containing IgG3 antibody to $GgOs_3Cer$ (group 5). The 1A1-G3 cells were cloned by limiting dilution at a density of one cell in every three wells, and the resultant clones were screened for binding to ^{125}I-labeled antibody to $GgOs_3Cer$. Three clones (Af7, BC11, and AG10) that showed minimal binding (data not shown) were expanded for chemical analysis. Neutral glycolipid fractions were obtained from cultured cells as previously described (34) and analyzed by TLC in a solvent containing chloroform, methanol, and water (65:25:4, by volume). Neutral glycolipids were visualized with orcinol spray reagent and quantitated by the comparative dilution method (56). The $GgOs_3Cer$ was present in these lymphoma cells as a triplet of orcinol-positive bands (34). The concentrations of $GgOs_3Cer$ are shown separately for the three bands.

	$GgOs_3Cer$ ($\mu g/10^7$ cells)			
Cell type	Fast band	Intermediate band	Slow band	Total
Subclone 1A1	4.0	1.5	1.2	6.7
Subclone 1A1-tu	1.8	1.3	0.5	3.6
Subclone 1A1-G3	0.4	0.2	0.0	0.6
Clone Af7	0.15	0.05	0.0	0.2
Clone BC11	0.1	0.05	0.05	0.2
Clone AG10	0.15	0.1	0.05	0.3

Furthermore, clones derived from the surviving cells contained 20-30 times less $GgOs_3Cer$ than did the 1A1 cells (Table 6). These results suggest that treatment with the antibodies to glycolipid resulted in the selection of glycolipid antigen-deficient tumor cells. It will be of interest to determine the enzymatic basis for the altered amount of $GgOs_3Cer$.

These studies indicate that antibodies specific for tumor cell glycolipid can protect host animals against inoculated tumor cells. Unlike most so-called "tumor-associated antigens" that are defined serologically, glycolipids offer the advantage of having chemical structures that can be completely defined.

Targeting Drugs to the Tumor Cells *in Vitro* and *in Vivo* with a Newly Designed Targeting System (55)

Since we have established ganglio-N-triosylceramide as a possible tumor cell surface marker of KiMSV sarcoma and L5178 lymphoma cells and have established specific polyclonal and monoclonal antibodies directed to the carbohydrate moiety of this glycolipid, we have endeavored to target drug-conjugated antibodies and liposomes covalently linked to antibodies to tumor cells. This approach is particularly relevant because antibodies, such as IgM, do not inhibit tumor growth *in vivo*, as described in the previous section.

Drug conjugation to antibody can result in inactivation of antibody as well as loss of drug activity. To avoid this situation, a new indirect targeting system was developed in which administration of biotinyl antiglycolipid antibody was followed by successive addition of 1) avidin and biotinyl drug conjugates (e.g., neocarzinostatin), 2) avidin and biotinylphosphatidylethanolamine/liposomes in which actinomycin D was encapsulated, and 3) drug encapsulated in liposomes covalently linked to avidin.

Targeting drugs *in vitro*. Successful targeting and killing of tumor cells expressing $GgOs_3Cer$ were observed in the *in vitro* system 1) above as shown in Fig. 6. Clearly, targeting required the presence of biotin on both the antibody and the drug. If biotin was absent from either molecule, or if the experiment was performed in the presence of excess free biotin, targeting was not seen (see legend, Fig. 6). Furthermore, the targeting of biotinyl neocarzinostatin to lymphoma cells was completely abrogated if the biotinyl anti-$GgOs_3Cer$ antibody was first absorbed with guinea pig erythrocytes containing $GgOs_3Cer$, whereas the targeting was not influenced by preincubation of the biotinyl anti-$GgOs_3Cer$ antibody with sheep erythrocytes not containing $GgOs_3Cer$ (see Fig. 7). Liposome targeting was successful in systems 2) and 3) above, but killing of the cells was not very dramatic because the targeted liposomes failed to fuse with the cells.

Targeting drugs *in vivo*. Since IgM antibody did not suppress tumor growth *in vivo* as described in the previous section, targeting

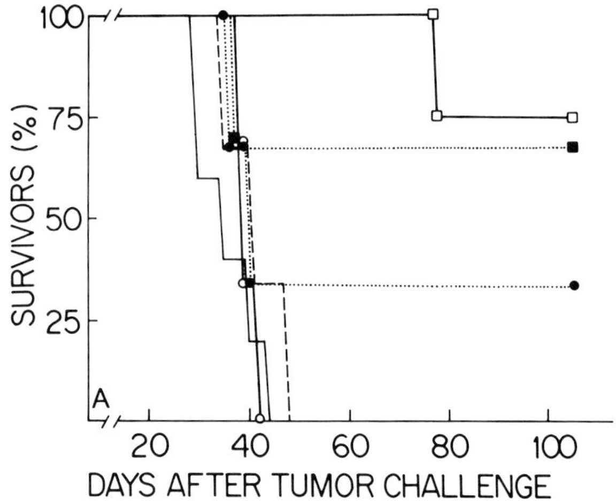

Fig. 5A

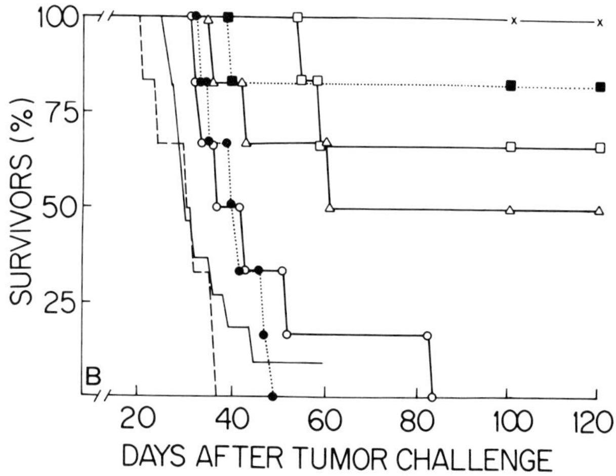

Fig. 5B

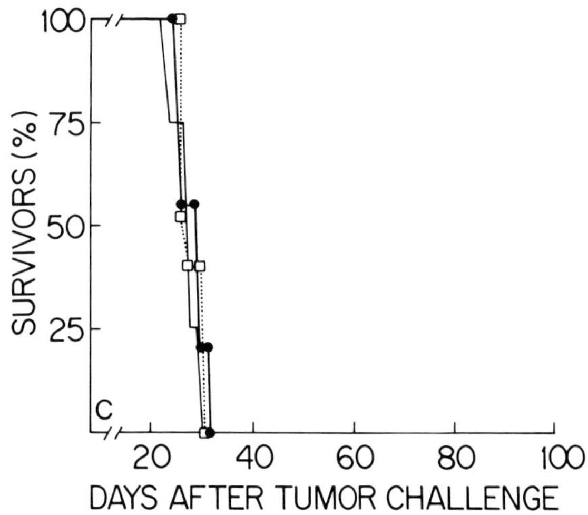

Fig. 5C

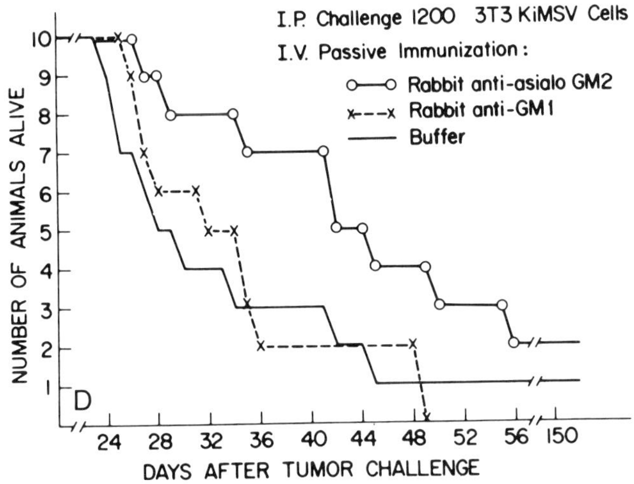

Fig. 5D

Fig. 5. Serotherapy of DBA/2 mouse L5178Y lymphoma cells with monoclonal antibodies to $GgOs_3Cer$.

(A) Male mice of strain DBA/2 were inoculated intraperitoneally with 10^6 subclone 1A1 cells on day 0. Group 1 (solid line), 5 untreated control mice; group 2 (broken line), 3 mice treated with guinea pig serum (as a complement source) alone; group 3 (open circles, solid line), 3 mice treated with ascites fluid containing IgM antibody to $GgOs_3Cer$ produced by clone 2D4; group 4 (closed circles, dotted line), 3 mice treated with 2D4 ascites fluid plus guinea pig serum; group 5 (open squares, solid line), 4 mice treated with ascites fluid containing IgG3 antibody to $GgOs_3Cer$ produced by clone D11G10; and group 6 (closed squares, dotted line), 3 mice treated with ascites fluid from clone D11G10 plus guinea pig serum. Treatment consisted of intraperitoneal injections of 100 µl of ascites fluid or guinea pig serum, or both, on days 1, 3, 7, and 10.

(B) Mice were inoculated intraperitoneally with 10^6 subclone 1A1 cells on day 0. Group 1 (solid line), 11 untreated control mice; group 2 (broken line), 6 mice treated with nonspecific ascites fluid containing monoclonal IgG3 produced by clone 3; group 3 (open circles, solid lines), 6 mice treated with ascites fluid containing IgM antibody produced by clone 2D4; group 4 (closed circles, dotted line), 6 mice treated with ascites fluid from clone 2D4 plus guinea pig serum; group 5 (open squares, solid line), 6 mice treated with ascites fluid from clone D11G10; group 6 (closed squares, dotted line), 6 mice treated with D11G10 ascites fluid plus guinea pig serum; group 7 (open triangles), 6 mice treated with D11G10 ascites fluid injected intravenously; and group 8 (crosses, solid line), 5 mice treated with purified IgG3 antibody to $GgOs_3Cer$. The treatment protocol was similar to that in (A) except for group 7, which received intravenous instead of intraperitoneal injections of ascites fluid.

(C) Mice were inoculated intraperitoneally with 10^5 clone 27AV cells (a variant that had no $GgOs_3Cer$) on day 0. Group 1 (solid line), 4 untreated control mice; group 2 (closed circles), 5 mice treated with 2D4 ascites fluid plus guinea pig serum; and group 3 (open squares, dotted line), 5 mice treated with D11G10 ascites fluid. The treatment protocol was the same as that in (A).

(D) Survival of mice injected with 3T3KiMSV tumor cells. Groups of 10 mice were challenged intraperitoneally with 1200 3T3KiMSV cells. After 2 h each group received a single intravenous injection of either rabbit polyclonal anti-asialo GM_2, rabbit polyclonal anti-GM_1, or buffer alone.

biotinyl drug derivatives with avidin was performed with a biotinyl IgM antibody. With this antibody the suppression of tumor growth by antibody alone would be minimal. The results of an experiment examining *in vivo* targeting with monoclonal IgM antibody are summarized in Table 7. Only animals treated with biotinyl-IgM anti-$GgOs_3Cer$ (256 hemagglutination units), avidin (150 μg), and biotinyl neocarzinostatin (2.4 μg) showed extended survival (group 7). Two out of five of these animals lived longer than 100 days. All other groups, including the one that received unsubstituted IgM (256 units), avidin (150 μg), and biotinyl neocarzinostatin (2.4 μg) (group 5), had survival times similar to the control group. These results suggest that the increase in survival seen in this experiment was due to the *in vivo* targeting of biotinyl neocarzinostatin to tumor cells (group 7) and not due to antibody-drug synergism (group 5).

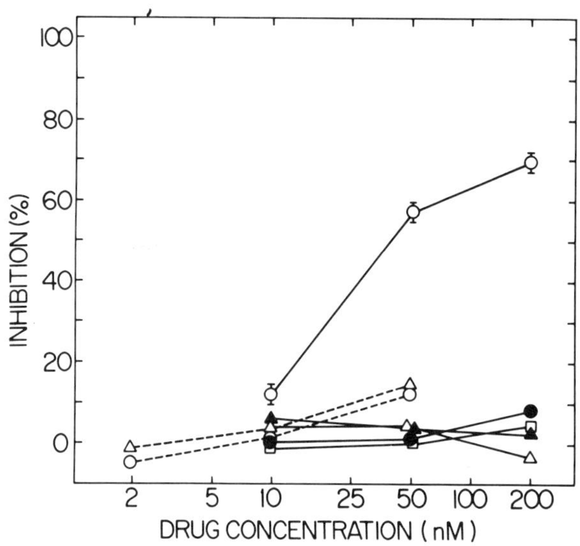

Fig. 6. Targeting of biotinyl neocarzinostatin to L5178c127 cells: Requirement for biotin on antibody and drug. O——O, biotinyl-anti-$GgOs_3Cer$ + avidin + biotinyl neocarzinostatin; □——□, biotinyl-anti-$GgOs_3Cer$ + avidin in 1 mM biotin + biotinyl neocarzinostatin; Δ——Δ, nonimmune serum + avidin + biotinyl neocarzinostatin; ●——●, unsubstituted anti-$GgOs_3Cer$ + avidin + biotinyl neocarzinostatin; ▲——▲, biotinyl-anti-$GgOs_3Cer$ + biotinyl neocarzinostatin (no avidin); O---O, biotinyl-anti-$GgOs_3Cer$ + avidin + unsubstituted neocarzinostatin; Δ---Δ, nonimmune serum + avidin + unsubstituted neocarzinostatin. Cell proliferation (increase in cell number) in all cultures without drug but with the different antibody and avidin treatments was more than 600%. No difference was seen between control cultures. The reproducibility of the assay is reflected by the standard error brackets (n:5) on the specific inhibition curve (O——O).

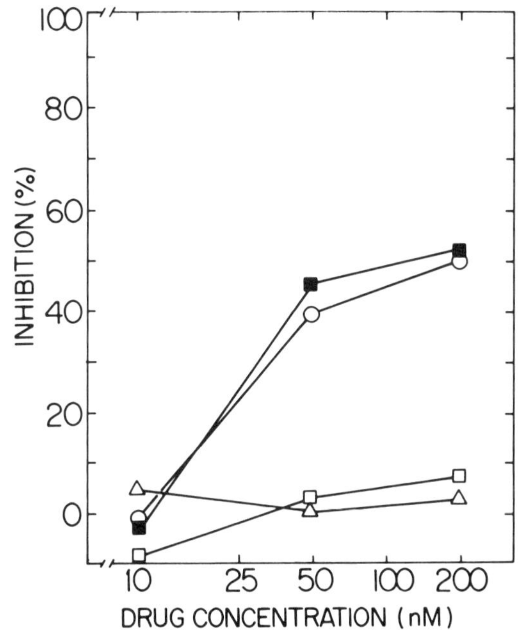

Fig. 7. Targeting of biotinyl neocarzinostatin to L5178c127 cells: Antigen specificity. O, biotinyl-anti-$GgOs_3Cer$ (not absorbed) + avidin + biotinyl neocarzinostatin; Δ, nonimmune serum + avidin + biotinyl neocarzinostatin; □ , biotinyl anti-$GgOs_3Cer$ (absorbed on guinea pig erythrocytes) + avidin + biotinyl neocarzinostatin; ■ , biotinyl anti-$GgOs_3Cer$ (absorbed on sheep erythrocytes) + avidin + biotinyl neocarzinostatin. Absorption of antibody was accomplished by incubating 125 µl of antibody with 200 µl of packed red blood cells for 1 h at room temperature followed by centrifugation to remove red blood cells.

Discussion

Glycosphingolipids are chemically well-defined antigens or cell surface markers that characterize certain types of cells. Our studies indicate that some glycolipids have been found in relatively high concentration at the cell surface of a certain type of tumor cell. The same glycolipid can be found in low concentration in other types of cells. However, the glycolipids at the tumor cell surfaces could be a useful target for immunological suppression by passive immunization with polyclonal or monoclonal IgG antibody and antibody-dependent drug targeting. One example of such an approach with ganglio-N-triosylceramide has been described in this paper. Glycolipid cell

Table 7. *In Vivo* targeting with monoclonal IgM anti-gangliotriosylceramide

Group	Therapy[a]			Days survived			Survivors	Therapeutic
	1	2	3	mean	SD	median	(> 80 days)	effect
1	NaCl/Pi	NaCl/Pi	NaCl/Pi	29	6.2	27	0/5	control
2	Avidin alone			34.8	1	35	0/4	-
3	Biotinyl IgM	NaCl/Pi	NaCl/Pi	32.4	6.3	35	0/5	-
4	IgM	Avidin	NaCl/Pi	33.4	7	35	0/5	-
5	IgM	Avidin	Biotinyl-NCS (2.4 μg)	36.8	13.3	35	0/5	-
6	Biotinyl-avidin IgM		NaCl/Pi	41.2	5.9	44	0/5	-
7	Biotinyl-avidin		Biotinyl-NCS (2.4 μg)	70	22	51	2/5	+

[a]Animals received 1 million L5178c1271A1 cells i.p. on day 0. Therapy was given on days 1 and 4 and consisted of 3 i.p. injections: 1) IgM monoclonal anti-gangliotriosylceramide (256 H.A. units), 2) avidin (150 μg), and 3) biotinyl drug (2.4 μg) with 30-min intervals between each injection. Group 2 received avidin (150 μg) alone in a single injection on days 1 and 4.

surface markers should meet either of the following requirements: 1) present at the cell surface of a specific type of cells in much higher concentration than other types of cells, a condition that can be caused not only by an enhanced synthesis or inhibited degradation of glycolipid but also by increased exposure of glycolipid at the cell surface; 2) presence of a glycolipid with a specific structure at the surface of target cells. This may require activation of a specific glycosyltransferase unique to the target cells. Glycolipid markers are chemically well-defined and available from other animal tissues, and they are usually not immunogenic to syngenetic hosts. This is in striking contrast to tumor-specific transplantation antigen (TSTA). If tumor cells contain a large quantity of a certain chemically-identified glycolipid, polyclonal or monoclonal antibody directed to this glycolipid will be available, and targeting to tumor cells by these antibodies is possible.

The monoclonal IgM anti-$GgOs_3Cer$ had no therapeutic effect on tumor-bearing animals but could be a potential targeting reagent. It is noteworthy that both IgG3 and IgM monoclonal antibodies can kill tumor cells *in vitro*. Interestingly, Bernstein et al. (58) found that serotherapy of Thy-1-positive tumors with monoclonal anti-Thy-1 antibodies was effected only with IgG antibodies; IgM was not effective. They suggested that the ineffectiveness of IgM may be due to 1) the inability of IgM to diffuse to tumors *in vivo* or 2) the inability of IgM to mediate antibody-dependent cellular cytotoxic (ADCC) mechanisms of cell killing. Since the therapy of lymphoma cells in our study was performed intraperitoneally, at a site where diffusion is possibly not a problem, perhaps the dramatic suppression by the IgG3 antibody was due to ADCC mechanisms.

Although we have presented a successful example of immune suppression and targeting drugs to tumor cells using glycolipid markers, there are a number of potential drawbacks to the serotherapy or antibody-directed drug therapy of tumors. First, a problem common to many anti-tumor strategies is that tumors are a heterogeneous population of cells, and it is possible that cells lacking the target antigen or resistant to the drug will be selected by the treatment. Indeed we found that the ascites cells from one animal treated with IgG3 anti-$GgOs_3Cer$ contained only 10% of the amount of $GgOs_3Cer$ present in the original lymphoma cells. Second, perhaps only certain tumors, those exposed to circulating antibody, will be susceptible to this type of therapy. Solid tumors, for example, could be highly resistant as demonstrated by Rosenberg and Terry (59). Most tumors encountered clinically are well established and cannot be compared with the model demonstrated in this paper. Third, many of the reagents administered in the course of therapy are foreign to the host, so that anaphylaxis and rapid elimination of materials from the host due to an active host immune response are possible. The major obstacle to performing serotherapy or targeting drugs to tumor cells has been the insufficiency of well-defined antibody directed to tumor cells. The problem has been partially solved by the discovery of tumor-associated glycolipid antigen and polyclonal or monoclonal anti-glycolipid antibodies. Further extensive studies along this line will certainly provide an important basis for the control of human cancer.

Acknowledgment

This work was supported by Research Grants CA 20026, GM 23100, and CA 27746 from the National Institutes of Health.

References

1. Hakomori, S (1981). GSLs in cellular interaction, differentiation and oncogenesis. Annu Rev Biochem **50**, 733-764.
2. Hakomori, S (1981). Blood group ABH and Ii antigens of human erythrocytes: chemistry, polymorphism, and their developmental change. Semin Hematol **18**, 39-62.
3. Marcus, DM, and L Cass (1969). Glycosphingolipids with Lewis blood group activity: uptake by human erythrocytes. Science **164**, 553-555.
4. Watanabe, K, S Hakomori, RA Childs and T Feizi (1979). Characterization of a blood group I-active ganglioside. Structural requirements for I and i specificities. J Biol Chem **254**, 3221-3228.
5. Niemann, H, K Watanabe, S Hakomori, RA Childs and T Feizi (1978). Blood group i and I activities of "lacto-N-norhexaosylceramide" and its analogues: the structural requirements for i-specificities. Biochem Biophys Res Commun **81**, 1286-1293.
6. Feizi, T, RA Childs, K Watanabe and S Hakomori (1979). Three types of blood group I specificity among monoclonal anti-I autoantibodies revealed by analogues of a branched erythrocyte glycolipid. J Exp Med **149**, 975-980.
7. Marcus, DM, M Naiki and SK Kundu (1976). Abnormalities in the glycosphingolipid content of human p^k and p erythrocytes. Proc Natl Acad Sci USA **73**, 3263-3267.
8. Siddiqui, B, and S Hakomori (1971). A revised structure for the Forssman glycolipid hapten. J Biol Chem **246**, 5766-5769.
9. Higashi, H, M Naiki, S Matsuo and K Okouchi (1977). Antigen of "Serum Sickness" type of heterophile antibodies in human sera: identification as gangliosides with N-glycolylneuraminic acid. Biochem Biophys Res Commun **79**, 388-395.
10. Merrick, JM, K Zadarlik and F Milgrom (1978). Characterization of the Hanganutzui-Deicher (Serum-Sickness) antigen as gangliosides containing N-glycolylneuraminic acid. Int Arch Allergy Appl Immunol **57**, 477-480.
11. Stein-Douglass, KE, GA Schwarting, M Naiki and DM Marcus (1976). Gangliosides as markers for murine lymphocyte subpopulations. J Exp Med **143**, 822-832.
12. Stein, KN, GA Schwarting and DM Marcus (1978). Glycolipid markers of murine lymphocyte subpopulations. J Immunol **120**, 767-779.
13. Schwarting, GA, and DM Marcus (1977). The reactions of antibodies to paragloboside (lacto-N-neotetraosyl ceramide) with human erythrocytes and lymphocytes. J Immunol **118**, 1415-1419.

14. Young, WW, Jr, S Hakomori, JM Durdik and CS Henney (1980). Identification of ganglio-N-tetraosylceramide as a new cell surface marker for murine natural killer (NK) cells. J Immunol **124**, 199-201.
15. Kasai, M, M Iwamori, Y Nagai, K Okumura and T Tada (1980). A glycolipid on the surface of mouse natural killer cells. Eur J Immunol **10**, 175-180.
16. Kato, PK, TJ Wang and WJ Esselman (1979). Radiolabeling and isolation of THY-1 active glycolipids from murine brain and lymphoma cell lines. J Immunol **123**, 1977-1984.
17. Willison, KR, and PL Stern (1978). Expression of a Forssman antigenic specificity in the preimplantation mouse embryo. Cell **14**, 785-793.
18. Stern, PL, KR Willison, E Lennox, G Galfre, C Milstein, D Secher and A Ziegler (1978). Monoclonal antibodies as probes for differentiation and tumor-associated antigens: a Forssman specificity on teratocarcinoma stem cells. Cell **14**, 775-783.
19. Kapadia, A, T Feizi and MJ Evans (1981). Changes in the expression and polarization of blood group I and i antigens in post-implantation embryos and teratocarcinomas of mouse associated with cell differentiation. Exp Cell Res **131**, 185-195.
20. Artzt, K, P Dubois, D Bennett, H Condamine, C Baninet and F Jacob (1973). Surface antigens common to mouse cleavage embryo and primitive teratocarcinoma cells in culture. Proc Natl Acad Sci USA **70**, 2988-2992.
21. Muramatsu, T, G Gachlein, M Damonneville, C Delarbre and F Jacob (1979). Cell surface carbohydrates of embryonal carcinoma cells: polysaccharidic side chains of F9 antigens and of receptors to two lectins, FBP and PNA. Cell **18**, 183-191.
22. Larraga, V, and M Edidin (1979). Immunochemical characterization of surface antigens of TerC, a teratocarcinoma-derived cell line. Proc Natl Acad Sci USA **76**, 2912-2916.
23. Hakomori, S, E Nudelman, S Levery, D Solter and BB Knowles (1981). The hapten structure of a developmentally regulated glycolipid antigen (SSEA-1) isolated from human erythrocytes and adenocarcinoma: a preliminary note. Biochem Biophys Res Commun **100**, 1578-1586.
24. Nagai, Y, T Momoi, M Saito, E Mitsuzawa and S Ohtani (1976). Ganglioside syndrome, a new autoimmune neurological disorder, experimentally induced with brain gangliosides. Neurosci Lett **2**, 107-111.
25. Fry, JM, S Weissbarth, GM Lehrer and MB Borenstein (1974). Cerebroside antibody inhibits sulfatide synthesis and myelination and demyelinates in cord tissue cultures. Science **183**, 540-542.
26. Hurby, S, EC Alvord, Jr and FJ Seil (1977). Synthetic galactocerebrosides evoke myelination-inhibiting antibodies. Science **195**, 173-175.
27. Schwarting, GA, SK Kundu and DM Marcus (1979). The reaction of antibodies that cause paroxysmal cold hemoglobinuria with globoside and Forssman glycosphingolipids. Blood **53**, 186-192.
28. Mullin, BR, AJ Montanaro, JD Reid and RN Nishimura (1980). Interaction of multiple sclerosis serum with liposomes containing ganglioside GM1. Ann Neurol **7**, 587-590.
29. Arnon, R, E Crisp, R Kelley, GW Ellison, LW Myers and WW Tourtellotte (1980). Anti-ganglioside antibodies in multiple sclerosis. J Neurol Sci **46**, 179-186.
30. Nagai, Y, K Sakakibara and T Uchida (1980). **In** Search for the cause of multiple sclerosis and chronic diseases of central nervous system, pp 127-138. 1st International Symposium of Hertie Foundation in Frankfurt/Main, Sept 1979. A Boese, ed. Verlag Chemie, Weinheim/Bergst.
31. Hirano, T, H Hashimoto, Y Shiokawa, M Iwamori, Y Nagai, M Kasai, Y Ochiai and K Okumura (1981). Antiglycolipid autoantibody detected in the sera from systemic lupus erythematosus patients. J Clin Invest **66**, 1437-1440.
32. Sundsmo, J, and S Hakomori (1976). Lacto-N-neotetraosylceramide ("Paraglobo-side") as a possible tumor-associated surface antigen of hamster NILpy tumor. Biochem Biophys Res Commun **68**, 799-806.
33. Rosenfelder, G, WW Young, Jr and S Hakomori (1977). Association of the glycolipid pattern with antigenic alterations in mouse fibroblasts transformed by

murine sarcoma virus. Cancer Res **37**, 1333-1339.
34. Young, WW, Jr, JM Durdik, D Urdal, S Hakomori and CS Henney (1981). Glycolipid expression in lymphoma cell variants: chemical quantity, immunologic reactivity, and correlations with susceptibility to NK cells. J Immunol **126**, 1-6.
35. Nakahara, K, T Ohashi, T Oda, T Hirano, M Kasai, K Okumura and T Tada (1980). Asialo GM_1 as a cell-surface marker detected in acute lymphoblastic leukemia. N Engl J Med **302**, 67-77.
36. Hakomori, S, S-M Wang and WW Young, Jr (1977). Isoantigenic expression of Forssman glycolipid in human gastric and colonic mucosa: its possible identity with "A-like antigen" in human cancer. Proc Natl Acad Sci USA **74**, 3023-3027.
37. Hakomori, S, J Koscielak, KJ Bloch and RW Jeanloz (1967). Studies on the immunological relation between the tumor glycolipids and blood group substances. J Immunol **98**, 31-38.
38. Häkkinen, I (1970). A-like blood group antigen in gastric cancer cells of patients in blood groups O or B. J Natl Cancer Inst **44**, 1183-1193.
39. Breimer, ME (1980). Adaptation of mass spectrometry for the analysis of tumor antigens as applied to blood group glycolipids of a human gastric carcinoma. Cancer Res **40**, 897-908.
40. Levine, P (1976). Illegitimate blood group antigens P_1, A and MN (T) in malignancy. Ann NY Acad Sci **277**, 428-433.
41. Magnani, JL, M Brockhaus, DF Smith, V Ginsburg, M Blaszczyk, KF Mitchell, Z Steplewski and H Koprowski (1981). A monosialoganglioside is a monoclonal antibody-defined antigen of colon carcinoma. Science **212**, 55-56.
42. Dippold, WG, KO Lloyd, LTC Li, H Ikeda, HF Oettgen and LJ Old (1980). Cell surface antigens of human malignant melanoma: definition of six antigenic systems with mouse monoclonal antibodies. Proc Natl Acad Sci USA **77**, 6114-6118.
43. Hakomori, S, and WT Murakami (1968). Glycolipids of hamster fibroblasts and derived malignant transformed cell lines. Proc Natl Acad Sci USA **59**, 254-261.
44. Gahmberg, CG, and S Hakomori (1975). Surface carbohydrates of hamster fibroblasts. I. Chemical characterization of surface-labeled glycosphingolipids and a specific ceramide tetrasaccharide for transformants. J Biol Chem **250**, 2438-2446.
45. Baumann, H, E Nudelman, K Watanabe and S Hakomori (1979). Neutral fucolipids and fucogangliosides of rat hepatoma HTC and H-35 cells, rat liver and hepatocytes. Cancer Res **39**, 2637-2643.
46. Holmes, E, and S Hakomori (1982). Isolation and characterization of a new fucoganglioside accumulated in precancerous rat liver and in rat hepatoma induced by N-2 acetylaminofluorene. J Biol Chem, in press.
47. Yang, H-J, and S Hakomori (1971). A sphingolipid having a novel type of ceramide and lacto-N-fucopentaose III. J Biol Chem **246**, 1192-1200.
48. Siddiqui, B, JS Whitehead and YS Kim (1978). Glycosphingolipids in human colonic adenocarcinoma. J Biol Chem **253**, 2168-2175.
49. Watanabe, K, T Matsubara and S Hakomori (1976). Alpha-L-fucopyranosylceramide, a novel glycolipid accumulated in some of the human colon tumors. J Biol Chem **251**, 2385-2387.
50. Gooi, HC, T Feizi, A Kapadia, BB Knowles, D Solter and MJ Evans (1981). Stage-specific embryonic antigen involves $\alpha 1 \rightarrow 3$ fucosylated type 2 blood group chains. Nature (Lond) **292**, 156-158.
51. Kawanami, J (1972). The appearance of Forssman hapten in human tumor. J Biochem (Tokyo) **72**, 783-785.
52. Hakomori, S, and WW Young, Jr (1978). Tumor associated glycolipid antigens and modified blood group antigens. Scand J Immunol **7**, 97-117.
53. Young, WW, Jr, EMS MacDonald, RC Nowinski and S Hakomori (1979). Production of monoclonal antibodies specific for distinct portions of the glycolipid asialo GM_2 (gangliotriosylceramide). J Exp Med **150**, 1008-1019.
54. Young, WW, Jr, and S Hakomori (1981). Therapy of mouse lymphoma with monoclonal antibodies to glycolipid: selection of low antigenic variants *in vivo*. Science **211**, 487-489.

55. Urdal, DL, and S Hakomori (1980). Tumor-associated ganglio-N-triosylceramide. J Biol Chem **255,** 10509-10516.
56. Siddiqui, B, and S Hakomori (1970). Change of glycolipids in minimal deviation hepatomas. Cancer Res **30,** 2930-2936.
57. Köhler, G, and C Milstein (1975). Continuous cultures of fused cells secreting antibody of predefined specificity. Nature (Lond) **256,** 495-497.
58. Bernstein, I, M Tam and RC Nowinski (1980). Mouse leukemia: therapy with monoclonal antibodies against a thymus differentiation antigen. Science **207,** 68-71.
59. Rosenberg, SA, and W Terry (1977). Passive immunotherapy of cancer in animals and man. Adv Cancer Res **25,** 323-388.

V
Applications to Bacteria, Viruses, and Parasites

GROUP B STREPTOCOCCAL MONOCLONAL ANTIBODY: DIAGNOSTIC AND THERAPEUTIC APPLICATIONS

Richard A. Polin
Mary Catherine Harris

Division of Neonatology
The Children's Hospital of Philadelphia
Philadelphia, Pennsylvania 19104

Streptococcus agalactiae, group B streptococcus (GBS), was first isolated in 1887 by Nocard and Mollereau from a case of bovine mastitis (1). In 1933, Lancefield demonstrated that hemolytic streptococci could be differentiated into five serological groups (A-E) based upon the presence of specific carbohydrates designated *C* substances (2,3). The following year group B streptococcus was further subdivided into three types (I-III) on the basis of newly discovered *S* substances (4). The serological scheme is based upon capillary precipitin tests with HCl-extracted antigens and hyperimmune type-specific rabbit antisera. Passive protection tests in mice have furnished confirmatory evidence of specific type classification (5). In 1938, type I was subclassified into types Ia and Ib (6), and in 1971 Wilkinson et al. identified an additional type, Ic (7). The current antigenic classification of group B streptococci is illustrated in Table 1.

In 1973, Franciosi and colleagues in Denver (8) and Baker and coworkers in Houston (9) delineated two clinical syndromes based upon the age of onset of symptoms. Streptococcal disease that begins in the first five days of life is labeled "early onset disease." Such infants frequently present with apnea, cardiovascular instability, or respiratory distress. The neonate acquires the organism during passage through the birth canal. Any of the group B streptococcal types may cause early onset disease. However, if the central nervous system is involved most isolates are type III. The mortality from GBS infection acquired at delivery exceeds 50%. Discrimination of this disease from hyaline membrane disease in the premature infant is exceedingly difficult and accounts for some of the mortality. No single test or battery of tests has been universally predictive of streptococcal infection. Late onset disease presenting as meningitis begins as early as the tenth day of life or as late as four months. Although the mortality rate is less than for early onset disease (20%), serious neurological sequelae are noted in as many as 50% of the survivors (10). Almost all isolates in late onset disease are type III.

When standard laboratory techniques are used, the isolation and identification of group B streptococci recovered from culture specimens require 24-48 h. The recent introduction of immunodiagnostic assays (Staphylococcal co-agglutination, latex particle agglutination, and counterimmunoelectrophoresis) has permitted rapid identification of streptococcal antigen in body fluid specimens or culture media containing mixed flora (11-13). Group B streptococcal antigen may be identified in 6-18 h from specimens containing mixed flora when selective media and one of the assays listed above are used. The minimal concentration of group B streptococcal antigen detectable with these assays has been 800 ng/ml (14). Two problems have been encountered with these procedures. Variations in the source of antisera used in the assays have decreased the sensitivity and specificity of the tests (15). In addition, most of the immunodiagnostic tests use antisera against group-specific determinants; therefore, rapid serotyping of group B streptococcal isolates is not generally possible.

Recent advancements in the technique of somatic cell hybridization by Köhler and Milstein have permitted isolation of hybrid myeloma (hybridoma) cell lines secreting homogeneous antibody of predetermined specificity (16). These cell lines are immortalized, and antibody may be harvested from cell culture supernatants (μg/ml quantities) or tumor-stimulated ascites fluid (mg/ml quantities). Polin and Kennett have isolated hybridomas secreting monoclonal antibodies specific for types Ia/Ic, Ib, II, and III group B streptococcus (17). Kasper has demonstrated that anti-GBS Ia/Ic, II, and III antibodies react with the polysaccharide determinant unique to each serotype (18).

The purpose of this report is to describe the clinical and therapeutic applications of the anti-group B streptococcal monoclonal antibodies: 1) detection of GBS colonization, 2) serotyping of bacterial isolates in the clinical microbiology laboratory, 3) identification of GBS antigen in body fluid specimens, and 4) protection against fatal GBS infection in mice.

Table 1. Antigenic composition of group B streptococcus

	Bacterial serotype				
	Ia	Ib	Ic	II	III
Antigenic determinants					
Protein antigen		Ibc	Ibc	Ibc*	Ibc*
Major carbohydrate antigen	Ia	Ib	Ia	II	III
Minor carbohydrate antigen	Iabc	Iabc	Iabc		

*Rarely

Production of Monoclonal Antibodies

Vaccines. Vaccines of formalinized group B streptococcus were prepared from the following Lancefield reference strains according to previously published methods (19): Type Ia-090/14; Type Ib-H36B/60/2; Type Ic-A909/14; Type II-18RS21/67/2; Type III-D136C.

Immunization. BALB/c mice were given three immunizations of formalinized bacteria at weekly intervals. The first immunization consisted of antigen (0.5 ml) in incomplete Freunds adjuvant administered intraperitoneally. The second dose (0.5 ml) diluted in saline was administered intraperitoneally and subcutaneously. The final injection (0.2 ml) was given intravenously in a tail vein.

Hybridoma production. Cell fusion and cloning were performed according to previously published methods (19). Hybridomas were tested for binding to types Ia, Ib, Ic, II and III GBS, and type XIV pneumococcus using a binding immunoassay in which monoclonal antibody bound to bacteria was detected with a sheep anti-mouse immunoglobulin conjugated to peroxidase. For the studies described below four monoclonal antibodies were chosen that exhibited a high affinity in the enzyme immunoassay for one of the GBS serotypes, anti-GBS Ia/Ic, Ib, II, III. The anti-GBS Ia/Ic, II, and III monoclonal antibodies were μk, whereas the anti-Ib monoclonal antibody was $\gamma 2_a k$.

Diagnostic Applications of Monoclonal Antibodies

The enzyme immunoassay was modified to identify GBS antigen in body fluid specimens and culture media, and to serotype bacterial isolates. This modification was termed the enzyme-linked monoclonal antibody inhibition assay (ELMIA). The specificity of each of the monoclonal antibodies used in this assay was checked to insure reactivity only with a single GBS serotype.

Enzyme Linked Monoclonal Antibody Inhibition Assay (ELMIA) (Fig. 1) (20)

Fixation of bacteria to polyvinylchloride plates. Fifty μl of a poly-L-lysine solution (0.001 gm/100 ml phosphate buffered saline), pH 7.2, were placed into each well of a 96-well, flat-bottomed polyvinylchloride plate and incubated 2 h at room temperature. The PLL was removed, and 2 x 6^{10} bacteria suspended in 50 μl PBS were added to each well. The plates were centrifuged (2,000 rpm x 5 min) and 50 μl of a 0.5% glutaraldehyde solution (Sigma Chemical Company) in cold PBS was placed into each well. Following a 15-min incubation at room temperature, all wells were washed twice by

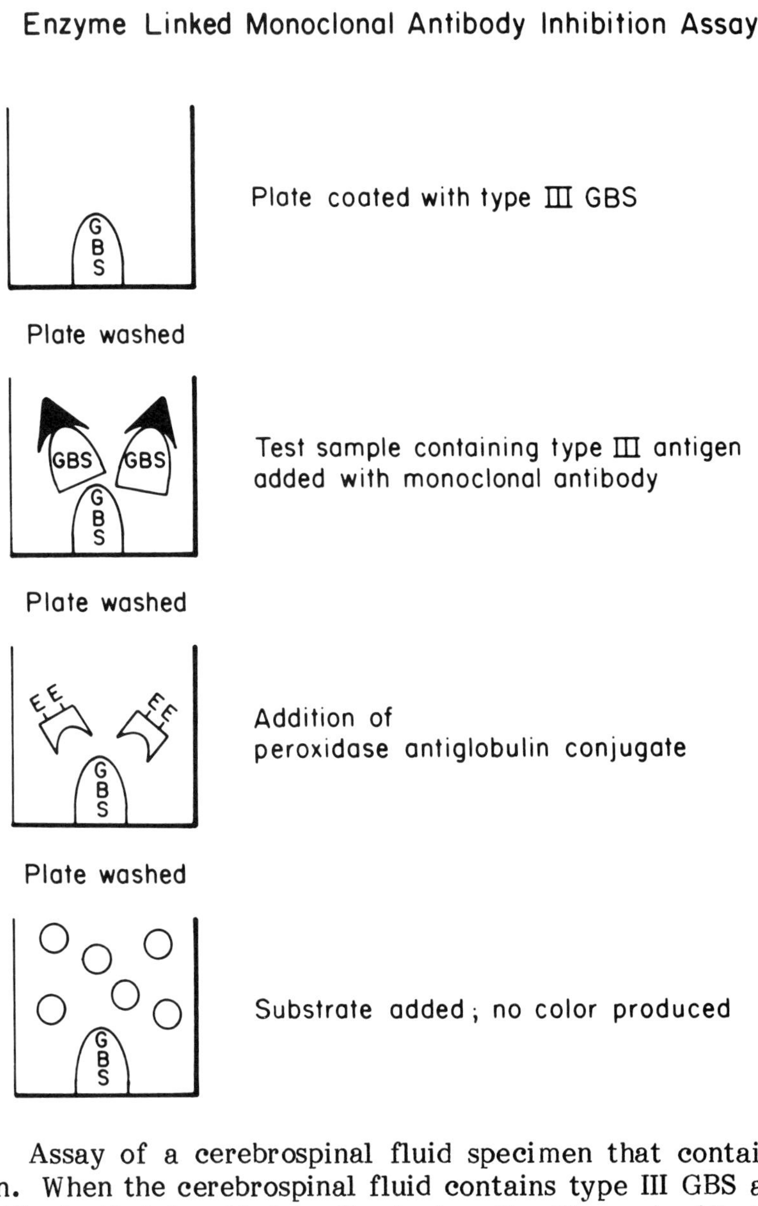

Fig. 1. Assay of a cerebrospinal fluid specimen that contains GBS antigen. When the cerebrospinal fluid contains type III GBS antigen, the antibody that is added to the test well will react with the CSF group B streptococcal antigen and will not react with the GBS antigen that has been preattached to the bottom of the well. Therefore, when the enzyme antiglobulin conjugate is added along with the appropriate substrate, no color reaction will result. If no antigen is present in the spinal fluid a strong color reaction will be produced as a result of the antibodies binding to the bacteria fixed to the plate. (Modified from Ref. 20.)

immersing in PBS and flicking the remaining fluid into the sink. Each well was then filled with a 100 mM glycine in 1% bovine serum albumin solution (pH 7.6) and incubated 30 min at room temperature. The plates were washed in PBS, dried under a heat lamp, and stored at room temperature until use within six months.

Assay. Twenty-five µl of PBS, or 25 µl of a body fluid specimen, bacterial isolate suspended in PBS, or culture media from an actively growing culture of GBS was placed in wells of a PVC plate coated with type-specific GBS. Serial dilutions of hybridoma supernatants containing type-specific GBS beginning at 1/4 were added to the wells. The plates were incubated 2 h at room temperature and washed three times in PBS by immersion flicking. One hundred µl of peroxidase-labeled anti-mouse IgG (Cappell 1/1000 in 1% BSA) was added to each test well and the plate incubated 2 h at room temperature. The wells were washed again six times and two drops of substrate added (10 ml citrate buffer, pH 4.5; 10 mg orthophenylene diamine (Sigma); 2 µl hydrogen peroxide). The color of each test well was evaluated 30 min after substrate was added. The reaction was stopped by adding 50 µl of 0.1 M NaF to each well. A specimen was interpreted as positive, i.e., containing type-specific GBS antigen, if it inhibited the binding of the type-specific GBS antibody to the bacteria attached to the wells. When antigen was present in the fluid tested and inhibition occurred, the optical density of the solution was significantly less than that of comparable wells containing only antibody. To obtain quantitative readings, all plates were read on an 8-channel photometer (Titertek-Multiscan).

Results

Detection of GBS antigen. The ELMIA detected group B streptococcal antigen in cerebrospinal fluid specimens from 20 infants with culture-proven group B streptococcal meningitis and in the knee aspirate from an infant with group B streptococcal arthritis. There were no false positive reactions noted with the control fluids. The concentration of type III antigen in the spinal fluids ranged from 0.8-12.8 µg/ml. However, the ELMIA can detect antigen at a concentration of 10 ng/ml (21), a value 80-100 times lower than is detectable with conventional assays. A sample printout from the Multiscan photometer illustrating an assay of four CSF specimens is shown in Table 2. The ELMIA has recently been used to identify GBS in selective culture media that has been artificially inoculated with type-specific group B streptococci. Starting with an inoculation of 10^6 bacteria/ml of selective media, the assay was positive within 4 h for types Ia, Ic, II, and III and within 6 h for type Ib. In addition, the assay has successfully identified numerous GBS isolates supplied by the Clinical Microbiology Laboratory at The Children's Hospital of Philadelphia.

Table 2. Analysis of a cerebrospinal fluid containing Type III Streptococcal antigen: Photometer printout.

Four spinal fluids were analyzed in this experiment. The photometer was programmed to compare the optical density of each test well to a reference optical density of substrate reaction mixture containing no enzyme activity. The numbers shown represent the amount of antibody remaining available for reaction with the glutaraldehyde-fixed type III GBS. Row A contained antibody dilutions ranging from 1/4–1/256 incubated without any spinal fluid. Row B contained spinal fluid from a proven case of GBS meningitis in addition to antibody dilutions, and Rows C, D, E contained antibody plus three spinal fluids from infants without any meningeal infection. In Row B there was a significant decrease in the optical density of wells 2 to 4. This spinal fluid was known to contain type III GBS antigen. (Ref. 20.)

	Antibody dilutions											
		Undiluted	1:4	1:8	1:16	1:32	1:64	1:128	1:256			
A. Antibody + PBS dilutent	0	6	6	5	4	2	1	1	1	0	0	0
B. Antibody + CSF (GBS +)	0	4	3	2	1	1	1	1	0	0	0	0
C. Antibody + control CSF	0	5	6	5	3	2	1	0	0	0	0	0
D. Antibody + control CSF	0	5	5	5	3	2	1	0	0	0	0	0
E. Antibody + control CSF	0	6	6	5	4	3	2	1	1	0	0	0
	0	0	0	0	0	0	0	0	0	0	0	0
	0	0	0	0	0	0	0	0	0	0	0	0
	0	0	0	0	0	0	0	0	0	0	0	0
Row number	1	2	3	4	5	6	7	8	9	10	11	12

Therapeutic Applications of Monoclonal Antibodies

Each monoclonal antibody was evaluated for its ability to agglutinate type-specific bacteria, fix complement, opsonize, and protect mice against lethal GBS infection.

Methods

Agglutination. Bacteria (10^6) suspended in 25 µl PBS-1% BSA (pH 7.2) were placed in each well of a 96-well, curved-bottom microtiter plate (Linbro). Twenty-five µl of the supernatants to be tested were pipetted into each well. The plates were covered, incubated 2 h at 37°C, and checked for macroscopic agglutination. Each hybrid myeloma supernatant was tested in duplicate on two separate occasions. Bacterial agglutination was performed with three different concentrations of each supernatant (undiluted, 1/5, 1/10). Each supernatant was incubated with types Ia, Ib, Ic, II, and III GBS. Control supernatants were obtained from actively growing cultures of SP2/O-Ag 14.

Complement fixation. Fifty µl of monoclonal antibody and 25 µl of a 1/40 dilution of serum (untreated, heat-treated or Mg EGTA-treated) were incubated in each well of PVC plates precoated with type-specific GBS of identical specificity to the antibody. The plates were incubated overnight at 4°C, and 25 µl of sheep red blood cells that had been sensitized with hemolysin were added to the test wells. Hemolysis was assessed macroscopically after 30 min.

Opsonization. Radiolabeled Bacterial Uptake Technique (22). Reference GBS strain D136C (GBS type III) was grown overnight in Todd Hewitt Broth containing 5 µci/ml of ^{3}H leucine. The bacteria were heat-killed, washed three times in phosphate buffered saline, resuspended at a concentration of 1.7 x 10^8 ml, and stored at -20°C. Prior to study this strain was opsonized by mixing 0.75 ml of the bacterial suspension with control serum diluted with either supernatant from an actively growing culture of SP2/O-Ag14, monoclonal anti-GBS type III, or Ia/Ic antibody. Monolayers of neutrophils prepared from leukocyte-rich plasma by dextran sedimentation were adhered to 15 mm x 15 mm glass cover slips at room temperature for 30 min. Non-adherent cells were washed off and 0.2 ml of the opsonized bacterial suspension placed on the cover slips. At intervals varying from 0 to 100 min the cover slips were washed in PBS and placed in scintillation vials with 10.0 ml of Aquasol and counted for 5 min. The number of neutrophils/cover slip was visually counted and results expressed as CPM/10^6 neutrophils.

Protection studies. BALB/c mice were given a subscapular injection of 5 x 10^5 hybridoma cells secreting monoclonal antibody with one of the following specificities: anti-GBS Ia/Ic, Ib, or II (type

III GBS does not infect adult mice). Tumors became visible within two weeks. After 14 days mice with tumors and an equal number of control mice were challenged with an intraperitoneal injection of 10^9 live GBS of identical specificity to the tumor. In addition, mice with tumors secreting antibody to type II GBS were challenged with Ia bacteria, and BALB/c mice with tumors making antibody to type Ia/Ic GBS were challenged with type II bacteria.

Results

Agglutination. As illustrated in Table 3 each of the monoclonal antibodies agglutinated GBS to which it corresponded in specificity but not GBS of a different serotype. Agglutination was positive at antibody dilutions ranging from undiluted to 1/10.

Table 3. Agglutination

	Group B streptococcal serotype				
Monoclonal antibody	Ia	Ib	Ic	II	III
Anti-GBS Ia/Ic	+[a]	-[b]	+	-	-
Anti-GBS Ib	-	+	-	-	-
Anti-GBS II	-	-	-	+	-
Anti-GBS III	-	-	-	-	+
SP2/O-Ag 14	-	-	-	-	-

[a]+, agglutination.
[b]-, no agglutination.

Complement fixation. Complement fixation results are shown in Table 4. All the monoclonal antibodies were complement-fixing. Pre-treatment of human sera with Mg EGTA (classical complement pathway inhibition) prevented complement fixation and resulted in hemolysis of the sensitized sheep red blood cells. This indicated that the monoclonal antibodies were interacting with the classical but not the alternate complement pathway. Heat inactivation of the sera destroyed complement and prevented hemolysis.

Opsonization. Figure 2 illustrates results of the opsonization studies with type III GBS using SP2/O-Ag14 control supernatant, anti-GBS Ia or III monoclonal antibody. Both monoclonal antibodies resulted in significantly greater phagocytosis of type III GBS than of control supernatant. This was true at 30, 60, 80, and 100 min for anti-GBS type III antibody ($p < .02$) and at 60 and 100 min for anti-GBS type Ia antibody ($p < .05$). In addition, phagocytosis was significantly greater with type III GBS monoclonal antibody than with the anti-Ia antibody ($p < .05$ at 60 and 80 min).

Mouse protection studies. Table 5 indicates the results of the protection studies. One hundred percent of tumor-bearing mice challenged with GBS of identical specificity to the tumor survived. All mice without tumors and the "tumor" mice challenged with GBS of a different specificity died. Surviving "tumor" mice had anti-GBS titers of > 1/10,000.

Discussion

Antisera directed against bacterial antigens, either raised in animals or harvested from human blood products, have been clinically applied in three different ways. First, they have been used in the diagnostic microbiology laboratory to identify bacteria that have been isolated from clinical specimens. Secondly, the antisera have been incorporated into immunoassays that detect bacterial antigen in body fluid specimens. Lastly, antisera have been administered to infants with life-threatening infections to decrease disease mortality and morbidity. This paper describes the application of monoclonal antibodies to each of these areas of clinical medicine.

Table 4. Complement fixation

	Serum		
Monoclonal antibody	Untreated sera	Mg EGTA treated sera	Heat inactivated sera
Anti-GBS Ia/Ic	+[a]	-[b]	*[c]
Anti-GBS Ib	+	-	*
Anti-GBS II	+	-	*
Anti-GBS III	+	-	*
SP2/O-Ag 14	-	-	*

[a]+, antibodies fixed complement; hemolysis absent.

[b]-, no complement fixation; hemolysis present.

[c]*, both complement pathways inactivated; hemolysis absent.

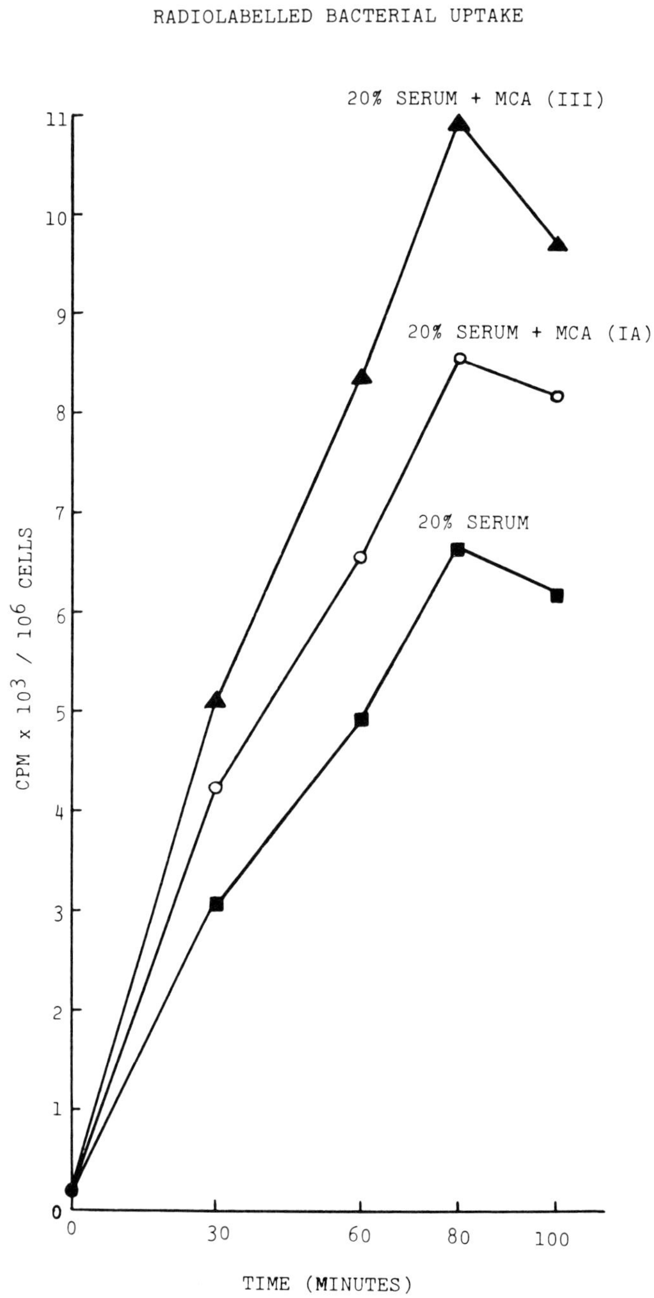

Fig. 2. Radiolabelled bacterial uptake: Type III GBS. Results of preincubation with anti-GBS type III or, monoclonal antibody versus 20% serum control.

Table 5. Mouse protection experiments

	No. of survivors/No. tested			
GBS serotype injected intraperitoneally	Ia	Ic	Ib	II
Antibody produced by tumor				
Anti-GBS Ia/Ic	5/5	5/5	--	0/5
Anti-GBS Ib	--	--	5/5	--
Anti-GBS II	0/5	--	--	5/5
Control mice (no tumors)	0/5	0/5	0/5	0/5

Three kinds of immunoassays have been developed to detect GBS antigen in body fluid specimens: staphylococcal co-agglutination (15), latex particle agglutination (14), and counterimmunoelectrophoresis (13). All of these assays rely on antisera raised in animals (sheep or goat) and frequently varying in quality between animals, and even with each bleed of the same animal. These tests are important because they permit rapid diagnosis of an infection with GBS before the organism is isolated in the microbiology laboratory. Unfortunately, many of these assays have not proven reliable because of variability in the source of antisera. In addition, the minimal concentration of antigen these assays can detect under the best possible conditions is 800 ng/ml. The ELMIA described in this paper can reliably identify GBS antigen at a concentration of 10 ng/ml.

A second important use of the ELMIA is the identification of women who are colonized with GBS during labor and delivery. Most neonates acquire group B streptococcus during passage through the birth canal. The sequence of events responsible for early onset infection has been designated the "ascending amniotic infection syndrome." Infection begins with colonization of the maternal genital tract. Pathogenic bacteria spread upward through the cervix into the amniotic cavity, resulting in amnionitis. Susceptible infants either inhale or swallow infected amniotic fluid and develop generalized infection. Recent attempts to decrease the incidence of the disease have focused upon the treatment of maternal GBS carriers with penicillin or penicillin derivatives. This approach has not been satisfactory because 1) it is difficult to predict which women will have genital colonization with GBS during labor or delivery, and 2) many investigators are reluctant to indiscriminately treat all women or infants regardless of their colonization with an antibiotic that has potentially serious side effects. The ELMIA should permit detection of GBS colonization within 6 h of obtaining a culture identifying women at high risk for delivering infants with invasive GBS disease.

The importance of antibody in the prevention of lethal GBS infection in mice was initially proven by Lancefield et al. Dr. Lancefield demonstrated that multiple mouse-protective antibodies can be produced in the sera of experimentally immunized rabbits. The human neonate is dependent on prenatal transfer of maternal antibody. Fortunately, a mechanism exists in the placenta for transport of maternal IgG to the fetus. Passively acquired antibody from the mother accounts for the rarity of neonatal infections with group A streptococcus. In 1978, Baker and Kasper compared antibody titers in mothers and infants who were asymptomatically colonized with GBS to a group of women who delivered septic infants, in an attempt to identify infants prone to develop type III group B streptococcal disease (23,24). Seventy-six percent of mothers who delivered asymptomatic infants had serum antibodies directed against GBS, whereas the seven infected neonates and their mothers had no demonstrable titer.

The newborn infant can be supplied with antibody either by active immunization of mothers with purified polysaccharide vaccines or through supplying of infants or mothers with preformed human antibody against group B streptococcal types. The majority of human volunteers given subcutaneous injections of purified type III group B streptococcal polysaccharide preparations develop antibody responses which are maximal by 2 weeks and remain positive for at least 21 weeks after immunization (25). An alternative to active immunization is administration of sera containing specific antibodies to GBS. Shigeoka et al. have administered fresh whole blood to 22 infants, 15 of whom had early onset of GBS sepsis (26). One hundred percent of infants transfused with blood containing opsonic antibody identical to their infecting strain survived. Many other authors have promoted the use of plasma or exchange transfusion to treat neonatal sepsis; however, controlled data is lacking. Somatic cell hybridization and hybridoma technology offer the possibility of making unlimited quantities of highly specific antibody against group B streptococcus. This antibody could be given prenatally to mothers who are known to lack serum antibody to GBS or could be used postnatally to treat infections in their infants. The present study demonstrates that these monoclonal antibodies possess the functional properties (agglutination, complement fixation, and opsonization) necessary to protect mice against experimental infection when they are challenged with large numbers of organisms. Although murine antibody could be purified for administration to infants, recent advances in hybridoma technology offer the possibility of developing a human hybridoma cell line producing human antibody to group B streptococcus.

References

1. Nocard, E, and A Mollereau (1887). Sur une mammitc contagicuse des vaches laitieres. Ann Inst Pasteur (Paris) 1, 109-126.
2. Lancefield, RC (1933). Serological differentiation of human and other groups of haemolytic streptococci. J Exp Med **57**, 571-595.
3. Curtis, SN, and RM Krause (1964). Antigenic relationships between groups B and G streptococci. J Exp Med **120**, 629-637.
4. Lancefield, RC (1934). A serological differentiation of specific types of bovine streptococci (group B). J Exp Med **59**, 441-459.
5. Lancefield, RC, M McCarty and WN Everly (1975). Multiple mouse-protective antibodies directed against group B streptococci: Special reference to antibodies effective against protein antigens. J Exp Med **142**, 165-179.
6. Lancefield, RC (1938). Two serological types of group B hemolytic streptococci with related but not identical, type-specific substances. J Exp Med **67**, 25-40.
7. Wilkinson, HW, and RG Eagon (1971). Type-specific antigens of group B type Ic streptococci. Infect Immun **4**, 596-604.
8. Franciosi, RA, JD Knostman and RA Zimmerman (1973). Group B streptococcal neonatal and infant infections. J Pediatr **82**, 707-718.
9. Baker, CJ, FF Barrett, RC Cordon and MD Yow (1973). Suppurative meningitis due to streptococci of Lancefield group B: A study of 33 infants. J Pediatr **82**, 724-729.
10. Horn, KA, RA Zimmerman, JD Knostman and WT Meyer (1974). Neurological sequelae of group B streptococcal neonatal infections. Pediatrics **53**, 501-504.
11. Feigin, RD, M Wong, PG Shackelford, BW Stechenberg, et al. (1976). Concurrent immunoelectrophoresis of urine as well as of CSF and blood for diagnosis of bacterial meningitis. J Pediatr **89**, 773-775.
12. Siegel, JD, and GH McCracken (1978). Detection of group B streptococcal antigens in body fluids of neonates. J Pediatr **93**, 491-492.
13. Edwards, MS, and CJ Baker (1979). Prospective diagnosis of early onset group B streptococcal infection by concurrent immunoelectrophoresis. J Pediatr **94**, 286-288.
14. Edwards, MS, DL Kasper and CJ Baker (1979). Rapid diagnosis of type III group B streptococcal meningitis by latex particle agglutination. J Pediatr **95**, 202-205.
15. Thirumoorthi, MC, and AS Dajani (1979). Comparison of staphylococcal coagglutination, latex agglutination, and counterimmunoelectrophoresis for bacterial antigen detection. J Clin Microbiol **9**, 28-32.
16. Köhler, G, and C Milstein (1975). Continuous cultures of fused cells making antibody of predefined specificity. Nature (Lond) **256**, 495-497.
17. Polin, RA, and R Kennett (1980). Use of monoclonal antibodies in an enzyme immunoassay for rapid identification of types II and III group B streptococcus. J Clin Microbiol **11**, 332-336.
18. Kasper, DL. Personal communication.
19. Polin, RA (1980). Monoclonal antibodies against streptococcal antigens. **In** Monoclonal Antibodies, pp 353-359. RH Kennett, TJ McKearn and KB Bechtol, eds. Plenum Press, New York.
20. Voller, A, A Bartlett and DE Bidwell (1978). Enzyme immunoassays with special reference to ELISA techniques. J Clin Pathol **31**, 507-520.
21. Polin, RA, and R Kennett (1980). Use of monoclonal antibodies in an enzyme linked inhibition assay for rapid detection of streptococcal antigens. J Pediatr **97**, 540-544.
22. Shigeoka, AO, RT Hall, VG Hemming, CD Allred and HR Hill (1978). Role of antibody and complement in opsonization of group B streptococci. Infect Immun **21**, 34-40.
23. Baker, CJ, and DL Kasper (1976). Correlation of maternal antibody deficiency with susceptibility to neonatal group B streptococcal infection. N Engl J Med **294**, 753-756.

24. Baker, CJ, and DL Kasper (1977). Immunologic investigation of infants with septicemia or meningitis due to group B streptococcus. J Infect Dis **136**, S98-S105.
25. Baker, CJ, MS Edwards and DL Kasper (1978). Immunogenicity of polysaccharides from type III group B streptococcus. J Clin Invest **61**, 1107-1110.
26. Shigeoka, SO, RT Hall and HR Hill (1978). Blood transfusion in group B streptococcal sepsis. Lancet **1**, 636-638.

THE USE OF MONOCLONAL ANTIBODIES TO IDENTIFY ANTIGENIC TARGETS OF IMMUNITY TO MALARIA

Joan Rener,* Louis H. Miller, and Richard Carter

Laboratory of Parasitic Diseases
National Institutes of Health
Bethesda, Maryland 20205

Malaria persists as a major disease in the tropical world, draining scarce financial resources available for health care. Because of the decreasing effectiveness of insecticides and anti-malarial drugs, efforts are now being made to develop vaccines directed against different stages of the malarial parasite's life cycle.

The malarial parasite is a unicellular protozoan of the genus *Plasmodium*. Of the four species producing malaria in man, *P. falciparum* causes the most virulent infection, lethal to a million children a year in Africa alone. Malarial infection in man begins with the bite of an infected anopheline mosquito. Sporozoites released into the bloodstream invade hepatic parenchymal cells, where each parasite divides into as many as 20,000 merozoites. Merozoites then enter the bloodstream and invade erythrocytes, where they divide asexually to form schizonts. When the schizonts mature, the erythrocyte ruptures to release new merozoites, each capable of invading a new erythrocyte. The synchronous release of merozoites and the "toxins" produced by the parasites cause the periodic fever and chills characteristic of malaria. Death from *P. falciparum* infection is caused in part by large numbers of infected erythrocytes obstructing capillaries in vital organs.

Some asexual parasites differentiate into gametocytes, sexual forms of the parasite that are infectious to mosquitoes. Ingested by a mosquito during a blood meal, gametocytes shed their erythrocytic membranes in the mosquito gut and develop into gametes. Fertilization occurs rapidly, and the parasite becomes established as an ookinete, a motile form that embeds in the gut wall to form an oocyst. Within 9-12 days sporozoites are formed, the oocyst ruptures, and the sporozoites migrate to the mosquito's salivary glands. At the next blood meal, sporozoites are inoculated into the blood stream, and a new round of infection begins.

Since each stage in the parasite's life cycle presents unique surface antigens, each stage is being studied separately to identify potential immunogens for induction of protective immunity. Supplementing research on vaccines are attempts to identify species-specific immunogens for immunodiagnostic tests.

*Present address: Hazleton Laboratories America, Inc., 9200 Leesburg Pike, Vienna, Virginia 22180.

Until the development of hybridoma technology, the identification of appropriate malarial antigens to use as immunogens was a formidable problem. Hybridomas now enable us to produce monoclonal antibodies against single malarial antigens. By screening for biological activity, i.e., ability to interfere with the parasite's life cycle, we can identify monoclonal antibodies whose target antigens are potential immunogens. Working with animal malarial systems or with human malaria parasites cultured *in vitro*, several laboratories have successfully used monoclonal antibodies to protect against infection or to identify stage-specific antigenic targets of immunity.

Monoclonal Antibodies Against Sporozoites

The use of irradiated sporozoites as antigens was initiated by Dr. Ruth Nussenzweig and her colleagues at New York University Medical Center. Promising results have been obtained in mice, monkeys, and man (1,2). Animals immunized in this way are completely protected against malarial infection induced with sporozoites of the same species but are not protected against blood-induced infections.

Sera from hosts immunized with sporozoites usually produce a large precipitate enveloping the surface of sporozoites and forming a long extension from the posterior end of the sporozoite. This circumsporozoite precipitin (CSP) reaction is species-specific and, in some cases, strain-specific and is used to identify anti-sporozoite antibodies. Monoclonal antibodies against sporozoites of *P. berghei*, a rodent malarial parasite, were screened by indirect immunofluorescence and the CSP test; those antibodies with CSP reactivity completely blocked *P. berghei*-induced infection of mice. In some cases, only 10 μg of antibody injected into a mouse afforded protection (3). Interestingly, Fab fragments were as effective as the intact antibody in neutralizing sporozoites (4); this indicated that the mechanism of protection was unrelated to complement activation, Fc binding to various cytotoxic cells, or agglutination of sporozoites. The target antigen for these hybridomas was a major sporozoite surface protein with an apparent molecular weight of 44,000.

A similar approach has been used successfully to define immunogens on sporozoites of malarial parasites infecting primates (5). The next step will be to identify the gene for this antigen and to obtain enough antigen to perform vaccine trials in animals.

Clearly, if a sporozoite-based vaccine were effective, an immunized individual would be completely protected against natural infection with malaria. However, if one sporozoite escapes immune surveillance, a fully virulent infection may occur because sporozoite immunity does not block development in the subsequent stages of the parasite's life cycle. For this reason among others, it is important to consider means of immunizing against subsequent stages of the malarial parasite's life cycle in its vertebrate host.

Monoclonal Antibodies Against Asexual Parasites

In the field of research in malaria vaccines the asexual erythrocytic parasite poses the greatest challenge to hybridoma technology. The problems of using monoclonal antibodies to identify functional antigens on asexual parasites reflect the complicated features of immunity to this stage, including the evolution in the parasite of such immune-evasive mechanisms as antigenic variation. Theoretically, antibodies can block merozoite invasion of erythrocytes either by interacting with a merozoite receptor for the red blood cell or by agglutinating merozoites as they emerge from a rupturing schizont. Monoclonal antibodies against merozoites can be screened first by indirect immunofluorescence and then for functional activity by their ability to block invasion *in vitro*. This approach has been only partially successful. Epstein et al. (6) identified two hybridomas against merozoites of *P. knowlesi*, a species causing malaria in primates, that block invasion of erythrocytes by agglutinating merozoites. These monoclonal antibodies must be present in high concentrations (1-2 mg/ml) and are probably not directed against a receptor molecule. Perrin et al. (7) identified monoclonal antibodies against *P. falciparum* that inhibited its intraerythrocytic development in culture. An unusual finding was that a hybridoma raised against *P. berghei* affected *in vitro* development of *P. falciparum*. Surprisingly, the effect of the antibody against *P. berghei* in mice was not reported. Freeman et al. (8) immunized mice against *P. yoelii* by infecting them with an avirulent strain of the parasite and then repeatedly infecting them with a virulent strain. Using the spleens from these mice, they produced several hybridomas against avirulent and virulent *P. yoelii*. In passive transfer experiments, only those monoclonal antibodies directed against merozoite antigens were protective against infection with the virulent strain. Subsequently, these workers have used *P. yoelii* antigen that has been affinity-purified with monoclonal antibodies to immunize mice against infection with *P. yoelii* (9).

Other targets in the asexual stage that may be identifiable with monoclonal antibodies are antigens expressed on the surface of infected erythrocytes. Antibodies against such targets may prove difficult to screen for functional activity, since immunity against infected erythrocytes in the host depends on the spleen and on cellular components of immunity in addition to antibody.

Monoclonal Antibodies Against Sexual Parasites

Antigamete immunity has been demonstrated in avian, rodent, and primate malarias (10-13). A vertebrate host immunized with gametes prior to infection with malaria does not infect mosquitoes. Circulating antigamete antibodies ingested by a mosquito during a blood meal will prevent fertilization by interacting with male and female gametes as they emerge in the mosquito midgut during gametogenesis.

Gametes are not present in naturally infected animals, and sexual parasites apparently have not evolved protective mechanisms such as antigenic variation. Experimental results with rhesus monkeys immunized with *P. knowlesi* gametes indicate that immunity against the Malaysian strain of *P. knowlesi* prevented transmission of the Philippine strain as well (13). This suggests that gametes associated with these strains of malarial parasites have shared antigens, although the sporozoites and asexual parasites are antigenically different. Antigamete immunity has been shown to be long-lasting in birds and monkeys. Rhesus monkeys were still non-infective to mosquitoes when challenged four years after immunization. Significantly, asexual infections in birds and monkeys boosted the levels of antigamete immunity.

To identify the antigenic targets of antigamete immunity, we have developed a number of hybridomas against gametes of *P. gallinaceum*, an avian malarial parasite (14). Two monoclonal antibodies have been identified that bind to the surface of live male and female gametes as determined by indirect immunofluorescence. Although each antibody caused a loose agglutination of male gametes, neither had any effect on the transmission of malaria to *Aedes aegypti* mosquitoes. When the monoclonal antibodies were mixed together they caused a tight, rope-like agglutination of male gametes, preventing their detachment from the residual body of the gametocyte. The mixture acted synergistically to reduce significantly the transmission of malaria to mosquitoes, although some transmission was always present. Total transmission-blocking immunity may require antibodies to multiple antigens on gametes. It is not known if antibodies block fertilization solely by agglutinating male gametes as they emerge during gametogenesis or if they work by blocking receptors for fertilization on either male or female gametes. The mixture of monoclonal antibodies that dramatically agglutinated male gametes *in vitro* also coated female gametes as shown by electron microscopy (15).

The antigenic target of one of the monoclonal antibodies, 11C7, has been identified as a protein with an apparent molecular weight of 230,000. This protein has been purified by affinity chromatography and used to immunize chickens. Sera from immunized birds agglutinate male gametes but are only partially effective in suppressing infectivity to mosquitoes. This result implies that polyspecific antiserum to a single gamete antigen may be no more effective in blocking transmission than a monoclonal antibody is against the same antigen. It may be, therefore, that fully effective transmission-blocking immunity involves the reaction of antibodies with other antigens on the gamete surface.

Conclusion

Hybridoma technology will help in the search for new tools to control and eradicate malaria. Monoclonal antibodies may first be used as immunodiagnostic reagents. Anti-malarial monoclonal antibodies of defined specificity will allow laboratories around the world access to unlimited amounts of an identical reagent. With such reagents, identification of an infection can be made with only a few circulating parasites as part of a quick, standardized screening procedure. Now, malaria surveillance within a community depends upon endless readings of hundreds of thousands of slides.

Vaccines against malaria will probably be derived from antigens identified with monoclonal antibodies. The antigens are likely to represent surface proteins from different stages of *P. falciparum* and other malarial species infectious to man. Such multivalent vaccines might combine sporozoite and asexual components to provide protection to the host, and an anti-gamete component to block transmission within a community.

References

1. Nussenzweig, RS (1977). Immunoprophylaxis of malaria; sporozoite-induced immunity. In Immunity to Blood Parasites of Animals and Man, pp 75-78. LH Miller, J Pino, J McKelvey, eds. Plenum Publishing Corp, New York.
2. Clyde, DF, VC McCarthy, RM Miller and DWE Woodward (1975). Immunization of man against *falciparum* and *vivax* malaria by use of attenuated sporozoites. Am J Trop Med Hyg **24**, 397-401.
3. Yoshida, N, RS Nussenzweig, P Potocnjak, V Nussenzweig and M Aikawa (1980). Hybridoma produces protective antibodies directed against the sporozoite stage of malaria parasite. Science **207**, 71-73.
4. Potocnjak, P, N Yoshida, RS Nussenzweig and V Nussenzweig (1980). Monovalent fragments (Fab) of monoclonal antibodies to a sporozoite surface antigen (Pb44) protect mice against malarial infection. J Exp Med **151**, 1504-1513.
5. RS Nussenzweig. Personal communication.
6. Epstein, N, LH Miller, D Kaushel, I Udeinya, J Rener, R Howard, R Asofsky, M Aikawa and RL Hess (1981). Monoclonal antibodies against a specific determinant on malarial (*Plasmodium knowlesi*) merozoites block erythrocyte invasion. J Immunol **127**, 212-217.
7. Perrin, L, HE Ramirez, PH Lambert and PA Miescher (1981). Inhibition of *P. falciparum* growth in human erythrocytes by monoclonal antibodies. Nature (Lond) **289**, 301-303.
8. Freeman, R, AH Trejdosiewicz and GAM Cross (1980). Protective monoclonal antibodies recognising stage-specific merozoite antigens of a rodent malaria parasite. Nature (Lond) **284**, 366-368.
9. Holder, AA, and RR Freeman (1981). Immunisation against blood stage rodent malaria using purified parasite antigen. Nature (Lond) **294**, 361-364.
10. Carter, R, and D Chen (1976). Malaria transmission blocked by immunisation with gametes of the malarial parasite. Nature (Lond) **263**, 57-60.
11. Gwadz, RW (1976). Malaria: Successful immunization against the sexual stages of *Plasmodium gallinaceum*. Science **193**, 1150-1151.
12. Mendis, KN, and GAT Targett (1979). Immunisation against gametes and asexual erythrocytic stages of a rodent malaria parasite. Nature (Lond) **277**, 389-391.

13. Gwadz, RW, and I Green (1978). Malaria immunization in Rhesus monkeys: a vaccine effective against both the sexual and asexual stages of *Plasmodium knowlesi*. J Exp Med **148**, 1311-1323.
14. Rener, J, R Carter, Y Rosenberg and LH Miller (1980). Anti-gamete monoclonal antibodies synergistically block transmission of malaria by preventing fertilization in the mosquito. Proc Natl Acad Sci USA **77**, 6797-6799.
15. Aikawa, M, J Rener, R Carter and LH Miller (1981). An electron microscopic study of the interaction of monoclonal antibodies with gametes of the malaria parasite, *Plasmodium gallinaceum*. J Protozool **28**, 383-388.

SCHISTOSOMAL GLYCOPROTEINS IMMUNOREACTIVE IN INFECTED HUMANS: CHARACTERIZATION BY MONOCLONAL ANTIBODIES

Mette Strand, William S. Aronstein, and Amy P. Norden

The Johns Hopkins University School of Medicine
Baltimore, Maryland 21205

Schistosomiasis, known as bilharziasis in Europe and as big belly disease in China, ranks as one of the most widespread and debilitating of tropical infections. Schistosomiasis is the pathological consequence of infection with sexually mature and reproducing adult worms of any one of several closely related species of digenetic trematodes. Schistosomes differ from all other digeneans in that the sexes are separate. These flat worms lead a complex life. Part of their life cycle must occur within a water-dwelling snail. The mobile larvae (cercariae) that emerge from the snail penetrate the intact skin of the definitive host and migrate to the mesenteric veins, where they mature sexually into inch-long male or female worms. They can live for up to 25 years paired in perpetual copulation producing eggs. A pair of worms can produce from 20-2000 eggs per day depending on the species. The eggs lodge in various tissues, provoking an intense inflammatory response and causing enlargement of the liver and spleen.

Previously, a variety of studies of schistosomiasis have shown that the worm-infected host contains circulating schistosome antigens (1-5), antibodies (6-12), and antigen/antibody complexes (13-17). The immunopathological basis of schistosomal disease has been appreciated for some time, but progress has been hampered by the lack of identification of biologically relevant antigens as well as by difficulties inherent in purification of individual antigens from an organism whose propagation depends upon passage in a mammalian host.

Our approach was to first identify the schistosomal proteins that are antigenic in infected humans. Therefore, we focused our attention on schistosomal membrane glycoproteins, because these proteins can be expected to play a significant role in the host's immune-mediated defense mechanisms and in the infectious process, because of their location and excretion (18-20). We have purified glycoproteins of cercariae, the infectious form of the organism, by lectin-affinity chromatography and have used these purified glycoproteins as antigens in preparing monoclonal antibodies. We report 1) the immunoreactivity of these isolated glycoproteins with sera of infected humans and 2) the use of three of the monoclonal antibodies to identify and characterize glycoproteins in different schistosomal developmental stages.

Results and Discussion

Identification of Cercarial Glycoproteins Reactive with Sera from Infected Humans or Mice

Cercarial glycoproteins purified by lectin-affinity chromatography were labeled with iodine-125 and analyzed by SDS-polyacrylamide gel electrophoresis (Fig. 1A). There were 15 major polypeptides ranging in mass from 190 kilodaltons to 9 kilodaltons. Sera of infected humans or mice precipitated all of these glycoproteins (Fig. 1B, lanes 2-10). No precipitation was observed with normal human or mouse serum (Fig. 1B, lanes 11 and 1).

Although the pattern of immunoprecipitated proteins was similar with sera from individual humans or mice, there were distinctive differences among some of these sera. The basis for these differences is not known.

Similar analysis of the proteins present in the fraction that did not bind to the lectin-affinity column showed that only a few polypeptides were reactive with serum of infected humans. By far, the predominant immunoresponse was directed against the glycoproteins, which were therefore used to immunize mice for hybridoma production (22,23).

Detection and Relative Antigen Concentration in Various Developmental Stages of the Schistosome

The relative concentration of antigen recognized by three different, cloned hybridomas (129A3/1/3, 130C3/2, 132C4A/4) was measured by direct binding assay. Equal amounts of schistosomal proteins extracted from eggs, female worms, male worms or cercariae were coated to a plastic surface (microtiter wells, Falcon Plastic, Oxnard, Calif.) and the amount of ^{125}I-labeled, purified monoclonal antibody bound was measured (Fig. 2). The antigens recognized by monoclonal antibodies 129A3/1/3 and 132C4A/4 were expressed in each of the developmental stages. In contrast, the antigen recognized by monoclonal antibody 130C3/2 was absent from egg protein extract. A monoclonal immunoassay for specific antigenemia of this glycoprotein should be particularly useful in diagnosis and management of schistosomiasis. Since severity of disease appears to correlate with worm pairs and not with fecal egg count (24), serum levels of this glycoprotein should accurately reflect the worm burden. The concentration of each of the three antigens recognized by the monoclonal antibody appeared to be three- to five-fold higher in cercariae and male worms than in female worms. The results also showed that the binding of each of the monoclonal antibodies was specific and that the antigenic sites were saturable.

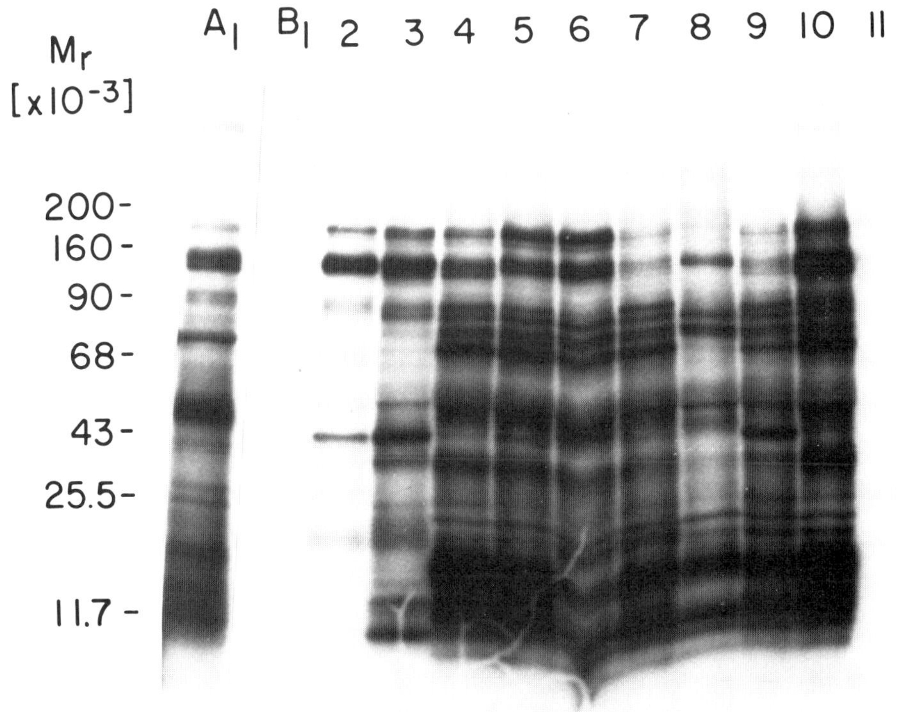

Fig. 1. Autoradiographs after one-dimensional gel electrophoresis of purified and ^{125}I-labeled cercarial glycoproteins before and after immunoprecipitation. Details of all materials and methods in this paper including purification, iodination, immunoprecipitation, gel electrophoresis, and autoradiography are described elsewhere (21,22). (A-1) Purified cercarial glycoproteins, ^{125}I-labeled. (B) The ^{125}I-labeled cercarial glycoproteins immunoprecipitated by 1) normal serum of six-month-old mouse; 2) serum of mouse three months post-infection; 3) serum of mouse eight months post-infection; 4) serum of patient No. 18; 5) serum of patient No. 25; 6) serum of patient No. 33; 7) serum of patient No. 42; 8) serum of patient No. 53; 9) serum of patient No. 54; 10) serum of patient No. 3496; 11) serum of normal human. Molecular weight standards, not shown, were cytochrome C, *M*r 11,700; chymotrypsinogen, *M*r 25,500; ovalbumin, *M*r 43,000; bovine serum albumin, *M*r 68,000; Sigma factor, *M*r 90,000; RNA polymerase, *M*r 160,000; myosin, *M*r 200,000.

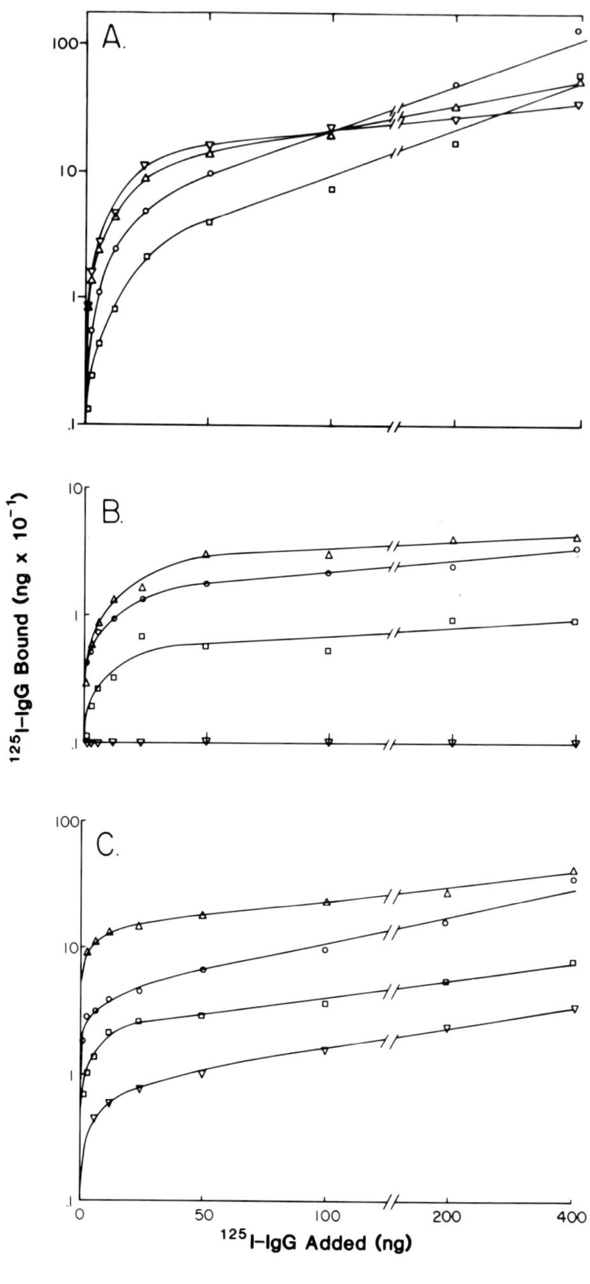

Fig.2. Binding of ^{125}I-labeled monoclonal antibodies (A) 129A3/1/3, (B) 130C3/2, and (C) 132C4A/4 to schistosomal protein extracts. Details of the plate binding assays are described elsewhere (21,22). The nonspecific binding of equivalent amounts of ^{125}I-labeled P3 have been subtracted. Five µg (A) or 25 µg (B and C) each of cercarial Triton X-305 protein extract (Δ), male worm protein extract (O), female worm extract (□), and egg protein extract (∇).

Antigen Recognized by Monoclonal Antibody 129A3/1/3 Was Immunoreactive in Infected Humans

Identification of the antigenic target for monoclonal antibody 129A3/1/3 was tested by analysis of immunoprecipitates of ^{125}I-labeled cercarial glycoproteins. Two polypeptides with apparent molecular weights of 35,000 and 20,000 were precipitated by this monoclonal antibody (data not shown, see below). These same two polypeptides were also present when analogous immunoprecipitates were analyzed on SDS-polyacrylamide gel without reduction, thus excluding their coprecipitation by disulfide bonding. Preliminary results from two-dimensional tryptic peptide mapping showed the presence of shared peptides, indicating the 35,000- and 20,000-dalton polypeptides were possibly derived by proteolytic cleavage (see below).

The serum of an infected human and the monoclonal antibody both appeared to precipitate glycoproteins with the same apparent molecular weight (data not shown). These immunoprecipitates were therefore further analyzed by two-dimensional gel electrophoresis to ascertain whether these were indeed the same protein (Fig. 3). The monoclonal antibody precipitated 14 isomorphs, pH 6.3-5.3, with molecular weights ranging from 32,000 to 35,000 and 2 isomorphs, pH 5.3-4.8, at 20,000 daltons. Each of these isomorphs was superimposable with polypeptides immunoprecipitated with serum of an infected human. Two-dimensional analysis of immunoprecipitates obtained with sera of other patients infected with schistosomiasis gave the same results. Sera of uninfected humans or mice were negative. Therefore, monoclonal antibody 129A3/1/3 has identified a glycoprotein that elicits an immune response in infected humans.

Female and Male Worm Antigens Recognized by Monoclonal Antibody 129A3/1/3

The protein molecules in male and female worms expressing antigenic determinants recognized by monoclonal antibody 129A3/1/3 were also identified by immunoprecipitation analysis (Fig. 4). Infected human serum precipitated over 15 glycoproteins of the female worms that were visualized as present in high concentration or intensely labeled. The pattern of glycoproteins immunoprecipitated from male worms was markedly different; only 9 glycoproteins present in high concentration or intensely labeled were visualized (lanes 4 and 5, respectively). One possible explanation for the differences in immunoreactivity between male and female worms is the presence of egg glycoproteins in the female worm extract, since eggs would be contained in the female worms when they were isolated from the mice. A protein of 170 kilodaltons (indicated by arrow) was immunoprecipitated from both male and female worms by

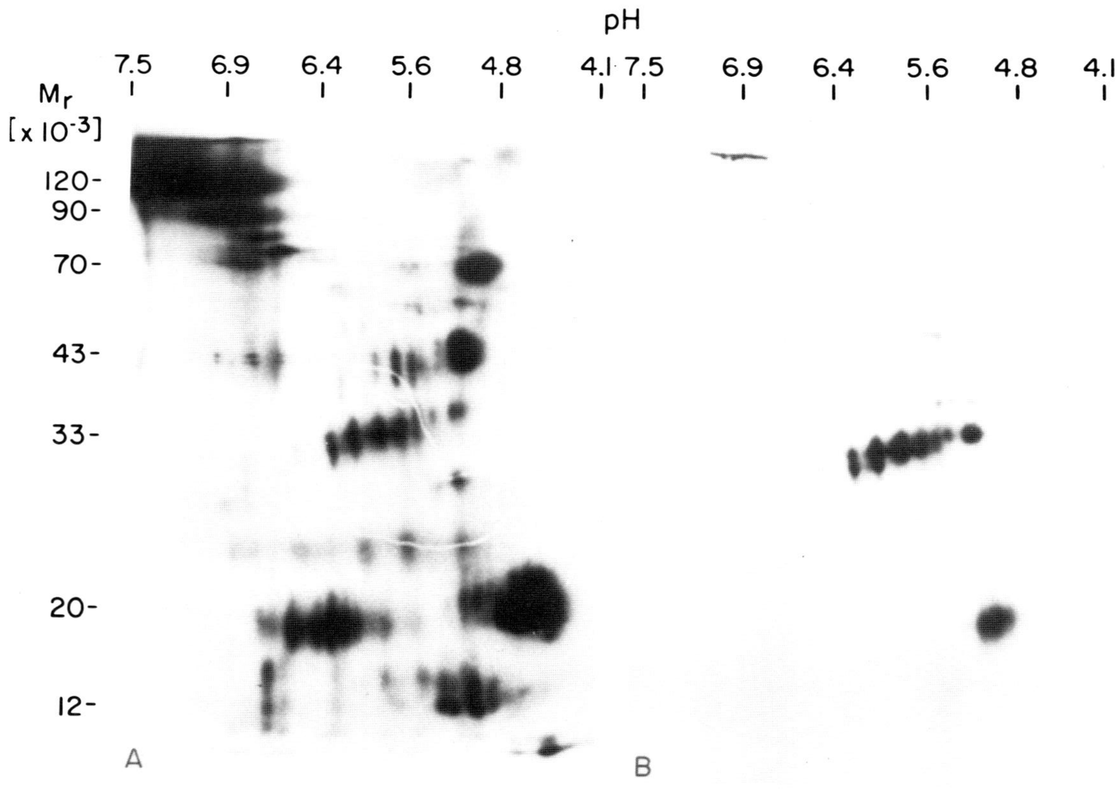

Fig. 3. Comparison of antigenic target recognized by monoclonal antibody 129A3/1/3 and serum of infected human. Autoradiographs after two-dimensional gel electrophoresis of immunoprecipitates of ^{125}I-labeled cercarial glycoproteins. The immunoprecipitated glycoproteins were fractionated by isoelectric focusing in the first dimension and by 10% SDS gel electrophoresis in the second dimension. (A) Immunoprecipitate with serum of infected patient No. 18. (B) Immunoprecipitate with monoclonal antibody 129A3/1/3.

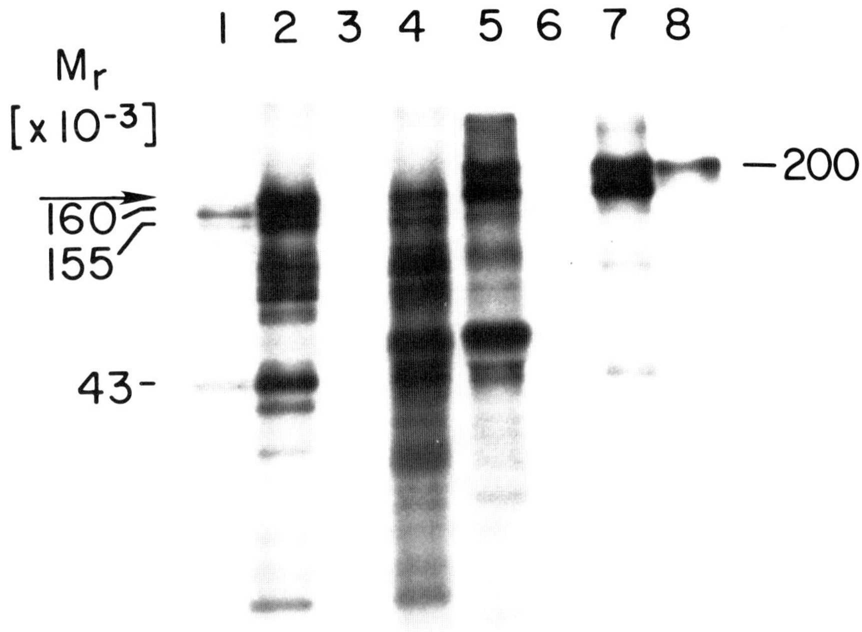

Fig. 4. Comparison of antigenic targets in male and female worms by monoclonal antibody 129A3/1/3 and serum of infected human. Analysis was conducted as described in Fig. 1. Autoradiography after one-dimensional gel electrophoresis of immunoprecipitates of ^{125}I-labeled glycoproteins of female worm (lanes 1-4), and male worm (lanes 5-8). Immunoprecipitates with monoclonal antibody 129A3/1/3, lanes 1 and 8; with serum of mice immunized with cercarial glycoproteins, lanes 2 and 7; with normal mouse serum, lanes 3 and 6; with serum of infected patient No. 18, lanes 4 and 5.

serum of infected humans and served as a marker for comparing the immunoprecipitated proteins.

Monoclonal antibody 129A3/1/3 also precipitated proteins from both male and female worms. A 200-kilodalton protein was precipitated from the male worm extract (lane 8), along with a minor component of 43 kilodaltons that was visible upon longer exposure of the radioautograph. The proportions of these two immunoprecipitated glycoproteins were variable, depending on the age of the worm extract. A second immunoprecipitation carried out six days later with the same ^{125}I-labeled male worm preparation showed that 60% of the precipitate was at 200 kilodaltons and 40% of the precipitate was at 43 kilodaltons. All the other proteins immunoprecipitated by the polyclonal sera showed no change, indicating that the glycoprotein recognized by clone 129A3/1/3 was susceptible to proteolytic fragmentation even in the presence of phenylmethylsulfonyl fluoride.

The antigenic targets of the female worm recognized by monoclonal antibody 129A3/1/3 differed from those recognized in the male worm extract. A 43-kilodalton polypeptide was also immunoprecipitated from the female worm, but in contrast to the 200-kilodalton male polypeptide, the female worm showed immunoprecipitation of proteins at 160 kilodaltons and 155 kilodaltons (lane 1). Whether these two proteins originated in eggs or female worms requires further study. At least one of the proteins is possibly an egg form, since this monoclonal antibody recognized antigenic determinants present in an egg extract, as measured by direct binding (shown above).

The pattern of proteins of male or female worms immunoprecipitated with serum of an infected human showed extensive similarity to that obtained with serum of mice immunized with cercarial glycoproteins (lanes 4 and 2 and lanes 5 and 7, respectively). However, several worm glycoproteins were uniquely precipitated with human serum, probably because these glycoproteins were not present in the cercariae used as the immunogen for the mice.

The relationship between the ^{125}I-labeled male worm glycoproteins precipitated with the monoclonal antibody or the infected human serum was also analyzed by two-dimensional gel electrophoresis. Immunoprecipitates with monoclonal antibody 129A3/1/3/ contained 13 isomorphs that were identical in charge (pI) and molecular weight to a protein immunoprecipitated by sera of infected humans (data not shown).

Antigen Recognized by Monoclonal Antibody 130C3/2 Was Immunoreactive in Infected Humans

The antigenic target of monoclonal antibody 130C3/2 was identified by immunoprecipitation of ^{125}I-labeled cercarial glycoproteins (Fig. 5). A polypeptide with an apparent molecular weight of 120,000 was precipitated. The serum of an infected human also precipitated a glycoprotein with the same apparent molecular weight. Normal mouse serum or nonrelevant immunoglobulin of the same class (IgG_1) showed no precipitation.

Analogous immunoprecipitations were also carried out with ^{125}I-labeled glycoproteins of either male or female worms. In both of these cases, monoclonal antibody 130C3/2 precipitated a polypeptide of 170,000 daltons (data not shown, see purification below).

Immunoprecipitates of ^{125}I-labeled glycoproteins of cercariae and adult worms were further analyzed by two-dimensional gel electrophoresis. Monoclonal antibody 130C3/2 precipitated seven isomorphs, pH 7.1-6.8, with molecular weights of 120,000 from cercariae and 170,000 from adult worms. Each of these isomorphs was superimposable with those immunoprecipitated with infected human serum (data not shown). Sera of uninfected humans or mice were negative.

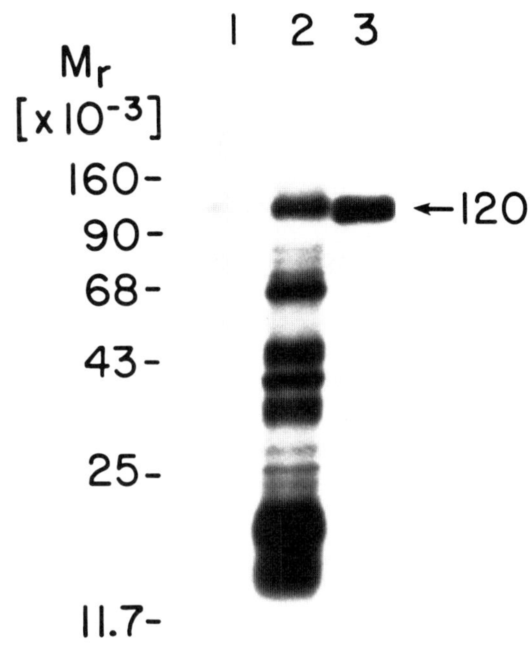

Fig. 5. Identification of cercarial antigen target recognized by monoclonal antibody 130C3/2. Autoradiograph after one-dimensional gel electrophoresis of immunoprecipitates of ^{125}I-labeled cercarial glycoproteins. Analysis was conducted as described in Fig. 1. 1) Serum of normal human. 2) Serum of infected human No. 18. 3) Monoclonal antibody 130C3/2.

The homology of the ^{125}I-labeled cercarial glycoprotein immunoprecipitated with monoclonal antibody 130C3/2 or sera of two different infected humans was established by two-dimensional tryptic peptide mapping (Fig. 6). The three tryptic peptide maps were indistinguishable. Thus monoclonal antibody 130C3/2 has identified a glycoprotein that elicits an immune response in infected humans.

Indirect Immunofluorescence Microscopy of Schistosomula with Monoclonal Antibodies 130C3/2 and 132C4A/4

The anatomic location of the antigens recognized by monoclonal antibodies 130C3/2 and 132C4A/4 was analyzed by indirect immunofluorescence microscopy. Artificially transformed schistosomula were examined because they represent a reproducibly prepared form of the larval stage which is the first to be contacted by the immune system of the vertebrate host (25).

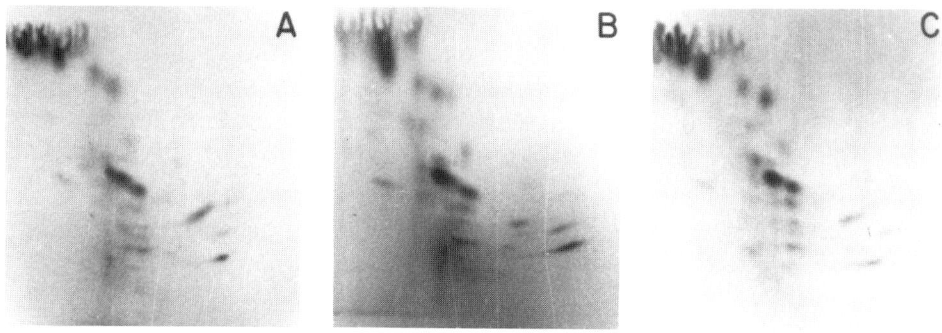

Fig. 6. Comparison of antigenic target recognized by serum of infected humans and monoclonal antibody 130C3/2. Autoradiographs of tryptic peptide maps of ^{125}I-labeled cercarial glycoproteins reactive with (A) serum of infected patient No. 18, (B) monoclonal antibody 130C3/2, and (C) serum of infected patient No. 25. Isolation and tryptic peptide analysis of the immunoprecipitated components were carried out as described elsewhere (21).

Schistosomula, both unfixed and after fixation with gluteraldehyde, were examined with normal mouse serum and purified myeloma P3 immunoglobulin (control) (Fig. 7A). Surface deposition of fluorescent label was limited to the points of attachment that had existed between the schistosomula body and the cercarial tail. The strong fluorescence at this location was occasionally observed with all antisera.

Monoclonal antibody 130C3/2 gave a punctuated fluorescence pattern that was restricted to the spines of the organism. These structures were present over the entire surface but were brightest and most clearly defined at the poles (Fig. 7B), which were covered with 20-25 rows of short spines. After gluteraldehyde fixation, the spines were more distinct and appeared to be about one micrometer in length, and, at the anterior end of the organism, to be oriented in an antero-posterior direction (Fig. 7C). In contrast, the antigen recognized by monoclonal antibody 132C4A/4 was seen as a striking pattern of narrow bands, punctuated by brighter regions suggesting cross-bridges, and running horizontally around the entire schistosomulum (Fig. 7D).

Direct Immunofluorescence Microscopy of Schistosomula and Adult Worms

The distribution of the antigenic targets recognized by antibodies 130C3/2 and 132C4A/4 on the tegument of adult worms was studied by direct immunofluorescence, because extensive amounts of murine

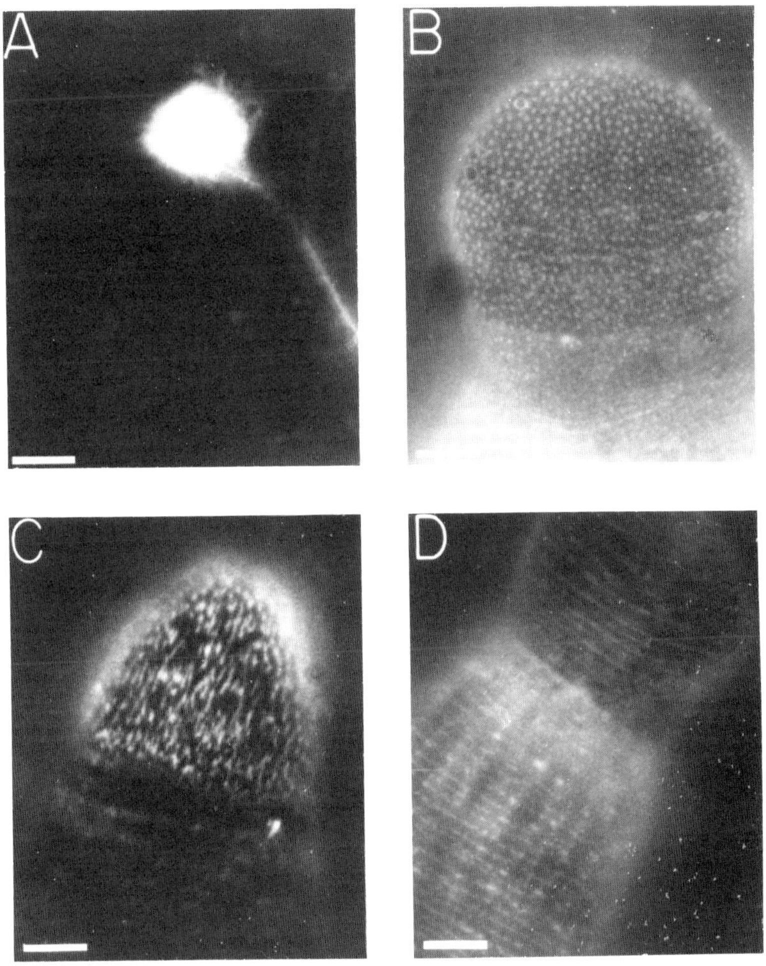

Fig. 7. Indirect immunofluorescent localization of the antigenic target recognized by monoclonal antibodies 130C3/2 and 132C4A/4. Details of primary and secondary incubations are described elsewhere (21). Bar = 10 μm. Primary incubations were (A) Fixed schistosomulum incubated with a 1:100 dilution of ascites fluid of negative control immunoglobulin P3. (B) Unfixed schistosomulum incubated with a 1:100 dilution of ascites fluid of monoclonal antibody 130C3/2. (C) Fixed schistosomulum incubated with a 1:100 dilution of ascites fluid of monoclonal antibody 130C3/2. (D) Unfixed schistosomulum incubated with a 1:25 dilution of ascites fluid of monoclonal antibody 132C4A/4. All secondary incubations were with a 1:250 dilution of fluoresceinated goat anti-murine IgG.

immunoglobulin on the parasite's surface precluded use of the indirect technique. Surface deposition of the negative control P3 immunoglobulin (Fig. 8A) was not detected, while male worms were extensively stained by antibody 130C3/2. The spines attached to the tubercles on the dorsum of the worm were brightly illuminated (Fig. 8B), and a few scattered spines were observed elsewhere. On female worms, spines were present mainly over the posterior surface and were similar in appearance to those concentrated on the male tubercles (Fig. 8C). Monoclonal antibody 132C4A/4 exhibited a fluorescence pattern on adult worms that was remarkably similar to that observed on schistosomula (Fig. 8D). In addition, the tubercles on the dorsum of the male worm were illuminated. Directly stained schistosomula exhibited a pattern identical to that of indirectly stained schistosomula. No deposition of rhodamine-conjugated control immunoglobulin was detected on the schistosomular surface.

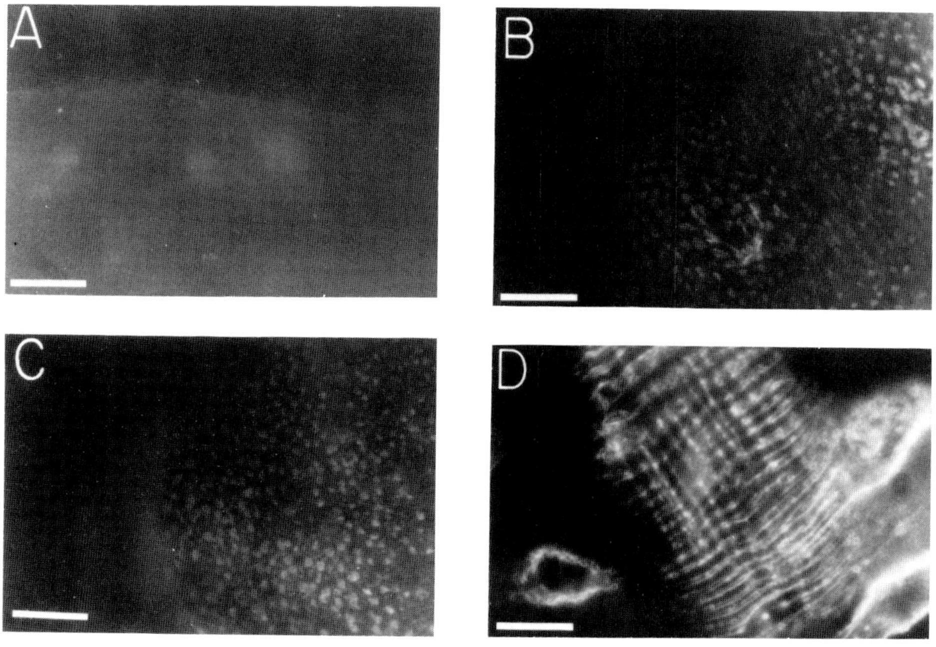

Fig. 8. Direct immunofluorescent localization of the antigenic target recognized by monoclonal antibodies 130C3/2 and 132C4A/4. Details of tetramethylrhodamine isothiocyanate (RITC) conjugation of immunoglobulins 130C3/2, 132C4A/4, and P3 (control) are described elsewhere (21). Immunoglobulins were used at a concentration of 0.05 mg/ml. Bar = 10 μm. (A) Male worm stained with control RITC-P3 immunoglobulin. (B) Male worm (dorsum) stained with RITC-130C3/2. (C) Edge of female worm (dorsum) stained with RITC-130C3/2. (D) Female worm stained with RITC-132C4A/4. Bar = 15 μm.

Immunoaffinity Purification of Male Worm Spine Glycoprotein

Immunoaffinity chromatography permitted a simple one-step purification of the spine glycoprotein (Fig. 9). A single band with an apparent molecular weight of 170,000 was observed following elution of the column with the chaotropic reagent, KSCN (lane B). The yield appeared to be maximal, since this glycoprotein was not visible in the column runthrough (lane C), whereas it was clearly seen in the glycoprotein mixture that was applied to the column (lane A).

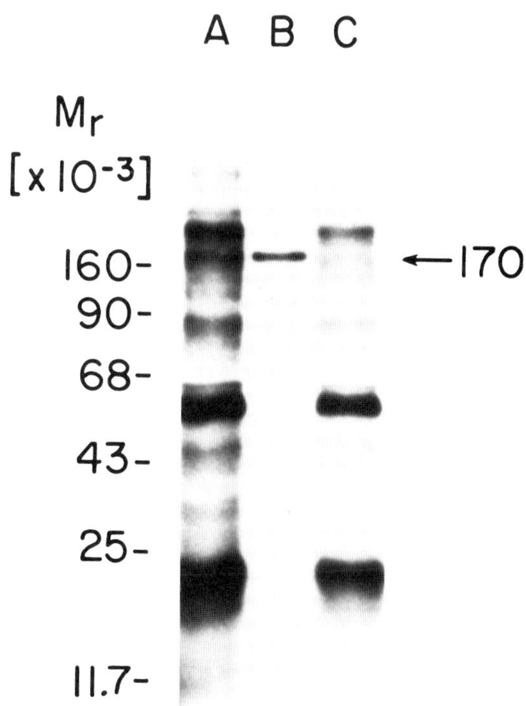

Fig. 9. Purification of ^{125}I-labeled male worm spine glycoprotein. Details of the preparation of the immuno-affinity column and the purification procedure are described elsewhere (21). (A) Aliquot of total glycoprotein extract applied to the column. (B) Aliquot of spine glycoprotein eluted with chaotropic reagent, KSCN. (C) Aliquot of glycoproteins that did not bind to the column.

Summary

In summary, we have shown that hybridoma antibodies prepared against a defined fraction of cercarial antigens can be used to identify, characterize, and purify to homogeneity glycoproteins that are antigenic in infected humans. In addition, these monoclonal antibodies are valuable probes in studies of differentiation of a highly evolved and complex organism.

Future work will be aimed at applying the monoclonal antibodies to clinical diagnosis and treatment of schistosomal infection.

Acknowledgments

We are indebted to Professor E. Bueding and Dr. J.G. Bourgeois for providing the cercariae. We thank A. George and A. McMillan for their excellent technical assistance, L. Cumor for secretarial assistance, and Dr. J. Ellner for infected human sera. W.S. Aronstein and A.P. Norden were supported by National Institutes of Health Training Grants 5 T32 GM07626-04 and 5 T32 CA09243-04, respectively.

References

1. Carlier, Y, D Bout, JC Bina, D Camus, JFM Figueiredo and A Capron (1975). Immunological studies in human schistosomiasis. I. Parasitic antigen in urine. Am J Trop Med Hyg **24**, 949-954.
2. Madwar, MA, and A Voller (1975). Circulating soluble antigens and antibody in schistosomiasis. Br Med J 1, 435-436.
3. Madwar, MA, and A Voller (1977). Serological investigations on patients with schistosomiasis with special reference to circulating antigen. Tropenmed Parasitol **28**, 310-315.
4. Santoro, F, R Borojevic, D Bout, P Tachon, JC Bina and A Capron (1977). Mother-child relationship in human schistosomiasis mansoni. I. Parasitic antigens and antibodies in milk. Am J Trop Med Hyg **26**, 1164-1168.
5. Santoro, F, B Vendemeulebrouke and A Capron (1978). The use of the radioimmunoprecipitation-peg assay (RIPEGA) to quantify circulating antigens in human and experimental schistosomiasis. J Immunol Methods **24**, 229-237.
6. Camus, D, Y Carlier, M Capron, JC Bina, JFM Figueiredo, A Prata and A Capron (1977). Immunological studies in human schistosomiasis. III. Immunoglobulin levels, antibodies, and delayed hypersensitivity. Am J Trop Med Hyg **26**, 482-490.
7. Deelder, AM, and W Van den Berge (1981). Detection of antibodies against circulating cathodic antigen of *Schistosoma mansoni* using the enzyme-linked immunosorbent assay. Z Parasitenkd **64**, 179-186.
8. Goodgame, RW, DG Colley, CC Draper, FA Lewis, ML McLaren and RP Pelley (1978). Humoral immune responses in human hepatosplenic schistosomiasis mansoni. Am J Trop Med Hyg **27**, 1174-1180.

9. Kelsoe, GH, and TH Weller (1978). Immunodiagnosis of infection with *Schistosoma mansoni*: Enzyme-linked immunosorbent assay for detection of antibody to circulating antigen. Proc Natl Acad Sci USA **75**, 5715-5717.
10. Lunde, MN, EA Ottesen and AW Cheever (1979). Serological differences between acute and chronic schistosomiasis mansoni detected by enzyme-linked immunosorbent assay (ELISA). Am J Trop Med Hyg **28**, 87-91.
11. Nash, TE, EA Ottesen and AW Cheever (1978). Antibody response to a polysaccharide antigen present in the schistosome gut. II. Modulation of antibody response. Am J Trop Med Hyg **27**, 944-950.
12. Salih, SY, A Bartlett and A Voller (1978). Detection of antibodies by enzyme-immunoassay in human *Schistosoma mansoni* infections: A clinical and chemotherapeutic study. Tropenmed Parasitol **29**, 409-412.
13. Bout, D, F Santoro, Y Carlier, JC Bina and A Capron (1977). Circulating immune complexes in schistosomiasis. Immunol **33**, 17-22.
14. Brito, E, F Santoro, H Rocha, M Dutra and A Capron (1979). Immune complexes in schistosomiasis. VI. Circulating IC levels in patients with and without nephropathy. Rev Inst Med Trop Sao Paulo **21**, 119-124.
15. Hiatt, RA, EA Ottesen, ZR Sotomayor and TJ Lawley (1980). Serial observations of circulating immune complexes in patients with acute schistosomiasis. J Infect Dis **142**, 665-670.
16. Lawley, TJ, EA Ottesen, RA Hiatt and LA Gazze (1979). Circulating immune complexes in acute schistosomiasis. Clin Exp Immunol **37**, 221-227.
17. Smith, MD, PJ Verroust, L Morel-Maroger, M Geniteau and JP Coulaud (1977). A study of the presence of circulating immune complexes in schistosomiasis. Trans R Soc Trop Med Hyg **71**, 343-348.
18. Kusel, JR, and PE Mackensie (1975). The measurement of the relative turnover rates of proteins of the surface membranes and other fractions of *Schistosoma mansoni* in culture. Parasitology **71**, 261-273.
19. Smithers, SR, DJ McLaren and FJ Ramalho-Pinto (1977). Immunity to schistosomes: the target. Am J Trop Med Hyg **26**, 11-19.
20. Wilson, RA, and PE Barnes (1977). The formation and turnover of the membranocalyx on the tegument of *Schistosoma mansoni*. Parasitology **74**, 61-71.
21. Norden, AP, WS Aronstein and M Strand (1982). *Schistosoma mansoni*: Identification, characterizaton, and purification of the spine glycoprotein by monoclonal antibody. Exp Parasitol, in press.
22. Strand, M, A McMillan and X Pan (1982). *Schistosoma mansoni*: Reactivity with infected human sera and monoclonal antibody characterization of a glycoprotein in different developmental stages. Exp Parasitol, in press.
23. Köhler, G, and C Milstein (1975). Continuous cultures of fused cells secreting antibody of predefined specificity. Nature (Lond) **256**, 495-497.
24. Cheever, AW (1968). A quantitative post-mortem study of schistosomiasis mansoni in man. Am J Trop Med Hyg **17**, 38-64.
25. Brink, LH, DJ McLaren and SR Smithers (1977). *Schistosoma mansoni*: a comparative study of artificially transformed schistosomula and schistosomula recovered after cercarial penetration of isolated skin. Parasitology **74**, 73-86.